THE CHILD CLINICIAN'S REPORT-WRITING HANDBOOK

ELLEN BRAATEN, PhD

Series Editor's Note by Edward L. Zuckerman

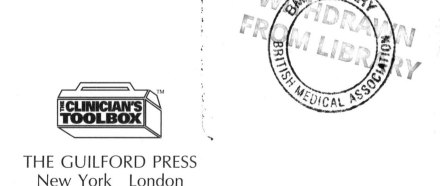

THE CLINICIAN'S TOOLBOX™

THE GUILFORD PRESS
New York   London

© 2007 The Guilford Press
A Division of Guilford Publications, Inc.
72 Spring Street, New York, NY 10012
www.guilford.com

Printed in the United States of America

This book is printed on acid-free paper.

Last digit is print number: 9 8 7 6 5 4 3

Library of Congress Cataloging-in-Publication Data

Braaten, Ellen.
    The child clinician's report-writing handbook / by Ellen Braaten.
      p. cm. — (The clinician's toolbox)
    Includes bibliographical references and index.
    ISBN-13: 978-1-59385-395-2 (pbk. : alk. paper)
    ISBN-10: 1-59385-395-5 (pbk. : alk. paper)
    1. Child psychiatry—Handbooks, manuals, etc. 2. Interviewing in child psychiatry—Handbooks, manuals, etc. 3. Neuropsychological report writing—Handbooks, manuals, etc. I. Title. II. Series.
    [DNLM: 1. Interview, Psychological—Handbooks. 2. Child. 3. Writing—Handbooks. WS 39 B794c 2007]
    RJ499.3.B73 2007
    618.92′89—dc22
                                                                        2006026727

THE CHILD CLINICIAN'S REPORT-WRITING HANDBOOK

THE CLINICIAN'S TOOLBOX™
A Guilford Series
Edward L. Zuckerman, Series Editor

*This book is dedicated to two mentors
who came into my life at just the right time:*

*Mitch Handelsman, PhD,
and Sheila O'Keefe, EdD*

*Thank you for supporting, guiding, and inspiring me
when I needed it the most.*

About the Author

Ellen Braaten, PhD, is an Assistant Professor of Psychology in the Department of Psychiatry at Harvard Medical School. She is also a child psychologist at the Massachusetts General Hospital, where she coordinates the Child Psychology Internship Program. Dr. Braaten is the coauthor of *Straight Talk about Psychological Testing for Kids* and has authored numerous scientific papers and chapters on child assessment, attention-deficit/hyperactivity disorder, anxiety, and learning disabilities. She lives with her husband and two children in the Boston area.

Series Editor's Note

The word "book" does not adequately describe *The Child Clinician's Report-Writing Handbook*. It is really a tool in the shape of a book—a tool for child clinicians that makes constructing and individually tailoring reports easier. It simply takes less mental "processing" to select the right word from a list (a recognition task) than to peruse one's memory (free recall). In addition, a report will be more tailored to the child when the author can sift through dozens of words and phrases and select exactly the right descriptor.

Based on her wide experience assessing and treating a large number and variety of children, Ellen Braaten offers all the words and phrases of American mental health that either the student or the senior clinician might need. Here "newbies" will find any descriptor they could possibly want (but they will still have to learn those terms' meanings). The experienced clinician can find new wordings to refresh a report style that may have become too repetitive or standardized.

Clinicians often struggle to avoid creating reports that seem "canned." Reports constructed with this book are unique for two reasons. First, their author is not constrained in any way. He or she can use the terms offered here or any others that come to mind or are preferred. In fact, authors may well find that reading the words here stimulates other even better choices (and should feel free to write them into the book to make recalling them easier). Second, the author of a report is not limited to the few hundred words that would on average be available to the clinician: the thousands offered here are very likely to exceed that number.

Dr. Braaten's work is comprehensive: words to fit every clinical phenomenon of interest, every setting, every age, and every stage of the evaluation and treatment process are here and are splendidly organized for easy access.

I am delighted to offer her work to my fellow clinicians. Read it and learn to be a more sensitive clinician; use it and become that rarity, a writer of reports that convey all of what we know and can use to help others.

EDWARD L. ZUCKERMAN, PHD

Acknowledgments

This book would not have been written without the encouragement, assistance, and support of a number of individuals with whom I had the privilege of working, most notably the staff at The Guilford Press. I will be forever grateful to Kitty Moore, who first approached me with this project; to Edward Zuckerman for his insightful comments along the way; to Barbara Watkins, who helped further develop this project into an actual manuscript; and to Anna Brackett for making sure the manuscript made it to print. This book was very much a collaborative effort between me and the editorial staff at The Guilford Press, and I am honored to have worked with such incredibly insightful and gifted individuals.

I would also like to express my gratitude to the colleagues who so willingly shared their experiences with child assessment and the training of child clinicians, particularly those of you who generously shared your reports with me. It is an honor to work at the Psychology Assessment Center at the Massachusetts General Hospital, and I am grateful to my colleagues for their support, particularly Dr. Mark Blais, Gretchen Timmel, Dr. Gretchen Felopulos, Dr. Amy Morgan, Dr. Cathy Leveroni, Dr. Lauren Polack, Dr. Janet Sherman, Dr. Lisa Blaskey, Dr. Margaret Pulsifer, and Dr. Dennis Norman. I would also like to thank Julie Sayer and Lucila Halperin, who assisted in the preparation of the manuscript, and the interns and fellows I have supervised over the years, whose questions and insights helped define the shape of this book.

Finally, I would like to give a huge thank you to my family, Eric, Hannah, and Peter, for their patience and support. They listened to my complaints when I had a stack of reports to write and still had to work on the book, and their loving faces never failed to encourage me.

* * *

The following copyright holders have generously given permission to reprint or adapt material from these copyrighted works:

From *Developmental Milestones: A Guide for Parents*, by Joyce Powell and Charles A. Smith, 1997 (Manhattan, KS: Kansas State University Cooperative Extension Service). Copyright 1997 by Kansas State University.

From *Wechsler Intelligence Scale for Children–Fourth Edition (WISC-IV)*, by D. Wechsler, 2003 (San Antonio, TX: Psychological Corporation). Copyright 2003 by Harcourt Assessment.

From *Neuropsychological Assessment* (3rd ed.), by Muriel Deutsch Lezak, 1995 (New York: Oxford University Press). Copyright 1976, 1983, 1995 by Oxford University Press.

From *Diagnostic and Statistical Manual of Mental Disorders* (4th ed., text rev.), by the American Psychiatric Association, 2000 (Washington, DC: Author). Copyright 2000 by the American Psychiatric Association.

From *Clinician's Thesaurus* (6th ed.), by E. L. Zuckerman, 2005 (New York: Guilford Press). Copyright 2005 by Edward L. Zuckerman.

From *Pocket Reference for Psychiatrists* (3rd ed.), by S. C. Jenkins, J. A. Tinsley, and V. A. Van Loon, 2001 (Washington, DC: American Psychiatric Press). Copyright 2001 by American Psychiatric Publishing, Inc.

From *Conducting School-Based Functional Behavioral Assessments*, by T. S. Watson and M. W. Steege, 2003 (New York: Guilford Press). Copyright 2003 by The Guilford Press.

Contents

Introduction

How *The Child Clinician's Report-Writing Handbook* Can Help You

The Child Clinician's Report-Writing Handbook provides terms, phrasings, concepts, report formats, and other practical information that clinicians working with children and adolescents use in their daily work. If you conduct evaluations or write diagnostic, personality, neuropsychological, or other testing-based reports, this book can make your life easier. It is organized to take you from the first meeting with a client to the final report and recommendations. It places particular emphasis on the reporting of test results, because testing is very often a crucial component of child and adolescent evaluations.

The Child Clinician's Report-Writing Handbook owes its inception, organizational format, and numerous borrowings (with permission) to Edward L. Zuckerman's well-loved *Clinician's Thesaurus*. Now in its sixth edition, the *Clinician's Thesaurus* is an essential resource for any clinician. The current volume, however, addresses in much greater depth the specific needs of practitioners who evaluate and report on children and adolescents.

If you are a beginning child (or adolescent) clinician, this book will help you collect the pertinent information you need from the young client and from parents/guardians, teachers, and/or other professionals. This book can then help you to organize this information into a high-quality report; to find the most precise terms to express your findings; to describe the tests used (if any); and to develop treatment plans and appropriate recommendations. If you are a seasoned clinician, you can use this book as a reference to refresh your skills, to get ideas about other tests or assessment instruments to use, to expand or be more succinct in your reports, and to develop diagnostic hypotheses about complicated cases. In other words, *The Child Clinician's Report-Writing Handbook* can help you do the following things:

- Structure your evaluations of children and adolescents, as well as interviews with their parents or guardians and professionals working with the children.
- Organize your information as you write or dictate your reports.
- Broaden your repertoire of terms and report-writing skills.
- Provide descriptions of tests used in evaluations.
- Make suggestions for treatment recommendations.

How This Book Is Organized

This book is organized in the same sequence that you would follow to conduct an evaluation and then to write the report.

Part I, "Questions for Conducting a Psychological Evaluation of a Child or Adolescent," offers a guide for interviewing parents or guardians, children, and teachers or other professionals.

- Chapter 1 provides **information on preparing for the interview**, establishing rapport, obtaining informed consent, and general questions for parents.
- Chapter 2 provides **specific questions for parents or guardians** to elicit information about particular disorders.
- Chapter 3 offers **questions that can be used to elicit information from children** of different ages, as well as information on observational assessments used with very young children.
- Chapter 4 provides general guidelines and **specific questions for eliciting information from children's teachers, psychologists, and other professionals**.
- Chapter 5 covers the traditional aspects of a **mental status examination** as practiced with children and adolescents.
- Chapter 6 offers suggestions for **ending the interview** with a child and parents.

Part II of this book, "Standard Terms and Statements for Wording Psychological Reports," is a guide for report writing. It begins with wordings for basic but necessary identifying information, including the referral reason and background information. It ends with recommendations and closing statements. In between, the chapters cover a wide range of possible areas and topics that might need to be addressed in a report. No single report is likely to include all these topics; rather, Part II presents a wide range of possibilities, so you can select those areas and terms most relevant to the writing task at hand.

- Chapter 7 covers **basic information** related to beginning a report, such as headings and dates, sources of information, and reliability statements.
- Chapter 8 presents wordings for possible **reasons for referral**, such as behavioral, cognitive, emotional, and family concerns.
- Chapters 9–12 cover phrases and wordings for **relevant aspects of history**, including the history of the current symptoms, medical and psychiatric background, developmental and family history, and academic history.
- Chapters 13–16 covers terms and phrases relating to the **child or adolescent in the evaluation**, such as behavioral observations; attitude toward the testing; and presentation of various affective, behavioral, and cognitive symptoms and syndromes that are first evidenced in childhood.
- Chapters 17–19 cover terms and descriptors for the **child or adolescent in the environment**, particularly home and family life, school situation, and social and recreation activities.
- Chapters 20–28 provide descriptions for the **most commonly used tests** for children and adolescents, as well as general guidelines for presenting test results in a report. Emphasis is placed on tests that are most frequently used (such as the Wechsler scales) and on tests that can be interpreted in multiple ways.
- Chapters 29–32 cover wordings for **ending the report**, including diagnostic statements, summary of findings, possible recommendations about particular disorders, and closing statements.

Part III of this book offers a chapter on the special circumstances of writing for the schools (Chapter 33), as well as chapters with a variety of useful resources. Coverage of the latter includes the following:

- Treatment-planning resources (Chapter 34).
- Formats and templates for clinical reports (Chapter 35).
- Lists of resources for professionals (Chapter 36) and for parents (Chapter 37).

- Lists of common medications (Chapter 38) and frequently used abbreviations (Chapter 39).
- Sample forms, such as a release of information form, a developmental history form, and teacher and school questionnaires (Chapter 40).

Understanding the Style and Format of the Chapters

As just described, the three parts of this book cover the questions that can be used in an evaluation (Part I); the wordings that can be used in a report (Part II); and special circumstances and resources (Part III). Each chapter is then subdivided into sections on more specific, useful topics. For example, Chapter 19, "Social and Work Relationships, Recreational Activities," has six main sections, each relating to a specific area of functioning, from general developmental aspects to friendships to work and recreational activities. Each of these main topics has its own section number (e.g., the fourth section of Chapter 19, "Peer Groups/Dating," is numbered 19.4). Cross-references are made throughout the book to these chapter and section numbers.

Within each numbered section, you may find the following different types of information:

- Introductory and explanatory comments.
- Cross-references to related sections of the book.
- References to standard works in the field or area.
- Descriptors, terms, and phrases for wording reports.

Figure 1 provides a quick visual guide to identifying the formats for these various types of information within a chapter. (It represents a composite of several pages, with some content omitted, so as to illustrate a wider range of information/format types.) It is from the descriptors that you may select the ones most appropriate for your report. The descriptors and phrasings in this book are standard American English usage. Because the terms are only rarely defined here, you may find a specialized psychiatric dictionary useful (e.g., Campbell, 2003; *Stedman's Medical Dictionary*, 2006; *Stedman's Psychiatry Words*, 2002).

Formats for Descriptors and Terms

The terms and descriptors offered in this book are printed in a **font different from the regular text and headings, to set them off.** They are arranged in several ways, ranging from an unordered group of related words or phrases to increasingly ordered arrangements, as follows:

1. **Unordered groups of similar but not synonymous words or phrases** in a line or paragraph. Example:

    Building is well/poorly maintained, clean/unkempt, is/is not wheelchair-accessible, is located in high-crime/unsafe/safe area, playground is well/adequately/poorly maintained, (no) outside play areas.

2. **An ordered spectrum of words or phrases,** indicated by a double-arrow graphic (↔), in a line or paragraph. Example:

    (↔ by degree) **No/avoided eye contact, stared into space, kept eyes downcast, poor, . . . looked only to one side, brief, flashes/fleeting, furtive/evasive, variable, appropriate, normal, expected, good, . . . penetrating, piercing, confrontative, challenging, stared without bodily movements or other expressions.**

3. **Groups of words or phrases sequenced by degree** (↔). Example:
    (↔ by degree) **These groups of descriptors are presented in order from strongest to weakest coping skills.**

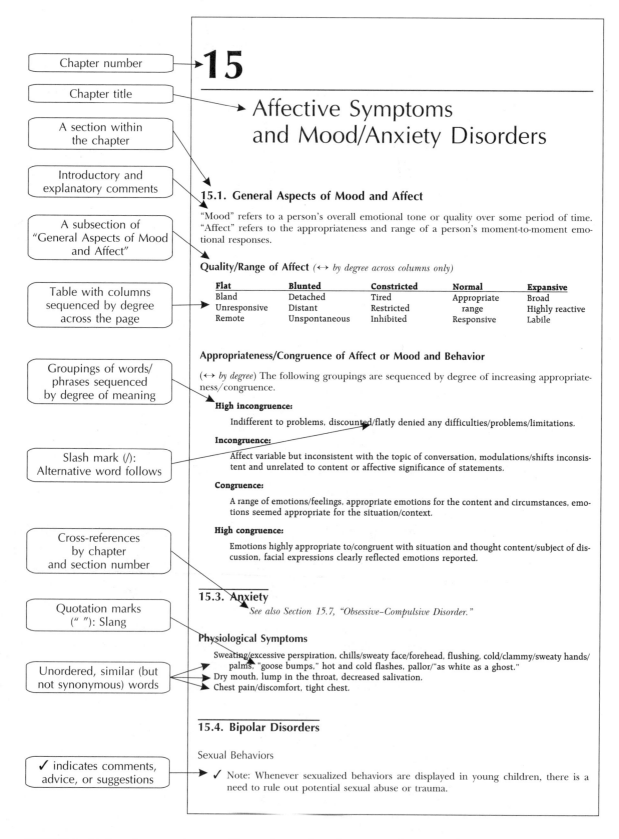

Chapter number

Chapter title

A section within
the chapter

Introductory and
explanatory comments

A subsection of
"General Aspects of Mood
and Affect"

Table with columns
sequenced by degree
across the page

Groupings of words/
phrases sequenced
by degree of meaning

Slash mark (/):
Alternative word follows

Cross-references
by chapter
and section number

Quotation marks
(" "): Slang

Unordered, similar (but
not synonymous) words

✓ indicates comments,
advice, or suggestions

15

Affective Symptoms and Mood/Anxiety Disorders

15.1. General Aspects of Mood and Affect

"Mood" refers to a person's overall emotional tone or quality over some period of time. "Affect" refers to the appropriateness and range of a person's moment-to-moment emotional responses.

Quality/Range of Affect (↔ *by degree across columns only*)

Flat	Blunted	Constricted	Normal	Expansive
Bland	Detached	Tired	Appropriate	Broad
Unresponsive	Distant	Restricted	range	Highly reactive
Remote	Unspontaneous	Inhibited	Responsive	Labile

Appropriateness/Congruence of Affect or Mood and Behavior

(↔ *by degree*) The following groupings are sequenced by degree of increasing appropriateness/congruence.

High incongruence:

Indifferent to problems, discounted/flatly denied any difficulties/problems/limitations.

Incongruence:

Affect variable but inconsistent with the topic of conversation, modulations/shifts inconsistent and unrelated to content or affective significance of statements.

Congruence:

A range of emotions/feelings, appropriate emotions for the content and circumstances, emotions seemed appropriate for the situation/context.

High congruence:

Emotions highly appropriate to/congruent with situation and thought content/subject of discussion, facial expressions clearly reflected emotions reported.

15.3. Anxiety

See also Section 15.7, "Obsessive–Compulsive Disorder."

Physiological Symptoms

Sweating/excessive perspiration, chills/sweaty face/forehead, flushing, cold/clammy/sweaty hands/palms, "goose bumps," hot and cold flashes, pallor/"as white as a ghost."
Dry mouth, lump in the throat, decreased salivation.
Chest pain/discomfort, tight chest.

15.4. Bipolar Disorders

Sexual Behaviors

✓ Note: Whenever sexualized behaviors are displayed in young children, there is a need to rule out potential sexual abuse or trauma.

FIGURE 1. Reduced composite page illustrating various formats and typographic conventions.

Good:

Did not appear frustrated by inability to solve a problem . . . , required only minimal encouragement when frustrated or distracted.

Adequate:

Often became discouraged by difficult items but persevered.

Poor:

Exhibited low frustration tolerance, gave up easily, . . .

4. **Tables of words ordered by degree across columns** (↔). Note that in these tables, the sequencing by degree is across columns *only*; words or phrases that happen to fall in the same row in such a table do not necessarily constitute a mini-sequence. Example:

Qualities of Clothing (↔ *by degree across columns only*)

Dirty	Disheveled	Neat	Stylish
Unclean	Messy	Well-groomed	Smartly dressed
Filthy	Unkempt	Neatly dressed	Chic
Grimy	Tousled	Clean	Elegant
. . .			

Typographic Conventions

Double arrow (↔): Indicates that terms or phrases are ordered along a spectrum of degree for the trait, quality, or behavior.

Slash mark (/): Indicates that an alternative word or words immediately follow. Example:

. . . presented as an attractive/handsome/pretty . . .

Quotation marks (" "): Indicates that a word is slang or inappropriate in a professional report. Examples:

"Tattling," baiting, provoking others, . . . "clowns around," "class clown."

Check mark (✓): Indicates comments, advice, cautions, and clinical tips. Note that these are intended *only* as aids to readers and should not be borrowed for a report.

Notes on Grammar and Usage

For simplicity and convenience, nouns, verbs, adjectives, and adverbs are sometimes mixed in a listing. Just modify a word as necessary to fit the sentence you have in mind.

The pronoun forms used throughout this book are intended to lessen sexist associations and implications whose harmful effects are well known. The book uses combinations such as "he/she" and "her/him" in varying order, or (much less often) alternates in turn between "he" and "she."

Finally, throughout the book, the term "parent" should be taken to mean biological parent, custodial parent, grandparent, foster parent, legal guardian, or any other caregiver/major attachment figure, even when alternative terms for "parent" are not provided. Also, the term "child" should be taken to mean "adolescent" whenever this is appropriate, even when the alternatives "child/adolescent" are not given.

A Functional Guide to Using This Book in Your Everyday Report Writing

The psychological report brings together not only test scores or other data, but the child's personality, behavioral observations, case history, family and school histories, and the child's individual strengths, weaknesses, and uniqueness. The construction of the report should actually begin long before you sit down at the computer or with the tape recorder to write or dictate your report. *The Child Clinician's Report-Writing Handbook* can be used to organize your thoughts before you meet the child and his/her family, as well as to help you express the results of the evaluation in a coherent fashion. The following discussion illustrates how this book can be used in these ways. Table 1 summarizes a generalized format for an evaluation and notes chapters or sections of this book that are relevant to each component.

Getting Ready for the Evaluation

Preparing for an evaluation of a child usually requires more "up-front" work than is required for adult work. Whereas adults most often arrive for their evaluation alone, children most often arrive with loved ones. Although adult clients and the adults who accompany children are typically prepared for a face-to-face discussion, this is not necessarily the case with the children. A child's age and developmental level significantly influence her/his approach to the evaluation. Younger children may be expecting to "play" with you, whereas adolescents would expect a more conversational approach. Thus it is essential to know the age of the child or adolescent before the first interview. In preparation, you will also want to ask yourself the following questions: "Who should attend the first session? How should I structure the interview? What toys, forms, or assessment instruments will I need? What questions do I need to ask of the parents or guardian, of the child, or of other professionals?" The following process may be helpful in preparing for the interview:

1. Consult Chapter 1 to get ideas about ways to structure the interview.
2. Chapter 40 provides forms you may want to use, such as a release of information form and a developmental history form. You will also need to have a consent form based on your state's and/or agency's guidelines. Make sure you have all pertinent forms at hand before you begin the interview.
3. Chapter 1 provides you with a list of general questions that can be asked of parents, while Chapter 2 provides a list of more specific questions for the parents or guardians. Based on the reason for the referral, you can tailor these lists to your specific focus. For example, if a child is coming for an appointment because he/she is said to be inattentive and hyperactive, you will want to ask the parent or guardian general questions found in Chapter 1 as well as questions found in Section 2.3, "Attention-Deficit/Hyperactivity Disorder (ADHD)." Based on the parent's responses, you may want to delve further into other areas, such as disruptive behavior disorders (Section 2.8) or learning disabilities (Section 2.11).
4. From Chapter 3, "Observation Procedures and Questions for Children and Adolescents," compile a list of questions appropriate for the age of the child. For example, if you are asked to assess an 11-year-old with symptoms of anxiety, you will want to pick some age-appropriate opening questions from Section 3.3; then ask age-appropriate questions about school (Section 3.4), home (Section 3.5), friends (Section 3.6), and interests (Section 3.7). You will also need to ask some specific questions about anxiety, obsessive behaviors, and mood (Section 3.9).
5. Either before or after the initial interview, you may need to talk with other professionals, such as the child's teacher, pediatrician, or psychologist. Use Chapter 4 as a guide to structure your conversation with these professionals. You can also provide a teacher with the form in Section 40.3 (a questionnaire that can be used to assess a child's classroom behavior

TABLE 1. Generalized Format for an Evaluation

Components of an evaluation	Chapters/sections of this book
Preparing for the evaluation	
Could include these:	
Advance preparation	Section 1.1
Structuring the interview	Section 1.2
Establishing rapport	Section 1.3
During the evaluation	
Could include these:	
General questions for parents	
Referral question	Section 1.6
Developmental, medical, and family histories	Sections 1.8–1.10
Relationships, interests, and school history	Sections 1.11–1.13
Additional questions for parents of adolescents	Section 1.14
Questions for parents related to the referral question	Chapter 2
General questions for the child or adolescent (questions in Chapter 3 are organized by age subject)	Chapter 3
Specific questions for the child or adolescent related to the referral question	Section 3.9
Writing the report	
Identifying information and other preliminary information	Chapter 7
Reason for referral	Chapter 8
History	
As it relates to the referral question	Chapter 9
Medical and psychiatric history	Chapter 10
Developmental and family history	Chapter 11
Academic history	Chapter 12
Behavioral observations	
Presentation	Chapter 13
Attitude toward the evaluation	Chapter 14
Clinical impressions	
Affective symptoms and mood/anxiety disorders	Chapter 15
Childhood behavioral and cognitive disorders	Chapter 16
Effects on presenting symptoms of:	
Home and family	Chapter 17
School	Chapter 18
Social relationships, etc.	Chapter 19
Test results	
Intellectual functioning	Chapter 21
Achievement	Chapter 22
Language functioning	Chapter 23
Memory	Chapter 24
Visual–spatial and motor skills	Chapter 25
Executive and neuropsychological functioning	Chapter 26
Emotional and personality functioning	Chapter 27
Behavioral and adaptive functioning	Chapter 28
Diagnostic statements (including DSM-IV-TR codes)	Chapter 29
Summary of findings	Chapter 30
Recommendations	Chapter 31
Closing statement	Chapter 32
After the interview or assessment	
You may want to:	
Interview the child's teacher or another professional working with the child	Chapter 4
Provide the teacher or other professional with forms to complete	Chapter 40
Provide the parents with additional resources	Chapter 37

and school functioning), or provide other professionals with the form in Section 40.4 (an assessment form with questions for such professionals).

6. If your evaluation includes formal testing, consult Chapters 21–28 for ideas on assessment instruments you may want to use, but please keep in mind that the lists of tests in these chapters are not exhaustive.

Writing the Report: A Suggested Outline

Once you have completed the assessment process and are ready to write the report, you can use the following outline to structure your results. The headings lettered A through D correspond to the subdivisions of Part II of this book.

A. Introducing the Report

IDENTIFYING INFORMATION

The first section of the report typically presents pertinent information about the child, including the child's name, identifying information (gender, date of birth, age, handedness), grade in school, and so forth. It also frequently includes statements about confidentiality, reliability, and self-sufficiency. The source or sources of the information are important to include as well. For example, did you interview one or both parents? Did the teacher provide information? How reliable were the informants, and were they willing participants in the assessment process? Chapter 7 provides you with information on how to present these findings within the report.

REASON FOR REFERRAL

Why did the child present for an evaluation? Who referred him/her, and what prompted the referral at this time? It is often helpful to restate the reason for the referral in a child's or parent's own language. However, it is frequently the case that the child or parent cannot succinctly state the reason for the referral, and Chapter 8 provides you with ways of describing this reason more succinctly.

B. History and Background

Chapter 9 covers the child's history as it relates to the referral question. This is often presented from a parent's (not the child's) viewpoint. For example, what is the parent's perception of the chief problem? When did it start? How has it progressed? Have the symptoms increased rapidly or gradually over time? Has anything been done to treat this problem? If so, how did it work? How much of an effect do these symptoms have on the child's functioning?

Other aspects of a child's background also need to be addressed. For example, what is the child's medical history? Has he or she developed appropriately? What is the family situation and living arrangements? Is the child doing well in school? If not, where are the difficulties? Does the child have more difficulties in one setting than in another (e.g., home vs. school)? How do these particular aspects of the child's history and background relate to the referral question? See Chapters 10, 11, and 12 for more information about these topics.

C. The Child or Adolescent in the Evaluation

Within the next section of the report, it is important to answer the following lists of questions.

OBSERVATIONS ABOUT BEHAVIOR AND ATTITUDE

- How did the child present during the evaluation? What is clinically relevant in her/his presentation? (Chapter 13)
- What was the child's attitude toward the evaluation? Was he/she a willing participant? Was rapport easily established? How was the child's effort and motivation? (Chapter 14)

CLINICAL IMPRESSIONS

- How was the child's mood? Did the mood change over the course of the evaluation? Were symptoms of anxiety, depression, or anger present? If so, did the child meet criteria for a formal mood or anxiety disorder? (Chapter 15)
- Did the child meet criteria for a formal childhood behavioral or cognitive disorder, such as attention-deficit/hyperactivity disorder (ADHD), a learning disability, or a developmental disability? How would you describe this child's unique presentation? How severe are these disabilities? (Chapter 16)

D. The Child or Adolescent in the Environment

What are the effects of the child's home and family (Chapter 17), school (Chapter 18), or social relationships (Chapter 19) on the presenting symptoms?

E. Test Results

Test results can be organized on a test-by-test, domain, or integrated basis. The way you choose to present the test results may depend on your referral source or on the audience who will be reading and using the report. What follows is a domain-based organizational strategy for presenting test findings.

Intellectual functioning (Chapter 21)
Achievement (Chapter 22)
Language functioning (Chapter 23)
Memory (Chapter 24)
Visual–spatial and motor skills (Chapter 25)
Executive and neuropsychological functioning (Chapter 26)
Emotional and personality functioning (Chapter 27)
Behavioral and adaptive functioning (Chapter 28)

F. Ending the Report

DIAGNOSTIC STATEMENTS/IMPRESSIONS

The diagnostic statement (Chapter 29) includes any relevant DSM diagnoses, as well as any rule-outs. It is generally recommended to include all five of the DSM axes in this statement.

SUMMARY OF FINDINGS AND CONCLUSIONS

In addition to a diagnostic statement, you will need to summarize the findings of the evaluation, integrating the results of the history, observations, interview, and test findings (Chapter 30). If formal testing has been completed, you should include a restatement of the reliability or validity of the findings (Chapter 20). A summary should always answer the referral question.

RECOMMENDATIONS

List the treatments or compensatory strategies that are most effective for the child's problems. Include whether follow-up evaluations will need to be pursued, such as a referral to an occupational therapist, neurologist, or psychiatrist (Chapter 31).

CLOSING STATEMENT

Thank the referrer, indicate your availability, provide a summary statement, and sign your report (Chapter 32).

Further Guidelines on Report Writing

- If you are writing with the intent of obtaining school services for the child (see Chapter 33), document whether—and why—the child *qualifies* for services. Don't simply say, "The child needs special education services."
- Write the report as soon as possible after the evaluation, so that you will be more likely to remember important details. If you are waiting for other results (e.g., teacher reports), write the history and behavioral observations as soon as possible, and add the additional data to the report once they have been collected.
- Be succinct in your writing. If information does not contribute to an understanding of the referral question or to the observed difficulties, the information is irrelevant and does not need to be included. Keep in mind the referral question and the resulting recommendations, and build a case for your findings. Information that does not contribute to this goal does not need to be included.
- Write reports that are understandable and useful to the persons or agencies that requested the report. Reports that are filled with jargon, are unrelated to referral concerns, or fail to address treatment are of little value to the referral source and to the child.
- Although you will want to report on the absence of symptoms (e.g., the child is not depressed/anxious/impulsive/etc.), the focus should be on the presence of a behavior.
- In excluding irrelevant information, be particularly careful to omit any such information that can be harmful to the child or to the family, particularly if the report will be read by school personnel. Such information may include a parent's (or adolescent's) sexual history or substance use, family living arrangements (e.g., separation), parental stress, parents' medical history, and so forth. In the course of the evaluation, you will probably learn much more about the child and the family than needs to be reported. It is your job as an evaluator to sift through this information and present *only* the information that will lead to appropriate diagnosis and treatment.
- The summary is arguably the most read section of the report. Make sure it is carefully written to emphasize those aspects of the evaluation that are most important to convey to your audience. At a minimum, it should include a restatement of the referral question, the major findings of the evaluation, their relation to the referral question, a possible diagnosis, and your conclusions.
- Knoff (1986) has indicated that the characteristics of a good report include the following: (1) The report clearly identifies the referral's concerns and answers these concerns directly in the report; (2) the report describes the most reliable behaviors that have been observed, and the information is described behaviorally, with all abstract information defined; (3) raw data are presented in context, so that readers are not asked to draw their own conclusions; (4) the child should be presented in a positive light, to the extent that this is possible; (5) the report should be concise, not omitting essential information or including irrelevant information; and (6) recommendations are described in a way in which they can be implemented.
- Proofread your report and use a spell-checker. This might seem obvious, but we've all read reports that were evidently not spell-checked. In addition, don't be afraid to get feedback on your reports from colleagues, and offer to review their reports as well. Reading and critiquing reports by other professionals will often have the effect of improving your own.

A Cautionary Note and Disclaimer

This book simply presents sample questions and lists of terms and descriptions that have been used in the field. Their presence here does not imply any endorsement by the author or the publisher.

These wordings are offered without any warranty, implied or explicit, that they constitute the only or the best way to practice as a professional or a clinician.

When individuals use any of the words, phrases, descriptors, sentences, or procedures described in this book, they must assume full responsibility for all the consequences—clinical, legal, ethical, and financial. The author and the publisher cannot, do not, and will not assume any responsibility for the use or implementation of the book's contents in practice or with any person, patient, client, or student. The author and publisher presume (1) that the users of this book are qualified by education and/or training to employ it ethically and legally, and (2) that users will not exceed the limits of documentable competence in their disciplines as indicated by their codes of ethical practice. If more than the material presented here is needed to manage a case in any regard, readers are directed to engage the services of a competent professional consultant.

Part I

Questions for Conducting a Psychological Evaluation of a Child or Adolescent

1

Beginning the Interview

1.1. Advance Preparation

Preparing the Parent(s) and Child for the Interview

See Chapter 2 regarding initial questions for parents.

Usually the initial contact with parents (or other caregivers) and children occurs on the phone. If so, the building of rapport begins even before a family arrives in the clinician's office. Use the phone call to determine whether the parents are anxious, hostile, eager, or ambivalent about being interviewed, and use this assessment as a way to approach the family in the actual interview.

- Discuss with the parent who has called you which family members should attend the first session (e.g., one or both parents, the child, etc.).
- Introduce yourself to the child's parent(s), using the name you would prefer the parents to use when speaking to you.
- Briefly describe what you will be doing with the child and what type of participation you will need from the parent(s).
- Give the parents an indication of how long the evaluation/intake will last and of how much the evaluation will cost.

Parents will often want the clinician's help in preparing their child for the first session. It is generally best for the child to know the reason for the interview or evaluation. Clear and simple statements can be used by parents to help their child understand the purpose of the evaluation—for example, "I know you've been struggling in school lately, and we want to find out how to make things better for you," or "You've seemed really sad lately, and we want to talk to someone about how we can help you feel better" These statements won't be misunderstood by the child as implying blame or be likely to distort your evaluation.

Preparing Yourself for the Interview

Be well prepared in advance of meeting a child and his/her family. Know the child's age, gender, and reason for referral. This will help you tailor your approach to each specific child. If you are scheduled to complete a testing evaluation, have all materials ready.

There are many good books for clinicians on conducting and structuring interviews with children and families. An excellent text is *The First Session with Children and Adolescents* (House, 2002).

Materials you will need for the initial session(s) include the following:

- Information regarding confidentiality and limits of privilege.
- Releases of information, multiple copies. (*See Section 40.1 for a release form.*)
- A form giving permission to evaluate or treat (to be completed by parents and/or child, depending on the child's age and state law).
- Behavior rating scales for parents and/or teachers/other professionals to complete.

1.2. Guidelines for Structuring the Interview Process

The interview is most often begun in one of the following ways:

- Parent(s) and child are interviewed together, after which time the parents or child will each be asked to respond to questions separately (with the other party out of the room).
- One or both parents are interviewed first, followed by an interview with the child, and then a joint interview.

Gathering Information from Multiple Sources

Ryan, Hammond, and Beers (1998) have suggested the following guidelines for gathering information from multiple sources:

For Inpatients

1. Observe the child's interactions with staff members.
2. Obtain information from the staff about the child's behavior and child–family interactions.
3. Evaluate whether formal assessment is appropriate.

For Outpatients

1. Obtain records from the referring professional and other relevant professionals.
2. Discuss the purpose of the evaluation with a family member (this is often done by phone).
3. Provide an opportunity for the child to speak to you, and speak plainly with the child about limits of confidentiality and what you can and cannot do.
4. Ask parents to bring school records to the evaluation.

Structured Diagnostic Interviews

Structured interviews range from highly structured to semistructured. In clinical practice, face-to-face structured interviews are most often used when there is a research component to the treatment. The more highly structured of these interviews are typically used by lay interviewers, as experienced clinicians typically find that they do not allow for latitude in clinical decision making. Semistructured interviews are designed to be administered by more extensively trained interviewers. Some clinicians will use a combination of structured and unstructured formats, such as administering a written evaluation form that will include structured questions, as well as conducting a less structured face-to-face interview. Examples of face-to-face structured interviews include the following (all of these interviews have both a parent and a child version):

- Diagnostic Interview Schedule for Children, Version IV (DISC-IV; Shaffer, 1996).
- Schedule for Affective Disorders and Schizophrenia for School-Age Children—Present and Lifetime Version (K-SADS-PL; Kaufman, Birmaher, Brent, Rao, & Ryan, 1996).
- Child Assessment Schedule (CAS; Hodges, 1993).
- Schedule for Affective Disorders and Schizophrenia for School-Age Children—Epidemiological Version 5 (K-SADS-E5; Orvaschel, 1995).
- Child and Adolescent Psychiatric Assessment (CAPA): Version 4.2—Child Version (Angold, Cox, Rutter, & Simonoff, 1996).

1.3. Establishing Rapport

The first few minutes of any interview are important. Suggestions for enhancing rapport include the following:

General Tips

- Greet the child by her/his first name and introduce yourself. Use the name you would prefer the child to call you. Some clinicians prefer to be called by their first names, while others prefer to use a title (e.g., "Dr."). Many clinicians use their first names with very young children but use a title when working with adolescents.
- Give younger children time to settle down. If they've brought something from home, use it as a way of making conversation.
- The things you say to a child and the first questions you ask should be flexible and geared to the particular child (see Chapter 3 for initial interview questions). However, these often include questions that a child can easily answer, such as "How old are you?" and "Do you have any pets?"
- Respond to the child with openness, warmth, empathy, and respect. Be attentive to the child's needs, such as hunger, need for physical activity, or use of the toilet. In contrast, know when it is appropriate to set limits on behaviors.
- Provide age-appropriate breaks as necessary.

With the Very Young Child (Ages 2½–6 years)

- Have a working knowledge of types of toys and activities that children of this age would enjoy. Know what is currently popular for the age group. You can then ask about and comment on a child's favorite toys and activities.
- Begin building rapport by talking about children's clothing, toys they may have brought to the office, toys they are playing with in the waiting room, how they got to the office, what the drive was like, how long it took them to get there, or the like.
- Be aware of a child's emotional state and respond appropriately to how he/she feels.
- Activities that enhance rapport with a very young child include drawing pictures of her/his choosing, playing structured games (Candy Land, Connect Four, Mancala, etc.), or playing with "open-ended" toys (Legos, modeling clay, dolls, etc.).

With the School-Age Child (Ages 6–12 Years)

- Children in this age group often enjoy talking about their hobbies, teachers, school, after-school activities, friends, video games, sports, clothes, shopping, "hanging out," and so forth.
- Have a working knowledge of activities, toys, TV programs, computer games, and the like that are of interest to this age group.
- Begin building rapport by talking about what the drive to the office was like; whether children are missing school or an activity for the appointment; any objects (e.g., Game Boy, iPod, MP3 player) or books they might have brought to the office; or similar topics.
- If an evaluation is being completed with the intention of beginning therapy, it is important to discuss the rules of therapy and of confidentiality in age-appropriate language. The "rules" of therapy vary by individual professionals or clinics, and frequently by individual cases as well. One such "rule" involves what type of information is shared by the therapist between parents and child (e.g., everything can be shared; nothing is shared, with the exception of topics the therapist is legally required to report; certain topics, such as boyfriends/girlfriends, are off limits; etc.). Other "rules" may include how frequently the parents will meet with the therapist; whether the child has a role in determining the frequency and con-

tent of these meetings; whether the treatment is to be individual or have a family component; and so on. It is important to make these "ground rules" clear to both the child and the parents. In some cases, the establishment of these rules becomes an important part of the therapy itself, opening the discussion of limit setting for parents and their children.

- Ask the child what he/she was told would happen. Decide where and how (e.g., in the presence of the parents, with the child alone, etc.) you will address this question, as it may be differently phrased, depending upon the age of the child. If you want a frank view from the child, it is frequently best to ask the child with the parents out of the room.

With Adolescents (Ages 12–18 Years)

- It is important to acknowledge an adolescent's feelings. Many adolescents are not happy at the prospect of an evaluation or therapy, and most will appreciate a clinician who validates their feelings.
- Adolescents also appreciate being treated as mature individuals. It is best to treat them as if they are adults, to the degree that this is reasonable. Of course, once adolescents reach the age of 18 they are legally adults, but it is the therapist's responsibility to decide to what degree they should be treated as adults. This is a central issue of adolescence; however, each child and family is different, so you will need to develop (and model) a balance that is logical, clear, acceptable, and therapeutically appropriate to all concerned.
- Discuss confidentiality and the "rules" of therapy (see above). Adolescents are typically much more involved in establishing these types of "rules," including who attends the sessions, what type of information will and will not be shared with the parents, how frequently sessions will be held, and so forth.

1.4. Informed Consent

Therapists are obligated to obtain informed consent before beginning assessment or treatment with any client. Although state regulations may vary somewhat, a clinician cannot treat or evaluate a minor without written consent from the minor's legal guardian. Although some state laws may differ, you can typically evaluate or treat a child from an intact family with the permission of either parent. When a minor's parents are divorced, it is essential to obtain the consent of the parent who has legal physical custody. If custody is shared, you will generally need to obtain permission from both parents. It is important to check your state's legal requirements regarding consent to treating a minor.

There is no "one size fits all" informed consent form, because different informed consent procedures are likely to be needed, depending on what a parent (and sometimes a child) wants and needs to hear (Braaten & Handelsman, 1997). Handelsman (2001) encourages professionals to follow these guidelines in providing informed consent:

- Obtaining informed consent should be thought of as a process and not a one-time event. For example, issues of confidentiality involving a minor can arise throughout the course of therapy, and such issues will need to be addressed as they arise.
- The informed consent process should be incorporated into the treatment of any child. In the case of a young child (below the age of 5 or 6 years), the "client" who needs to be kept informed is typically one or both parents; for a school-age child or an adolescent, the "client" typically includes both the child and the parent(s).
- Provide information that, in your opinion, "[children] or their loved ones would want" (Handelsman, 2001, p. 457).
- Solicit assent even from those who are not competent (or of age) to consent.

- Provide information that a "reasonable person would want to know" (Handelsman, 2001, p. 454).
- Document the consent process, including the initial conversation as well as ongoing ones.
- Make your forms readable and personalized to your practice.
- Give the client (see the definitions of "client" in the second point above) a copy of the form.
- Review the initial information as needed throughout the professional relationship.

Wiger (1999) has identified several areas of confidentiality that should be addressed with the client (again, see the definitions of "client" above):

- A professional must report abuse of children and vulnerable adults.
- A professional has a duty to warn and protect when a client indicates she/he has a plan to harm self or others.
- Parents and legal guardians have the right of access to their children's psychotherapy and testing records, unless doing so would be harmful to the children.
- The client should be informed if someone other than the therapist types the child's reports.
- A professional is required to report admitted prenatal exposure to controlled substances.
- A therapist is required to release records in the event of a court order.
- Professional misconduct by a health care provider must be reported.
- Professionals should inform clients about their policy regarding the use of collection agencies. Clinicians have a right to use such an agency, if a client is informed that some aspects of the treatment (such as number of sessions) can be shared with a collection agency in the interest of obtaining unpaid fees.
- Information about third-party payers should be provided, such as what type of information (e.g., diagnosis, progress reports, etc.) you are required to give to a client's insurance company in order for insurance to cover the claim.
- The client should be informed about the role of professional consultations.
- The therapist should provide clear guidelines regarding the keeping of information in child, family, and relationship counseling.
- The client should be provided with information regarding telephone calls, answering machines, and voice mail.

Here are some final points to keep in mind regarding consent with children and adolescents:

- Discuss the issues of confidentiality involved in treating minor patients with the client. The discussion should include how you intend to balance the child's need for confidentiality against the parents' need for essential information.
- Consider writing a formal agreement regarding this discussion. Although the agreement would not be legally binding, it is often helpful to have a clearly written understanding of this policy.
- Working with minors often entails communicating with other professionals (e.g., teachers, etc.), which can present dilemmas for clinicians. Therapists and evaluators need consent from parents in order to share information with school personnel, and a therapist or evaluator should be aware that the information thus shared may not necessarily be entirely confidential.
- *The Paper Office* (Zuckerman, 2003) provides a wealth of data regarding informed consent to treatment and assessment, including some forms.
- Clinicians should always consult the state statutes that govern their profession.

1.5. Obtaining Identifying Information from Parents

"What is the child's name? Address? Phone number? Date of birth? Age?"
"What is your family's living arrangement? Who lives with your child?"
"What school does your child attend? What grade is she/he in?"

"What language is spoken in the home/the school/the neighborhood?"
"How would you describe your family's racial or ethnic identity?"

1.6. Eliciting the Chief Concern/Problem from Parents

"What is your reason for seeking this evaluation/consultation?"
"Tell me in your own words what you feel your child's main problem is."
"Tell me what has been going on with the child."
"What are your specific concerns?"
"What concerns you most?"
"What are your hopes for this evaluation/consultation/treatment?"
"What are your hopes for the child?"

Eliciting the Parents' Understanding of the Chief Concern/Problem

"Do you have any ideas about what might have caused the child's problem?"
"Do you think anything particular triggered or contributed to your child's problems?"
"What do you think are the most important aspects of the child's history in light of the chief concern?"
"Do you think that any aspects of the family's medical or psychological history may have played a role in the problem?"

Dimensionalizing the Concern/Problem

"When did you first notice the child's difficulties?" (duration)
"How long has this been happening?" (duration)
"How often does this happen?" (frequency)
"How intense or mild is it usually? (intensity)
"How difficult is the problem for the child?" (intensity)
"Where are the child's difficulties most apparent? (At home? At school? In friendships?)" (setting)

Determining Earlier Efforts to Deal with the Concern/Problem

"How have you, as parents, dealt with the problem?"
"How has your family adjusted to the child's problem(s)? What types of accommodations have been made in the school?"
"Has your child been previously diagnosed with a psychological or academic difficulty? (If yes:) What was the diagnosis? Who made the diagnosis? When was the diagnosis made?"
"Did you agree with the diagnosis? Why or why not?"
"What is the child's teacher's view of his/her problem(s)?"

1.7. Prenatal, Birth, and Neonatal History   *See Chapter 10 for descriptors.*

Prenatal History

"Did you experience any difficulties during pregnancy, such as preterm labor, medical complications, or psychosocial stressors? (If yes:) What types of difficulties did you experience?"
"Did you receive prenatal medical care? Beginning at what month?"
"Was the child exposed to any prescription or nonprescription drugs during pregnancy? (If yes:) What were they, and how often were they taken?"
"Did you/the child's mother smoke during pregnancy? (If yes:) How much?"

Delivery

"Was the pregnancy full-term, or was the child born prematurely? (If prematurely:) At how many weeks' gestation?"

"How much did the child weigh at birth?"

"Was the delivery normal, or were there complications?"

"What was the child's general health at the time of the delivery?"

"What were the child's Apgar scores?"

Infant Temperament

"What type of baby was the child?"

"What was the child's activity level? Level of alertness?"

"Was it easy or difficult for you to soothe/calm the child? Could the child soothe/calm him-/herself?"

"Would you say that the child was a generally happy baby? A generally fussy baby?"

"How did the child respond to you as an infant?"

"Did the child experience any feeding difficulties in infancy? Sleeping difficulties? Other problems?"

Adoption

"At what age was the child adopted?"

"Where did the child's adoption take place?"

"What do you know of the child's prenatal and birth history?"

"With whom was the child living at the time of the adoption?"

"Describe the terms of the adoption (e.g., open adoption, international adoption, etc.)."

"Are there any issues regarding the child's adoption that are important to consider in light of her/his current difficulties? (If so:) What are they?"

1.8. Developmental History

See Section 40.2 for a developmental history form that can be used to elicit information. For developmental history descriptors, as well as lists of milestones in specific developmental areas, see Chapter 11.

Ask the parent or guardian whether the child reached key developmental milestones at the appropriate ages. The following lists, adapted from one by Powell and Smith (1997), gives various milestones by average age.

List of Developmental Milestones

By 3 Months of Age

MOTOR SKILLS

- Lift head and chest when lying on his/her stomach.
- Follow a moving object or person with her/his eyes.
- Grasp rattle when given to him/her.

SENSORY AND THINKING SKILLS

- Turn head toward the sound of a human voice.
- Recognize bottle or breast.
- Respond to the shaking of a rattle or bell.

LANGUAGE AND SOCIAL SKILLS

- Make cooing, gurgling sounds.
- Communicate hunger, fear, discomfort (through crying or facial expression).
- React to "peek-a-boo" games.

By 6 Months of Age

MOTOR SKILLS

- Reach for and grasp objects.
- Play with toes.
- Explore by mouthing and banging objects.
- Move toys from one hand to another.
- Sit with only a little support.
- Roll over.

SENSORY AND THINKING SKILLS

- Imitate familiar actions a caregiver performs.

LANGUAGE AND SOCIAL SKILLS

- Babble, making almost sing-song sounds.
- Know familiar faces.
- Smile at her-/himself in a mirror.

By 12 Months of Age

MOTOR SKILLS

- Drink from a cup with help.
- Feed him-/herself finger foods (e.g., raisins or bread crumbs).
- Grasp small objects by using thumb and index finger/forefinger.
- Put small blocks into and take them out of a container.
- Sit well without support.
- Crawl on hands and knees.
- Pull her-/himself to stand or take steps holding onto furniture.
- Stand alone momentarily.

SENSORY AND THINKING SKILLS

- Try to accomplish simple goals (e.g., seeing and then crawling to a toy).
- Look for an object he/she watched fall out of sight (such as a spoon that falls under the table).

LANGUAGE AND SOCIAL SKILLS

- Say her/his first word.
- Respond to another's distress by showing distress or crying.
- Show mild to severe anxiety at separation from parent.
- Show apprehension about strangers.
- Understand simple commands.

By 18 Months of Age

MOTOR SKILLS

- Pull off hat, socks, and mittens.
- Turn pages in a book.
- Stack two blocks.
- Scribble with crayons.
- Walk without help.

SENSORY AND THINKING SKILLS

- Identify an object in a picture book.
- Look for objects that are out of sight.
- Follow simple one-step directions.

LANGUAGE AND SOCIAL SKILLS

- Say 8–10 words a caregiver can understand.
- Ask specifically for his/her mother and father.
- Use "hi," "bye," and "please," with reminders.
- Asks for something by pointing or by using one word.
- Become anxious when separated from parent(s).
- Play alone on the floor with toys.
- Recognize her-/himself in the mirror or in pictures.

By 2 Years of Age

MOTOR SKILLS

- Drink from a straw.
- Feed him-/herself with a spoon.
- Toss or roll a large ball.
- Open cabinets, drawers, boxes.
- Walk up steps with help.

SENSORY AND THINKING SKILLS

- Like to take things apart.
- Point to five or six parts of a doll when asked.

LANGUAGE AND SOCIAL SKILLS

- Have a vocabulary of several hundred words.
- Use two- to three-word sentences.
- Say names of toys.
- Listen to short rhymes.
- Take turns in play with other children.
- Apply pretend action to others (e.g., pretending to feed a doll).
- Refer to self by name and use "me" and "mine."
- Verbalize desires and feeling (e.g., "I want cookie").
- Laugh at silly labeling of objects and events (e.g., calling a nose an ear).
- Point to eyes, ears, or nose when asked.

By 3 Years of Age

MOTOR SKILLS

- Feed her-/himself (with some spilling).
- Hold a glass in one hand.
- Hold a crayon well.
- Fold paper, if shown how.
- Throw a ball overhead.
- Dress him-/herself with help.
- Use the toilet with some help.
- Walk up steps, alternating feet.
- Kick a ball forward.
- Pedal a tricycle.

SENSORY AND THINKING SKILLS

- Remember what happened yesterday.
- Know some numbers (but not always in the right order).
- Understand "now," "soon," and "later."
- Look through a book alone.
- Match circles and squares.
- Match an object to a picture of that object.
- Match objects that have similar functions (e.g, putting a cup and plate together).
- Count two to three objects.
- Follow simple one-step commands.

LANGUAGE AND SOCIAL SKILLS

- Use three- to five-word sentences.
- Use plurals ("dogs," "cars," "hats").
- Name at least one color correctly.
- Ask to use the toilet almost every time.
- Demonstrate some shame when caught in a wrongdoing.
- Play spontaneously with two or three children in a group.
- Understand "I," "you," "he," and "she."
- Answer whether she/he is a boy or girl.

By 4 Years of Age

MOTOR SKILLS

- Feed him-/herself (with little spilling).
- Hold a pencil.
- Draw a circle.
- Draw a face.
- Try to cut paper with blunt scissors.
- Brush teeth with help.
- Build a tower of seven to nine blocks.
- Put together a simple puzzle of 4–12 pieces.
- Pour from a small pitcher.
- Use the toilet alone.
- Catch a bouncing ball.
- Walk downstairs, using a handrail and alternating feet.

SENSORY AND THINKING SKILLS

- Understand "big," "little," "tall," "short."
- Sort by shape or color.
- Count up to five objects.
- Distinguish between the real world and the imaginary or "pretend" world.

LANGUAGE AND SOCIAL SKILLS

- Have a large vocabulary and use good grammar often.
- Use regular past tenses of verbs ("pulled," "walked").
- Ask direct questions ("May I?", "Would you?").
- Understand "next to."
- Separate from a parent for a short time without crying.
- Help clean up toys at home or school when asked to.
- Like to play "dress-up."
- Often prefer playing with other children to playing alone, unless deeply involved in a solitary task.
- Share when asked.

By Childhood Years (Ages 6–12)

SOCIAL AND EMOTIONAL DEVELOPMENT

- Have an average five good friends and at least one "enemy," who often changes from day to day.
- Act nurturing and commanding with younger children, but follow and depend on older children.
- Begin to see the point of view of others more clearly.
- Define her-/himself in terms of appearance, possessions, and activities.
- Develop and practice inner control each time decisions are made.
- At around age 6–8, may still be afraid of monsters and the dark; these are replaced later by fears of school or disaster and confusion over social relationships.
- Often become attached to an adult (teacher, club leader, caregiver) other than parents, and quote the new "hero" or try to please him/her to gain attention.

PHYSICAL DEVELOPMENT

- Recognize differences between boys and girls.
- Develop muscle coordination and control (uneven and incomplete in the early stages, but almost as good as adults by the end of middle childhood).
- Lose baby teeth and begin acquiring permanent ones.
- Reach visual maturity (both size and function).

MENTAL DEVELOPMENT

- Begin to read and write early in middle childhood, and should be skillful in reading and writing by the end of this stage.
- At first, can rarely sit for longer than 15–20 minutes for an activity; attention span gets longer with age.
- Can talk through problems to solve them.
- Can focus attention and take time to search for needed information.
- Can develop a plan to meet a goal.
- Develop greater memory capability, because many routines (brushing teeth, tying shoes, bathing, etc.) are automatic now.

Questions about Developmental Milestones/Delays

"How old was the child when he/she started to crawl? Walk? Talk? Use the toilet? Dress him-/herself?"

"Was the child delayed in reaching any of these milestones?"

(If yes:) "Did the child receive treatment for any of these delays/difficulties?"

(If yes:) "What were the treatments, and did you feel they were successful?"

"Were there any significant events in the child's early life that may be related to her/his current difficulties? (If so:) What were these events?"

1.9. Medical History   *See Chapter 10 for descriptors.*

"Tell me about the child's medical or health history."

"Has the child experienced any difficulties with the following: Allergies? Asthma? Frequent ear infections? Epilepsy? Enuresis/bedwetting? Encopresis/soiling? Eczema? Head injury? Hypoxia/oxygen deprivation? Neonatal jaundice? Meningitis? Problems with vision or hearing?"

"Has the child experienced any significant illnesses (If so:) What were they, and when did they occur?"

"Has the child had any surgeries? (If so:) What were they, and when did they occur?"

"Has the child ever been hospitalized? (If so:) When and why?"

"Has the child been exposed to toxins such as lead? Do you know whether your house has lead paint, and, if so, have you discussed this issue with your pediatrician?"

"Does the child currently take any medications? (If so:) What are the medications, and do these have any significant side effects?"

"In the past, has the child ever taken medications for an extended period of time? (If so:) What were the medications, and why were they prescribed?"

"Has the child been prescribed glasses/hearing aids? (If so:) Does the child consistently wear them?"

"Were there any significant medical problems in the child's life that may be related to his/her current difficulties? (If so:) What were these events?"

1.10. Family History   *See Chapter 11 for descriptors.*

"Tell me what your home is like."

"Who lives in your home? What is each person's relationship to the child?"

"Has the child moved frequently/recently? (If so:) What were the reasons for the moves?"

"Has your family experienced any recent stresses that may be affecting the child's behavior?"

Information about Siblings

"Where is the child's place in your children's birth order?"

"Do any of the child's siblings have any significant medical problems or psychiatric problems? (If so:) What is the effect of these problems on the child?"

Information about Parents

"Are you single, married, divorced, or living with a partner?"

(If married:) "Is your spouse the child's natural/birth mother/father? How many years have you been married? How would you describe the quality of your relationship?"

(If divorced:) "When did you separate? What was the effect of the divorce on the child's behavior? How would you describe your current relationship with the child's mother/father? Who has custody? How often does the child visit his/her noncustodial parent?"

"How old were you when the child was born?"

"How old was your spouse/partner when the child was born?"

"What is your/your spouse's/partner's current occupation?"

"What is the effect of your job/your spouse's/partner's job on the family?"

"Does either of your families have a history of drug or alcohol abuse? Learning disabilities? Medical problems? Psychiatric difficulties?"

(If living with a partner:) "How long have you been living with your current partner? How would you describe your child's relationship with your partner? How would you describe your partner's relationship with your child's father/mother?"

Adoption Issues

"Does the child know he/she is adopted?"

"Does the child have contact with her/his birth parents? (If so:) What kind of contact, and how frequently does it occur?"

1.11. Relationships

For descriptors, see Section 11.7 (relationships with parents); Section 11.8 (relationships with siblings); and Sections 19.3 and 19.4 (friendships and peer groups, respectively).

With Peers

"Does the child have friends? (If no:) Why do you think the child doesn't have friends?"

"How well does the child get along with his/her friends?"

"Do you like his/her friends?"

"What kinds of opportunities does the child have to make friends?"

"How do other children treat/react to the child?"

With Siblings

"How does the child get along with her/his brothers/sisters? What do they do that the child likes/dislikes?"

With Parents and Other Adults

"How would you describe the quality of your relationship with your child? Is it different from the quality of the relationship with your other children?"

"How does the child show affection for you? Anger toward you?"

"What family member is the child most like? Why?"

"How does the child interact with other adults? Is there anything about these relationships that concern you?"

"How is discipline handled in your home? Is it effective? Who usually administers the discipline?"

1.12. Interests and Routines

Interests

"What kinds of things does the child like to do in her/his free time?"

"What does the child like to do when he/she is alone? With friends/sisters/brothers/other family members?"

"How much television does the child watch? Do you feel happy with that amount? What kinds of TV shows does she/he like to watch?"

"What kinds of music does the child like to listen to?"

Routines

"Do you have any particular routines (such as bedtime, homework, etc.) that you typically follow? (If so:) Can you describe these for me?"

"What happens to your child when you're not able to follow the routines on a particular day?"

"Does the child do any chores? (If so:) What are they?"

1.13. Academic History   *See Chapter 12 for descriptors.*

Current Placement

"What type of school does the child attend (e.g., private, public, Montessori, etc.)?"

"How long has the child attended this school?"

"What grade is the child in?"

"What type of classroom setting is this (e.g., traditional, multiple ages, etc.)? How many teachers are in the classroom? How many students?"

"How do you feel about the school? About the child's current teacher(s)?"

School Experiences

"Describe the child's school experiences, beginning with preschool."

"At which ages or grades (if any) did the child begin experiencing difficulties?"

"What types of difficulties were observed?"

"What type of special services (if any) did the child receive?"

"Has the child ever been on an Individualized Education Plan or a Section 504 plan?"

General Academic Functioning

"How do you feel school is going for the child?"

"What does the child like/dislike about school? What are his/her best/worst subjects?"

"How satisfied is the child with his/her progress or performance in school?"

1.14. Additional Questions about Adolescents

"Does your teen date? What does she/he generally do on a date? Do you approve?"

"Do you think that your teen may be sexually active? Have you discussed appropriate sexual behavior with him/her? (If yes:) What have you talked about?"

"Do you have any concerns about drug/alcohol use? (If yes:) What kind of drugs/alcohol do you think your teen may be using? Has the teen been in trouble because of drug/alcohol use? How does she/he pay for/get drugs/alcohol? Have you ever sought treatment for her/his alcohol/drug use? (If yes:) What type of treatment? Was it effective?"

"Does the teen have a job? (If yes:) What does he/she do? Do you approve of his/her working?"

2

Questions for Parents on Signs, Symptoms, and Behavior Patterns

Chapter 1 has offered general questions for gathering background information and history, as well as for eliciting the referral reason. This chapter suggests further questions to ask parents (or other guardians) depending upon the specific referral reason or chief concern. These questions are meant only as a guide; no interviewer will ask all of these questions. The clinician should focus on those areas of concern to the particular child, as well as on the parents' or guardians' concerns and goals for the assessment.

2.1. Anger and Aggression

See also see Section 2.8, "Disruptive Behavior Disorders." See Section 15.2 for descriptors.

"What does the child do when he/she gets angry?"
"When your child gets angry, what behaviors concern you most?"
"When the child gets angry, does a tantrum usually follow? And does anger usually accompany tantrums?"
"Where does this anger behavior happen most often (e.g., home, school, etc.)?"
"When does this behavior most often happen? Are there particular times?"
"Can the child get over her/his angry feelings without adult help?"
"Who are usually the targets of the child's angry behavior?"
"Are there particular things that set off the child's angry behavior? Or can anything set the child off?"

2.2. Anxiety *See Section 15.3 for descriptors.*

General Anxiety Symptoms

"Does your child worry a lot? Appear nervous or tense?"
"Does your child complain about how he/she feels? (If so:) Does he/she experience sweaty palms or excessive perspiration? Dry mouth? Frequent nausea or upset stomach? Shaking or dizziness? Muscle tension? Rapid heart beat or respiration?"
"When the child was young, was she/he frequently clingy?"

"As a baby or toddler, did the child have trouble being separated from you/the parents?"
"Does your child have any nervous habits, such as nail biting, tics, or repetitive movements?"
"Has the child's anxiety/nervousness affected his/her relationships with other children? With you?"

Panic Attacks

"Do you think your child has ever had a panic attack—intense fear, rapid heartbeat, shortness of breath, sweaty palms, without an obvious trigger for the event? (If yes:) How did the child act? What made you most concerned? When did the panic attack happen? Has there been more than one? How frequently does your child have them?"
"Are the panic attacks linked to any specific situation, such as riding in a car or taking a test?"
"Has your child ever been treated for panic attacks? (If yes:) Did the treatment help?"
"Do you do anything to help your child during a panic attack? (If yes:) What works? What doesn't work?"

2.3. Attention-Deficit/Hyperactivity Disorder (ADHD)

See Section 16.1 for descriptors.

There are several standardized questionnaires that can be used with parents when the referral question relates to ADHD. These are the most common:

ADHD Rating Scale–IV (DuPaul, Power, Anastopoulos, & Reed, 1998)
Behavior Assessment System for Children, Second Edition (BASC-2; Reynolds & Kamphaus, 2004)
Behavior Rating Inventory of Executive Functions (BRIEF; Gioia, Isquith, Guy, & Kenworthy, 2000)
Conner's Rating Scales–Revised (CRS-R; Conners, 1997)

"How well does your child pay attention to tasks? Is the child easily distracted? Does he/she frequently daydream? How well is he/she able to screen out background noise or details?"
"Is your child often forgetful? (If yes:) Can you give me an example?"
"Does your child have difficulty remembering to do things?"
"Does your child have problems with memory in general? (If yes:) Can you give me an example?"
"Does your child have any chores at home? (If yes:) Is he/she able to complete these chores?"
"Does your child complete her/his homework? Is the homework usually done well? Is it hard for her/him to complete assignments? How much help do you need to provide? Does your child make careless errors on assignments? (If yes:) What types of errors?"

"How active is your child? Is it hard for him/her to sit still? (If yes:) What is this like? Does it ever seem as if he/she is driven by a motor that you can't shut off? Does he/she have an excessive amount of energy? Does your child talk excessively? Does she/he frequently interrupt others? Does he/she have difficulty awaiting his/her turn?"
"Does your child often act 'in the moment' without thought to the consequences? Does she/he have trouble controlling her/his response in different situations? (If yes:) Can you think of an example? Would you describe her/him as a risk taker?"
"Has your child had any serious problems at school? Expulsion? Suspensions? Poor grades? Poor attendance?"
"Is your child easily frustrated? What types of things typically frustrate her/him?"
"How frequent are the problems you've described?"

"Does the child see that he/she has problems? (If yes:) What does he/she think of them?"

"Has anything ever been done to treat these problems (at school or through medication)? (If yes:) How successful were these efforts?"

"What are your greatest concerns about your child's behavior? Do both parents agree with each other? Does the child's other parent agree with you about these problems?"

2.4. Bipolar Disorders   *See Section 15.4 for descriptors.*

"Does your child ever seem to be out of control? For instance, does she/he show extreme silliness? Extreme irritability? Impatience to the point of being highly agitated? A disregard for authority? Aggressive behaviors? (If yes to any:) Can you give me an example?"

"Does your child ever have a decreased need for sleep? (If so:) Can you give me an example of what that is like?"

"Does your child ever show unusual sexual behaviors? For example, does he/she engage in doctor play abnormal for his/her age? Show inappropriate interest in sexual manners? Expose him-/herself to other children? Engage in increased masturbation?"

(For an adolescent:) "Does your teen show an excessive interest in sex or pornography? Make frequent and/or unwelcome sexual overtures to others? Have increased sexual activity and/or masturbation?"

✓ Note: If sexual symptoms are endorsed, the examiner should thoroughly rule out the possibility of sexual abuse.

"Is there any family history of bipolar disorders/manic–depressive illness?"

2.5. Communication Disorders   *See Section 16.2 for descriptors.*

"How well does your child understand spoken language/what people say?"

"Does she/he have trouble understanding if long or complex sentences are used?"

"Do you have any concerns about the child's ability to speak or express him-/herself in words? How well does the child use language to express his/her thoughts/ideas?"

"Does the child have problems saying certain words or sounds? (If yes:) Can you give me an example?"

"Does your child have problems finding the right word? Do you think the child uses words like 'you know,' 'stuff,' or 'thing' when she/he can't come up with the right word? Does the child often use the wrong word for something, such as 'fork' for 'spoon'?"

2.6. Depression   *See Section 15.5 for descriptors.*

"Does your child ever have periods of depressed/low mood or extreme sadness? (If yes:) How long do these periods last?"

"Does your child ever feel too sad to get out of bed in the morning? Does he/she smile rarely or cry frequently? Is the child uncommunicative?"

"Have you noticed any problems with the child's appetite—either overeating (being hungry all the time, can't stop eating) or not feeling like eating at all? (If yes:) Is this a change for her/him?"

"Does your child complain about low energy level, feeling tired all the time, intestinal distress, stomach cramps, or just not feeling right?"

"Have these symptoms affected the child's academic performance? Social relationships and friendships? Family relationships?"

"Does the child seem harder on him-/herself these days? More self-critical than usual? Does the child have feelings of low self-esteem? Is there a preoccupation with death? Is the child overly sensitive to criticism?"

✓ Note: If depression is suspected, but typical symptoms are not endorsed, screen for symptoms of "masked" depression: anger, irritability, and/or hyperactivity.

2.7. Developmental Disorders, Pervasive   *See Section 16.9 for descriptors.*

"How does the child relate to others? Does the child share interests or pleasures with others? Or does she/he prefer to play alone?"

"How well does your child make eye contact with others? As a baby, did the child avoid looking at others? Was the child an unresponsive infant in other ways? Did he/she smile appropriately as a baby?"

"Did you notice any problems in the child's development of language? How well does he/she understand language? Jokes?"

"Does the child ever repeat what others say in a robotic way? Do you ever notice that the child reverses pronouns, such as referring to him-/herself as 'you,' or referring to others as 'I' or 'me'?"

"Is the child able to carry on a conversation?"

"Does the child repeat any actions or behavior patterns over and over again? (If yes:) What are they? How does the child react when someone tries to interfere with these repeated actions?

"Does the child talk on and on and on about a particular topic?"

"Is the child ever fascinated with parts of objects? Is the child more interested in objects than people? Is the child obsessively fascinated with unusual things for his/her age?"

"Describe how the child plays. What kinds of things does she/he do?"

"Does the child have any particular patterns of body movements (spinning, hand flapping, rocking, twirling, etc.)?"

"Does the child have any difficulties moving arms or legs? Using his/her large muscles? Does he/she have any difficulty making small, precise movements, such as in drawing or writing?"

"What is the child's attention like?"

"Has the child ever been either insensitive or oversensitive to noise, touch, foods, smells, light, or pain?"

2.8. Disruptive Behavior Disorders   *See Section 16.3 for descriptors.*

"Does your child defy or oppose you or other adults? (If yes:) How? Arguing? Refusing to do what you ask? Refusing to follow rules? Deliberately annoying others? Losing her/his temper?"

"How does the child explain his/her behaviors? Does he/she blame others?"

"Has the child ever done any of the following (if yes, ask parent to explain): Theft? Running away from home? Truancy from school? Setting fires? Writing graffiti? Violating curfew? Drug use? Sexual activity? Gang membership? Frequently getting into fights?"

"How would you describe your child's mood generally? Is she/he generally angry, resentful, irritable? Does the child have a short fuse? Feel bad about her-/himself?"

2.9. Eating Problems and Disorders

For descriptors, see Section 16.4 (eating disorders) and Section 16.5 (intake disorders).

"Has your child had any eating difficulties? Is he/she a finicky eater? Does he/she overeat? Does he/she eat unusual substances? (If yes:) Please describe."

"Is your child cutting down on the amount of food she/he eats, or refusing to eat? Have you noticed any fixed patterns of behavior about eating? Does the child have a preoccupation with food or dieting?"

"Has the child experienced any physical consequences from his/her eating problems, such as heart difficulties? Hair loss? Low blood pressure? Reduced body temperature? (For an adolescent girl:) Problems with menstrual irregularity?"

"How would you describe your child's personality? Is she/he perfectionistic, self-disciplined to a fault, or too eager to please others?"

"How would you describe your child's normal body size? Average? Thin? Overweight? What is his/her current body weight?"

"Does the child exercise? (If yes:) Describe her/his exercise routine. Do you feel this is excessive?"

"Do you know whether your child uses laxatives, diuretics, or appetite suppressants?"

"When it comes to food, does your child seem to have trouble thinking clearly or rationally? (If yes:) How? Can you give me an example?"

"Does the child have any other emotional difficulties, such as depression, anxiety or mood swings? Is he/she oversensitive to criticism from others? Does the child suffer from poor self-esteem?"

"Have the child's eating problems affected her/his relationships in the family? With friends? At school? At work?"

2.10. Elimination Problems   *See Section 16.5 for descriptors.*

"Has your child had any difficulties with toileting, such as problems with toilet training, bedwetting, or severe constipation? (If yes:) Can you give me an example?"

"Does the child have any medical conditions, or is he/she currently taking any medicines that could account for his/her difficulties?"

2.11. Learning Disabilities   *See Section 16.6 for descriptors.*

General Questions

"How would you describe your child's learning ability? Describe her/his greatest learning challenges."

"Does your child have any of the following difficulties in the classroom: Problems with work completion? Failing to turn in homework? Problems taking notes? Difficulty taking certain kinds of exams, such as essay exams?"

"What kinds of materials seem to make it easier for the child to learn? How many of these kinds of materials are offered in his/her current classroom?"

"What is homework like for the child? Are certain types of homework more difficult than others?"

"Does the child suffer from any other symptoms, such as anxiety, depression, problems with attention, or impulsivity?"

"What are the effects of the child's learning difficulties on his/her social relationships? On family relationships?"

✓ Note: if learning disabilities are suspected, ask parents for copies of report cards and standardized test scores.

Reading

"How does your child's teacher describe her/his reading ability? What kind of grades does your child receive in reading? Has your child ever received any special education support for reading? (If so:) What was it?"
"Did the child have difficulty learning to read or learning letters or letter sounds?"
"How well does the child spell? Does he/she often misspell common words?"

Math

"Does the child do well at math? Have problems with math? (If so:) What kind of problems?"
"What are the child's typical grades in math?"
"Does the child ever misread operational signs, such as plus, minus, or division signs? Does she/he have difficulty understanding basic operations, such as addition, subtraction, multiplication, or division? Problems learning basic math facts, such as multiplication tables?"
"Does he/she transpose/switch numbers?"
"Does the child have trouble with story/word problems?"

Written Expression

"What does your child's teacher say about your child's writing ability?"
"Does the child have trouble expressing her-/himself in written words?"
"Does the child have problems with grammatical errors? Problems with spelling? Trouble thinking of ideas or things to say about an idea?"

Nonverbal Learning Disability

"Has your child had any problems with muscle or physical coordination?"
"Does the child dislike being touched or touching certain textures?"
"Does the child have problems with reading comprehension? Math reasoning? Social relationships?"

2.12. Mental Retardation   *See Section 16.7 for descriptors.*

"How would you describe the child's ability to take care of his/her daily needs, such as dressing and other self-care skills?
"Is the child able to manage money? Use the telephone? Tell time?"
"Can your child be left alone at home or in the backyard?"
"How does your child get along with others? Does the child have friends? (If yes:) Who are some of her/his friends?"
"Does the child act aggressively? Have frequent tantrums? Harm him-/herself? Is the child verbally or physically abusive?"
"Does the child have any physical disabilities, such as problems with walking, running, coordination, or paralysis?"
"Does the child behave inappropriately? Does she/he seem to have fetishes? (If yes:) Can you give me an example?"

2.13. Movement and Tic Disorders   *See Section 16.8 for descriptors.*

"Does the child have any muscle twitches or verbal tics? (If yes:) What are they? How often do you observe these behaviors? Are there certain situations that seem to trigger these tics?"

"Have you tried to control these behaviors? (If yes:) How has this worked?"

2.14. Obsessive–Compulsive Disorder   *See Section 15.7 for descriptors.*

Obsessions

"Does your child seem unusually focused on any particular situation or topic?"

"Does your child seem particularly interested or concerned with cleanliness? Excessively worried about things that children his/her age don't frequently worry about, such as the future? World events?"

"How concerned is the child with this topic or situation? Mildly? Moderately? Extremely?"

"Are there other subjects or topics the child often talks on and on about?"

"How frequently does the child get caught up in and seem stuck on a subject?"

"Once the child seems stuck on a particular topic, how easy or difficult is it to get the child interested in something else?"

Compulsions

"Does the child have any quirky, repetitive behaviors? For instance, does she/he seem to check on the same thing a lot? Wash hands often? Count things?"

"Does the child need to have his/her things in a certain order? Books? Toys? Clothes? What does the child do when things are out of order?"

2.15. Phobias   *See Section 15.3 for descriptors.*

"Does the child have any extreme fears? (If yes:) What are they?"

"Do these fears affect the child's behavior? Social relationships? Family relationships? (If yes:) In what ways?"

"Does the child do anything to cope with these fears? (If yes:) Is the coping effective?"

2.16. Schizophrenia and Other Psychotic Disorders
See Section 16.10 for descriptors.

Cognitive Symptoms

"Does the child's thinking seem confused or disordered? Does she/he seem disoriented in time or place? Does the child have bizarre ideas or illogical thinking? (If yes to any:) Can you give me an example?"

Delusions and Hallucinations

"Does the child ever seem to have an exaggerated sense of his/her abilities, such as putting thoughts in other people's minds? Does he/she think anyone can read his/her mind?"

"Does the child talk to imaginary people? Complain of hearing voices in her/his head? Smell things that aren't there?"

Affective Symptoms

"Does the child seem to have problems with emotion? Have you noticed extreme mood changes? Does the child's emotion sometimes seem inappropriate to the situation? Does the child sometimes seem to have no emotion at all? Does he/she seem indifferent? Euphoric or extremely happy? Agitated or nervous? Very sad or depressed?"

"Have you noticed any changes in the child's ability to communicate or speak, such as disorganized or bizarre speech content? Mumbling? Inappropriate responses to questions? Difficulty finishing a thought? Becoming very still and unresponsive?"

"Have any of these emotions or behaviors had an effect on social relations with friends? The child's functioning at school? Family relationships?"

2.17. Suicidality   *See Section 15.8 for information and descriptors.*

"Has your child ever mentioned having suicidal thoughts to you or anyone else? (If yes:) What did the child say? How often has the child mentioned this? How likely do you think it is that she/he would act on these thoughts?"

"Has your child seemed much more withdrawn lately? (If yes:) How so? Has he/she lost significant interest in recreational or social activities?"

"Has your child ever done anything intentionally to harm her-/himself? (If so:) What did the child do? Was there anything that could have triggered this incident?"

"Do you know whether your child uses drugs or alcohol? (If yes:) What kinds? How often?"

"Has your child had any stresses or crises recently? A breakup with a boyfriend/girlfriend? Rejection in school, sports, or other recreation? Stresses in the family?"

"Is there any family history of suicide attempts, completed suicides, or incidents of self-harm? (If yes:) What happened? How much does your child know about those incidents?"

3

Observation Procedures and Questions for Children and Adolescents

3.1. General Advice for Questioning Children

Format and Content of Questions/Comments

The format and content of an initial interview will vary considerably, depending on a child's age and presenting problem(s). The following are important points to keep in mind when you are questioning children.

- "Why" questions don't typically work well with children, because they are often beyond the children's developmental capacity. Such questions can make them feel threatened or inferior. For example, asking a question such as "Why do you have trouble staying in your seat at school?" is unlikely to yield any useful information. Instead, ask questions such as "What is it about staying in your seat at school that is hard for you?" or "What do you like best and least about sitting in your classroom at school?"
- It is important to begin with questions that are open, more general, and less threatening before proceeding to more specific questions. One rule of thumb is to start with an "essay" question, move to a "multiple-choice" question if the first approach is not productive, and finally try a "true–false" format if neither of the previous approaches is productive.
- Keep in mind that some topics may be sensitive for a child. For example, a child with a learning disability may be sensitive about topics relating to academics. It is usually best to leave these sensitive topics until rapport has been established and the child understands why you are asking about this.
- Make positive comments on a child's ongoing behavior, such as "Wow, that's a great picture," or reflect feelings, such as "You seem really angry."
- Use praise liberally; avoid critical statements, but set clear boundaries as to what is appropriate and inappropriate behavior.
- Use age-appropriate terms, pacing, and sentence structure.

Ascertaining the Child's Point of View

Nuttall and Ivey (1986) have provided the following suggestions for learning about a child's point of view during an initial assessment interview:

- Try to "get into the child's shoes" by focusing on the child's construction of the world.
- Discover the child's perception of the problem, and be able to state what the child thinks is wrong, using his/her words.
- Note the key words that the child uses.
- Assess the child's construction of her/his environment (e.g., socioeconomic and housing issues).
- Avoid stereotypes, and be aware of how your theoretical constructs may get in the way of your ability to conduct a successful evaluation.
- Determine the child's goals through the use of questions such as "Imagine the perfect day. What would your life look like if everything were just the way you wanted it to be?" or "How could things be worse? What's the worst thing you can imagine happening?"

Play-Based Interviews

In evaluations of young children, play interviews are sometimes performed (in contrast to adhering to a list of questions). In a play interview, the clinician takes the child's lead, becoming an observing participant. Young children are often more comfortable telling a story, or sharing their inner emotional experience with toys and through fantasy. Morrison and Anders (2001) have suggested a number of strategies that can be used to engage a child in a play interview (many of these are used outside the play context and are elaborated throughout this chapter):

Engagement—refers to building a relationship with the child, and includes techniques such as letting the child determine the pace of the interview and choose what materials will be used.

Exploration—refers to attempts to elicit information from the child, using the play themes as a starting point.

Continuing/deepening—refers to attempts to expand a child's exploratory themes through commenting on his/her drawings, play, and so on.

Remembering-in-play—refers to interpretations or acknowledgments of behaviors that the child may not be aware of, "possibly because they occurred at a developmental stage prior to the onset of verbal language" (Morrison & Anders, 2001, pp. 43–44). These are typically used sparingly and almost never in an initial evaluation.

Limit setting—refers to establishing the "boundaries" of the therapeutic relationship, such as treating play materials with respect, cleaning up the office at the end of the session, and so forth.

3.2. Observing the Very Young Child (Ages Birth to 2½ Years)

For a very young child, the interview will be conducted primarily with at least one parent (or guardian/caregiver) who will provide the clinician with historical information (*see Chapters 1 and 2*). However, the clinician should attend to the following:

- Observe how the child interacts with the parent or caregiver. Note mutual gaze behavior, social responsiveness.
- How does the child react to separation from the adult? What is the reunion like when the adult returns?
- Is there a difference in the child's behavior when accompanied by father, by mother, or by another caregiver?
- How does the child communicate with the adult? How does the adult respond?
- Does the child smile often? When the child is distressed, can she/he be consoled?
- Does the child appear secure or clingy, distant, withdrawn, or resistant?
- Observe developmental behaviors: language, motor skills, handedness, affect regulation.

3.3. Opening Statements and Questions

The Preschool-Age Child (Ages 2½–6 Years)

The evaluation of a preschool-age child is usually carried out in part with at least one parent (or other caregiver) present, and in part with the child alone. Evaluation of the preschool child is frequently elicited through play and observation of behavior. It is usually less structured than an evaluation of an older child. As in earlier stages of development, most of the information will come from the parent (*again, see Chapters 1 and 2.*) When observing the child directly, you will want to attend to the following:

- How does the child relate to you, and how does it differ from the way the child relates to the parent or caregiver?
- What is the child's approach to the appointment/evaluation? Is he/she negative, compliant, relaxed, tense, inhibited?
- Does the child watch the adult to discover whether her/his answers or behaviors are appropriate?
- How confident is the child's play or responses? What is the general tone of the child's play (aggressive, cooperative, etc.)?
- How well does the child attend? Is the behavior appropriate for his/her age? Does (or how much does) the child's interest vary, depending on the task or play materials?

✓ Children this age respond well to initial questions that are factual and easy for them to answer, such as:

"How old are you?"
"Who came with you today?"
"Where do you live?"
"Who do you live with?"
"What kinds of things to you like to do?"

The School-Age Child (Ages 6–12 Years)

Opening Statements

You will want to begin the interview by introducing yourself and establishing rapport. With a child within this age range, if you use the title "Dr.," it is often helpful to explain what kind of "doctor" you are (e.g., you won't be giving shots, taking blood, etc.). Here are some possible opening statements:

"Hi, [name], I'm Dr. [name]. I'd like to spend some time getting to know you."
"Hi, [name], I'm Dr. [name]. Your mom/dad/grandmother/guardian told me that you're having a hard time at school, but I'd like to hear about what's going on at school from you."
"Hi, I'm Dr. [name]. You must be [name]. Come on in."
"Hi, I'm [name], it's nice to meet you. Please come in."

Opening Questions

Opening questions can include the following:

"Why do you think you're here today?"
"What did your parents tell you about me?"
"How old are you?"

The Adolescent (Ages 12–18 Years)

Opening Statements

An opening statement for an adolescent (especially when a parent is present) should be simple and casual:

> "Hi, [name], I'm Dr. [name]. Thanks for coming in today."

It is important to establish the limits of confidentiality with an adolescent early in the interview and to obtain her/his assent. It is also necessary to explain what you're going to do (e.g., whether you're going to talk to the adolescent first, parents alone, etc.) and to establish "ground rules" for the evaluation process—such as how much (and what types of) information will be considered privileged, how often you will talk to the parents, whether the parents' conversations with you will be discussed with the adolescent, and so forth. The exact "ground rules" may vary considerably, based on the referral question and family dynamics (*see Chapter 1*). The important point is to have a discussion with everyone involved and to come to a clear agreement as to what would be most helpful in a particular case.

Opening Questions

When you and the adolescent are alone, opening questions can include the following:

> "What did your parents tell you about this?"
> "What brought you here today? Who suggested that you come here? Do you agree with their idea that you come here? Why/why not?"
>
> "Tell me what a typical day would look like for you, from when you get up in the morning until you go to bed at night."

3.4. School-Related Questions

The Preschool-Age Child (Ages 2½–6 Years)

> "What day care center/(pre)school do you go to? What do you like about it?"
> "What is your teacher like?"
> "Do you have friends at day care/school? (If yes:) What are their names?"

The School-Age Child (Ages 6–12 Years)

> "What school do you go to?"
> "Who is/are your teachers? Tell me about him/her/them."
> "What do you like most about school this year? What kinds of things do you dislike about school this year?"
> "Who helps you with your homework?"
> "Are you doing poorly in any subjects? (If yes:) Do you have any ideas why you might be having trouble in this area (i.e., with math, reading, etc.)?"

> ✓ Note: If a child endorses difficulty with school, consider probing further about ADHD (*see Section 3.9*).

The Adolescent (Ages 12–18 Years)

> "What grade are you in?"
> "What's a typical day like at your school? What time do you have to be there? How do you get to school? How do you get home?"

"What do you do after school? Are you involved in any sports/clubs/activities?"
"Do you have a lot of homework?"
"Are you having any difficulties in school? (If so:) What are they? Do you have any ideas about why you're having trouble?"

3.5. Home- and Family-Related Questions

The Preschool-Age Child (Ages 2½–6 Years)

"Who is in your family?"
"How do you get along with your mom/dad? With your brothers/sisters?"

Depending on a child's language and cognitive development, a clinician may want to use a few questions from the list below that is targeted for the school-age child.

The School-Age Child (Ages 6–12 Years)

A clinician will probably not ask all of the questions from the following list, but can choose some of these questions to elicit information from the child.

"Who do you live with?"
"What does your mom/dad do?"
"How many brothers or sisters do you have? What kinds of things do you do together? What kinds of things do you fight about?"
"What does your family do for fun?"
"What is dinnertime like in your house?"
"What do you like best about your mom/dad? Which parent do you get along with better?"
"If you wanted to make your mom or dad really mad, what would you do?"
"How do people in your family show each other that they appreciate them?"
"What does your house look like? Do you have your own room?"
"Pretend you were showing me around your house. What would you like to show me?"
"What would the perfect family look like to you?"
"Does your family take vacations? (If yes:) Where do you go?"
"Have you ever felt like running away (or have you ever run away) from home? What made you feel like that?" (Assesses for externalizing problems.)
(For a child of divorced parents:) "When you visit your dad/mom, how does that go? What types of things do you do with him/her?"

The Adolescent (Ages 12–18 Years)

See the questions above for a school-age child, as well as the following:

"Tell me about your family."
"Tell me about your brothers/sisters. Do they look up to you? Do you look up to them?"
"How do your parents get along? Have you ever heard them fight?"
"When people argue in your family, what do they usually argue about?"
"What do you usually do when people in the house are arguing?"
"Does your family get together at mealtimes?"
"When you want something from your parents, how do you usually get it?"
"Describe a typical day in your house."
"What do your parents do when they find out you've done something they don't want you to do?"
"How do your parents discipline you? Do they hit you? Did they ever hit you in the past?"

✓ Note: If abuse is suspected, probe further (see Section 3.9).

3.6. Questions about Friends

The Preschool-Age Child (Ages 2½–6 Years)

"Do you have friends you like to do things with? What kinds of things do you like to do?"
"Do you have a best friend? (If yes:) What is her/his name? What do you like to do together?"

The School-Age Child (Ages 6–12 Years)

"What do you like to do with your friends?"
"Do you have a lot of friends, or do you wish you had more?"

✓ Note: If child is reporting few or unsatisfying friendships, consider probing further about depressive symptoms (*see Section 3.9*).

"Do you have a best friend? (If yes:) What is he/she like? What are your other friends like?"
"Do you go on sleepovers? (If yes:) What do you do at sleepovers?"

The Adolescent (Ages 12–18 Years)

"What are your friends like? What do you like to do together?"
"Do you date? (If yes:) What age did you begin dating? What do you generally do on dates?"
"Do you currently have a boyfriend/girlfriend?"

3.7. Interests

The Preschool-Age Child (Ages 2½–6 Years)

"What kinds of things do you like to play with?"
"What's your favorite toy?"
"What TV shows do you like?"
"Do you take any special classes, like art class or gymnastics?"
"Do you have any pets?"
"What did you do on your last birthday?"

The School-Age Child (Ages 6–12 Years)

"What types of activities do you like to do? Do you play any sports, like soccer?"
"Do you like to watch TV?"
"Do you have any collections (e.g., dolls, cards, etc.)"
"What kinds of toys do you like to play with?"
"Do you have a bedtime routine? (If yes:) What it is it? What other types of family routines do you have?"
"Do you get an allowance? (If yes:) What do you like to spend your money on?"

The Adolescent (Ages 12–18 Years)

"What do you like to do in your free time?"
"Are you involved in any extracurricular activities? (If yes:) What kinds?"

3.8. Adolescent-Specific Questions

Areas that are not included in interviews with young children, but are typically covered in adolescent assessments, are as follows:

- Substance use (tobacco, alcohol, drugs)
- Gang involvement or conduct problems
- Sexual experiences; birth control; knowledge of sexually transmitted diseases and AIDS
- Developmental tasks of adolescence: adjustment to changing body and sexuality; separation from family; goals for the future

Substance Use

"Do you smoke cigarettes? (If yes:) How often? When? Does it cause you any problems?"

"Have you ever tried alcohol? (If yes:) How frequently do you use alcohol? Does it cause you any problems?"

"Have you ever tried marijuana? PCP? Cocaine? Heroin? LSD? Mushrooms? Speed? Steroids? Others? (If yes:) How frequent is your drug use? What kinds of problems does it cause you?"

Conduct Problems

"Have you ever gotten in a physical fight with someone? Been beaten up?"

"Have you ever been in trouble with the law? Been truant from school? Run away from home? Stolen property?"

Development

"At what age did you begin developing (ask about voice change for boys, first menses for girls, etc.)?"

"What would you like to do after high school? What kinds of careers interest you?"

"Are you dating? Do you have a boyfriend/girlfriend? (If no:) Do you wish you did, or are you happier without one? (If yes:) What is your relationship like?"

3.9. Specific Questions Related to Psychiatric Symptoms

The following are questions to be selected on the basis of the referral question and the parents' and child's answers to the preceding questions. When you suspect specific problems or psychiatric disorders, you can choose questions from this list to probe further.

Mood Symptoms

"How do you feel right now? How do you usually feel when you're at school? At home?"

"What kinds of things make you mad? Sad? Happy? Scared? Bad? Glad? Really happy?"

"What kinds of things are easy for you to do? What kinds of things are hard?"

"Would you like to change anything about yourself?"

Depressive Symptoms

Physiological Symptoms

"What has your appetite been like lately?"

"Do you ever have stomachaches? Other aches and pains? Have you been feeling sort of sick?"

"Do you ever find you don't have much energy? Have you been feeling really tired lately?"

Behavioral Symptoms

"Do you ever have trouble getting out of bed in the morning?"
"Do you cry a lot? (If yes:) What do you cry about?"
"Have you had difficulty concentrating?"
"Have you had trouble completing work at school?"

Social Effects

"How have you been getting along with your friends? Do you feel supported by them?"
"Do you feel lonely? Do you have people who will listen to you when you need to talk to them?"

Cognitions

"When you look into the future, what do you see?"
"Do you ever feel guilty about things?"
"Is it hard for you to make up your mind about things?"
"Do you think about death? (If yes:) What kinds of things do you think about?"
"Do you ever feel helpless?"

Violence, Suicidality, Homicidality

"Have you ever wished you were dead?"
"Have you ever tried to hurt yourself or kill yourself?"
"Have you ever tried to hurt someone else?"

✓ If history is positive for suicidal thoughts, ask the following questions:

"What did you consider doing?"
"What stopped you (or is stopping you) from following through with these ideas?"
"When did you last have these thoughts?"
"How often do these thoughts come? Is it hard to control them?"

Worries/Anxiety

"Do you ever feel really scared or anxious?"
"Are there certain things that make you worried? (If yes:) What are they like?"
"Do you ever feel so nervous that you're sick to your stomach? Do you ever feel shaky, dizzy, or tense? Does your heart ever pound really hard? Do you sweat?"

Obsessive–Compulsive Behaviors

"Do you ever have to do things over and over again?"
"Do you ever have things that you need to check on all the time?"
"Are you very neat? Do you need to have things arranged in a certain way? (If yes:) Like what?"
"Do you ever get really upset when things in your room are moved?"
"Are there things you feel you have to do before you can get to sleep at night?"
"Do you ever feel you have to touch certain things whenever you see them?"
"Do you ever feel you have thoughts or actions that you can't control?"

(If yes to the questions above:)

"How do you feel when you do these behaviors?"
"How does doing these things affect you in school? At home? With your friends?"

Disruptive Behavior Disorders

ADHD, Inattentive Symptoms

"Do you have trouble paying attention at school?"
"When someone asks you to do something, do you have trouble remembering what he/she asked you to do?"
"Do you have trouble doing your homework? (If yes:) What's hard about it?"
"Do you have a tendency to lose things?"

ADHD, Impulsive Symptoms

"Do you sometimes have trouble controlling your behavior?"
"Do you often get in trouble for interrupting others? Not waiting your turn? Being disruptive?"

ADHD, Hyperactive Symptoms

"Do you ever feel like you're driven by a motor or are on the go all the time?"
"Is it hard for you to sit still?"
"Do you have trouble falling asleep at night?"

Other Disruptive Behaviors

"Do you have problems with other kids at school? Do you ever get into trouble at school?"
"Have you ever run away from home? Been truant from school? Violated curfew? Stayed out all night? Driven a car without a license?"
"Do you lose your temper a lot? (If yes:) What causes you to lose it?"
"Do you get into a lot of fights? (If yes:) Who do you usually fight with? What kinds of things do you fight about?"
"Do you find that you're always in trouble? (If yes:) What kinds of things do you get in trouble for? What happens to you when you get in trouble?"
"Have you ever set fires? Used spray paint/made grafitti? Shoplifted? Forged checks? Broken into someone's home/store/car? Committed an armed robbery?"
"What kinds of drugs/alcohol have you tried or do you use? How frequently do you use drugs/alcohol?"
"Are you a member of a gang?"
"Do you engage in unsafe sexual practices?"

Thought Disorders

"Do you ever hear voices that other people don't hear? See things that other people don't see?"
"Do you ever have times when you're feeling way too good—so terrific it's almost scary? During these times, do you find you need to sleep less?"

Eating Disorders

Behavioral Symptoms

"What do you eat?"
"How frequently do you exercise?"
"Do you ever eat in secret? Binge-eat? Make yourself vomit? Use laxatives inappropriately?"

Cognitive Symptoms

"Are you happy with the way you look?"
"How much do you think about food? What kinds of things do you think about food?"
"Do you have any fears of getting fat? Are there certain foods you fear or avoid?"

Abuse

"Has anyone ever hit you too hard or hard enough to leave a bruise or a mark? (If yes:) Tell me about it. Who did this, and when did it happen?"
"Has anyone ever touched you in a way that made you really uncomfortable? (If yes:) Tell me more about this."
"Are you afraid of anyone? (If yes:) What did this person do to make you afraid of her/him?"

3.10. Questions Used in Projective Assessments

Often, the interview with a child or adolescent is used to gain information about the youngster's hopes, dreams, and wishes. The following is a collection of questions or activities that can be used for this purpose.

Wishes/Fantasies

"If you had three wishes, what would they be?"
"Are there some things about you that your mom/dad don't know about? (If yes:) Would they be surprised if they knew this about you?"
"What is the best age to be?"
"When you dream at night, what kinds of things do you dream about?"
"If you could change something about yourself, what would it be?"
"What do you want to do when you grow up?"
"What is something you remember that happened a long time ago?"
"If you could change three things about you (your life, your family, etc.), what would they be?"
"If you were forced to live for a year on an abandoned island and could only take three people with you, who would they be? Why?"

Draw-A-Person

When a child is completing the Draw-A-Person task, it is useful to ask the child questions about the person, such as these:

"Is this person anyone in particular? (If yes:) Who?"
"What types of things makes this person happy? Sad? Angry? Scared?"
"What kinds of friends does the person have?"

3.11. Closing Questions

"Is there anything important we didn't talk about?"
"How do you feel about the time we've spent talking?"
"Where should we go from here? What would be helpful for you?"

4

Questions for Teachers
or Other Professionals

This chapter suggests questions for eliciting the basic information you may want from a child's teacher or other professional who works with the child. See Chapter 40 for a sample teacher questionnaire (Section 40.3) and a sample assessment form for other professionals (Section 40.4).

4.1. General Guidelines

Obtaining information from a child's teacher is frequently done over the course of an assessment or treatment. It not only provides supplemental information about how the child copes and performs in school, but also provides the opportunity to establish rapport and a collaborative relationship with the teacher. Less frequently, the clinician may desire to obtain information from other professionals who know the child well. For example, a football coach may know more about an adolescent's depressive symptoms than any classroom teacher does. When there is a medical issue involved in treatment, it is often important to discuss these issues with the child's physician, as well as to obtain a release for the child's medical records.

When interviewing a child's teacher or other professionals (such as psychiatrists, pediatricians, coaches, clergy, or guidance counselors), you will ask many of the same questions that you ask the parents. (See the questions for parents about specific disorders in Chapter 2.) However, you will also want to get their unique perspectives about the child's problems, such as how the child performs in the school or other settings. In many cases, these types of interviews are conducted over the phone and are often brief. Thus it is often helpful to focus on the specific areas of concern.

4.2. Areas to Cover in Interviewing Teachers and Other School Personnel

Teachers and other school system personnel are key people in a child's life, and their input is often essential to evaluating or treating a child. In addition, they are in the unique position of helping you develop remediation strategies. A collaborative approach is often most successful, and the following strategies can be used to enhance collaboration:

- Solicit the teacher's input by making a phone call, paying a classroom visit, and/or asking him/her to fill out brief questionnaires or rating forms (see the end of this chapter).
- Give the teacher a description of the assessment procedure or treatment plan.

- If recommendations include classroom interventions, discuss with the teacher the necessary accommodations or other changes, and help her/him to develop procedures for implementation.
- Offer to remain available for future consultation.

What follows are suggested general areas to cover when you are talking to a teacher, followed by specific questions to elicit information in each area. Remember that you must obtain written permission from the parents before contacting a child's teachers or other professionals. As noted above, Section 40.3 provides a questionnaire that can be used to assess a teacher's perceptions of a child's classroom behavior and school functioning. It can be used by the clinician to record a phone interview with a teacher, or it can be sent to the teacher to complete as a self-report. If it is sent to the teacher, compliance will be enhanced by inclusion of a self-addressed stamped envelope for return of the form.

Child's Major Problem

"What do you see as the child's major problem?"
"Tell me about his/her problems in the classroom."
"How often are these problems a concern to you?"
"How long has this been going on?"
"When it happens, how long does it last?"
"How serious do you think the child's problem is?"
"Are there any specific situations that trigger the problem behavior?"
"How do other kids react when she/he behaves in this way?"

Cause of the Problem

"Do you have any ideas about why the child has this particular problem?"
"What do you think might be causing this difficulty?"

Teacher's Reaction to Child's Problem

"How have you reacted to the child's problem?"
"How have you tried to help the child's problem? Was it successful? Why or why not?"
"How do you feel about the child in general?"

Peer Relations

"How well does the child get along with peers?"
"How does the child get along with his/her classmates?"
"In school, how many friends does the child have? Many? A few? None?"
"Is she/he liked by other children? (If no:) What causes other children to dislike her/him?"
"What do other children do when the child engages in the problem behavior?"
"What does the child do during recess or free-play times?"
"Are there any other children in the class with similar problems?"

Academic Performance

"How would you characterize the child's academic performance?"
"What was the child's highest grade on the last report card?"
"What was the child's lowest grade?"
"What kinds of academic problems does the child have in the classroom?"
"Does the child have any difficulties in reading? Math? Spelling? Language? (If yes in any area:) What types of difficulties?"
"Does the child perform differently with different teachers/adults?"

"Does the child have any learning disabilities? (If so:) What are they?"
"Does the child receive special tutoring or support? (If so:) What?"
"Does the child have an individualized education plan (IEP)?"
"Has the child ever had special testing in school? (If so:) Please explain."

Strengths and Weaknesses

"What do you see as the child's emotional and social strengths and weaknesses?"
"What are the child's academic strengths and weaknesses?"
"In what situations is the child most likely to display his/her strengths and weaknesses?"
"Do you think it is possible to build on the child's strengths to help treat her/his difficulties? (If so:) How?"

Teacher's Perception of Child's Family

"How would you describe the child's family?"
"How often do you see the child's family?"
"What is your perception of the child's family?"
(If the child has difficulties:) "How does the family cope with the child's difficulties?"
(If the family has difficulties:) "How is the family coping with its difficulties?"

General Classroom/School Behavior

"Does the child appear motivated for school?"
"How does the child generally behave in the classroom?"
"Is the child in school regularly?"
"Is the child usually in class on time?"
(If not:) "How frequently is he/she late? What is the excuse given for being late?"
"Does the child usually complete her/his homework? (If so:) How well is it usually done?"
"What are the child's attention and concentration skills like?"
"Do you see any difficulties with memory? Problems with motor activity? Behavioral issues?"
"Does the child participate in extracurricular activities? (If so:) What?"

Teacher's Expectations/Hopes for Child

"What expectations do you have for this child?"
"What hopes do you have for this child?"
"What about the child would you like to see change as a result of this evaluation/treatment?"

Thoughts on What Might Help

"Do you have any ideas about what might be most helpful for the child?"
"Is there anything in particular you'd like to see happen as a result of this evaluation/treatment?"
"Is there anything else about the child that would be helpful to know?"

4.3. Areas to Cover in Interviewing Health or Mental Health Professionals

When you are interviewing a health or mental health professional, such as the child's psychologist, neurologist, or pediatrician, it is often best to focus closely on the areas of concern. Contacts with such professionals are often brief. The key areas to cover include the following:

Child's Problem

"What do you see as the child's major problem?"
(If this is the referring professional:) "Why did you make the referral at this time?"
"Do you have any ideas why this problem has emerged?"

Professional's Perception of Child's Family

"What is your perception of the child's family?"
"How do you view the family's role in the child's difficulties?"
"How has the family reacted to this problem?"

Medical Issues (for Medical Professionals)

"Are there any neurological or other medical conditions that might affect this child's behavior?"
"Is this child on any medications that might affect his/her behavioral or emotional functioning?"

Professional's Expectations

"What would you like to see happen in the course of this evaluation/treatment?"

As noted earlier, a questionnaire that can be used to interview these professionals is provided in Section 40.4. It can be either used to guide phone interviews or sent to them to complete and return; in the latter case, enclosing a copy of a signed release and a self-addressed stamped envelope for return will expedite a response. Again, remember that health and mental health professionals must have the parents' written permission to speak with you.

4.4. Teacher Report Measures of Functioning in Children and Adolescents

Direct interviewing of teachers is often supplemented by the use of teacher-completed questionnaires. You may want to ask a teacher to complete such a questionnaire before you meet or talk to her/him, as it may give you ideas about areas that deserve further inquiry. These questionnaires can provide quantifiable information about the severity of a child's symptoms (as compared to peer norms), the situations in which the behaviors occur, and the extent to which these behaviors interfere with school functioning. These measures can also elicit information about the quality of peer relationships, social skill strengths and weaknesses, and academic strengths and weaknesses. However, these measures should be used sparingly and thoughtfully, as teachers and other school personnel have many responsibilities and overloading them with unnecessary paperwork is obviously not recommended.

- Academic Competency Evaluation Scale (DiPerna & Elliott, 2000)
- Academic Performance Rating Scale (DuPaul, Rapport, & Perriello, 1991)
- ADHD Rating Scale–IV (DuPaul, Power, Anastopoulos, & Reid, 1998)
- Behavior Assessment System for Children, Second Edition–Teacher Rating Scale (BASC-2-TRS; Reynolds & Kamphaus, 2004)
- Brown Attention-Deficit Disorder Scales (Brown ADD Scales; Brown, 2001)
- Conners' Teacher Rating Scale–Revised (CTRS-R; Conners, 1997)
- Devereux Scales of Mental Disorders (DSMD; Naglieri, LeBuffe, & Pfeiffer, 1994)

- Revised Behavior Problem Checklist (RBPC; Quay & Peterson, 1996)
- School Situations Questionnaire (SSQ; Barkley & Murphy, 2006)
- Social Skills Rating System (SSRS; Gresham & Elliott, 1990)
- Student Behavior Survey (SBS; Lachar, Wingenfeld, Kline, & Gruber, 2000)
- Teacher's Report Form (TRF; Achenbach & Rescorla, 2001)
- Walker–McConnell Scale of Social Competence and School Adjustment (Walker & McConnell, 1988)

5

The Formal Mental Status Exam with Children and Adolescents

5.1. Differences between Adult and Juvenile Mental Status Exams

The formal mental status exam is used to help determine the precise nature and degree of a child's or adolescent's abnormal functioning through the observation of demeanor, thought processes, speech, memory, affect, and mood. It is used less often with children than with adults, but is often helpful in cases of traumatic brain injury, substance use disorders, or confusion in general psychological functioning (e.g., psychotic disorders).

Morrison and Anders (2001) have described the following differences between an adult's and a child's mental status exam:

- Because child and adolescent development encompasses a wide spectrum of behavior, the examiner must have a firm knowledge of normal behavior at all ages.
- The evaluation of a young child is usually completed with the parent(s) in the room.
- Depending on the child's age, appropriate toys or projective material should be available to elicit behaviors and facilitate communication.

5.2. Contents of a Juvenile Mental Status Exam

A mental status exam with a child or adolescent often includes the following areas:

1. Appearance and behavior
   a. Apparent age as compared to chronological age and physical characteristics (e.g., height, weight, cleanliness, nutrition); any physical abnormalities
   b. Dress, hairstyle, body ornamentation (jewelry, piercings, tattoos)
   c. Eye contact
   d. Level of activity and motor movements; gait; posture; stereotyped behaviors
   e. Appropriateness of behavior for child's age, education, and socioeconomic status
2. Alertness/cognition
   a. Orientation with regard to time and place (appropriate for age/level of development)

    b. Awareness of what is going on (e.g., reason why child is at clinic; what is occurring in her/his family)

    c. Alertness; ability to concentrate

    d. Congruence of vocabulary and fund of information with child's educational and socio-economic background

3. Demeanor/attitude
   a. Level of cooperation
   b. Rapport with examiner
   c. Facial expressions (sample descriptors: **happy, tense, tearful, relaxed, smiling**) and appropriateness of facial expressions to affect, conversational topics, and content of the interview

4. Thought processes
   a. General descriptors: **normal, concrete, confused, psychotic**
   b. Content of information discussed (particularly information spontaneously given by child)
   c. Recurrent themes
   d. Evidence for delusions, hallucinations, fantasies, fears, worries, phobias, obsessions, compulsions

5. Speech
   a. General descriptors: **normal, pressured, fast/slow, apraxia, appropriate/inappropriate for age**
   b. Expressive language: **normal, delayed/advanced for age, echolalia, anomia, perseverations, mutism**
   c. Verbal fluency: **normal, problems with word finding, aphasia**
   d. Receptive language: **appropriate/delayed/advanced for age**
   e. Articulation
   f. Relationship between verbal and nonverbal communication

6. Sensory–motor functioning
   a. Intactness/unaided functioning of senses (hearing, sight, touch, smell, taste)
   b. Fine and gross motor functioning: **normal, uncoordinated, slow performance speed, tics, tremors**
   c. Performance on copying tasks (draw a person, clock, house; write name)

7. Mood (description of child's pervasive, sustained emotional states)
   a. Sample descriptors for mood: **normal, depressed, "miserable," unhappy, "down," glum, anxious, euphoric, angry**
   b. Comments on what the child says about his/her mood and feelings
   c. Fluctuations of mood

8. Affect (observed expressions of emotion)
   a. Sample descriptors for affect: **flat, inappropriate, labile, congruent/incongruent with mood, broad, blunted, restricted**
   b. Match of affect with speech content
   c. Fluctuations in affect

9. Vegetative signs
   a. Weight gain/loss
   b. Energy level/sleep habits

10. Insight/judgment
    a. Level of insight
    b. Ability to articulate problems
    c. Child's belief about why he/she has come for interview
    d. Self-awareness of her/his problem
    e. Judgment in carrying out everyday activities

11. Memory
    a. General descriptors: **normal, fair, poor, impaired**
    b. Impairments in immediate, recent, or remote memory
    c. Common ways of assessing memory: Ask about the child's recent and early history, including details such as names, dates, events; digits forward and backward; serial subtraction; recall of words (immediate and delayed)
12. Suicidal ideation
13. Homicidal ideation

6

Ending the Interview

6.1. General Guidelines

It is important to have a clear idea of when and how to conclude the interview. Make sure you leave enough time to have adequate opportunity to summarize the important points and end the session without feeling rushed. Be sure to conclude the interview with both the child and the parents, whether they are seen separately or together. If anyone is visibly upset, you want to make sure that the individual has time to regain his/her composure. When you are conducting a play-based interview with a young child, leave time for the child to help you clean up the room, as this can facilitate the transition out of the interview.

- Give parents and child some indication of the approaching end by mentioning the length of time left:

    "We only have 5 minutes left."
    "Our time is almost up."

- Leave time at the end so that the child or adult has time to add information that was not previously covered, or to ask questions:

    "Is there anything else that you'd like me to know/understand?"
    "Are there any questions that you'd like to ask me?"

- Summarize the main points regarding the referral questions, and/or recap the problem that occasioned the referral.
- State whether you can confirm the existence of the problem, or whether you suggest further evaluation.
- Offer details about what you learned about the child as a result of the evaluation.
- Give the child/parents an idea of the next step in the process.

6.2. Ending Statements for the Child

General

"Our time is almost up, but I can see you still have a lot to talk about. Let's make another appointment so we can continue our discussion."
"Thank you for taking the time to come here and talk to me."
"I know that it took a lot of courage to come here today and talk about your concerns, and I want you to know that I really appreciate it."

"Thanks for coming here today. I'm going to try to do all I can to help you, and the information you've given me will be very helpful."

"Is there anything else you want to add/tell me?"

Next Step

"Do you have any ideas about what you'd like to do next?"

"I think our next step should be _____."

Summary

"I really appreciate your cooperation today. It sounds like you're having problems in _____, and it's my job to figure out how best to help you. When we're finished with the evaluation, I'll have a better idea of how to do that."

6.3. Ending Statements for the Parent

"You will need to make an appointment with _____ for _____."

"You brought Bobby to me because you are worried that he may be depressed. Now that I've talked to you and Bobby, it does appear to me that he is feeling very sad and hopeless. His behavior is similar to that of a depressed child, in that he is having difficulty sleeping and eating. His mood and behaviors are also consistent with a depressive episode. I'd like you to make another appointment with me/make an appointment for a psychopharmacological evaluation/(etc.), so that we can help him."

"Do you have any questions about what we have done today/about this evaluation/about the report I will be writing?"

"You have some significant concerns about Cindy's performance in school and are worried that a learning disability may underlie the problems she's having. I suggest performing some testing to determine the extent of her difficulties. After we complete this, I'll have a better idea about the specific nature of her difficulties."

Part II

Standard Terms and Statements for Wording Psychological Reports

A. Introducing the Report

7

Beginning the Report

This chapter covers the basic information with which you would begin any report. Reasons for referral are covered in Chapter 8, while report formats are covered in Chapter 35.

7.1. Heading and Dates for the Report

Use stationery that includes your full name; degree(s); title(s); addresses (office and mailing, if different); phone number(s); and, when appropriate, affiliations, supervisor, license number, and agency.

Title or head the report to fit its contents. Most report titles are combinations of two words, one describing the discipline or activity, and one describing the kind of document:

Discipline/Activity

Neuropsychological, Psychological, Psychosocial, Psychoeducational, Educational, Intellectual, Personality, Behavioral, Multidisciplinary, Social Work, Psychiatric.

Intake, Forensic, Diagnostic, Home Observation, Classroom Observation, Custody, Clinical Interview, Testing, Treatment, Progress, Rehabilitation, Mental Status, Discharge, Closing, Termination.

Document Type

Evaluation, Assessment, Report, Summary, Plan, Note, Formulation, Consultation, Update.

Date the report itself. Also include all dates and locations for interviews, testing and evaluations; if relevant, include total testing and/or duration of each testing session. For example, near the top of the report, state:

Child was seen on 1/1/07.

Then, under "Other Sources of Information," state:

Teacher was interviewed on 2/2/07.

In terms of insurance/reporting issues, the "date of the report" should be the date the child or adolescent was evaluated/seen, with other dates given in the body of the report itself.

7.2. Identifying Information about the Client

The headings below represent possible types of identifying information. You are not likely to use all of these areas in describing a child or adolescent.

Name

Always give the child's given name and surname. A nickname or preferred name may also be included as follows:

Prefers to be called _____.

Other Identifying Information

Give the family's address and phone number; the child's case number and medical record number; and the referral source.

Date of Birth and Chronological Age

Give the month, day, and year of the child's birth, as well as the child's chronological age on the day when the evaluation was completed. Use a year-and-month format (e.g., 10 years, 5 months—not 10.5). For a child below the age of 3 years, include an adjusted chronological age if the child was premature by more than 3 weeks and showed delays.

Gender

Do not use the term "sex"; use "gender," and specify "male" or "female." For a younger child, the term "girl" or "boy" is acceptable.

School

Include the name of the school, as well as the child's grade in school. If the child does not yet attend school full-time, indicate school/preschool/day care schedules, as in these examples:

Brittany attends the Peter Pan Preschool 2 days a week for 3 hours each day.
Taguan is cared for by his maternal grandmother at her home from 8 A.M. to 4 P.M. weekdays while his mother works.

If the child is in a special class, indicate:

Mary is enrolled in a 2nd-grade self-contained classroom at the Milton Elementary School.

Note whether the child has changed schools in the last 18 months or has had frequent school changes.

Handedness

Include handedness (right, left, ambidextrous) when appropriate, and eye and foot preferences if relevant.

Previous Diagnoses

If the child has a well-documented learning disability or psychiatric disorder, identify and describe it briefly.

Nationality, Language Spoken in Home, and Immigrant/Refugee Status

When this information is relevant to the case, report the child's nationality and the language(s) spoken at home. If English is the child's second language, indicate his/her degree of proficiency in English, as in this example:

> Maria was adopted from Mexico. She speaks both Spanish and English, although Spanish is her first language and she is not yet as fluent in English as in Spanish.

If the child is not a U.S. citizen and that fact is relevant, indicate the country of citizenship:

> Ahmed is a Saudi citizen currently in school at Garfield Academy.

If the child and family are immigrants/refugees from another country, indicate which country and the circumstances of their arrival:

> Alisa was born in Bosnia-Herzegovina, where she lived with her parents and sister until she was 3 years old, at which time the family fled the country because of persecution and moved to the United States.

Race/Ethnicity

Be consistent in reporting race/ethnicity across reports; do not report it only for minorities. If you are in doubt, it is best to ask older children and adolescents (or parents) which term they prefer in describing their race/ethnicity. Race is not simply skin color. The following is a list of commonly used terms.

> African American, Caucasian/Euro-American/European American/"white"/"Anglo," Asian American/Asian, Pacific Islander, Hispanic/Latino/Latina, Native American, Inuit, biracial/multiracial/of mixed races.

Child's Familiarity with Examiner

When relevant, indicate if the child has a previous history with the examiner, as in this example:

> Dan was familiar with the testing evaluator from a therapeutic relationship.

Living Arrangements

Indicate others with whom the child lives, and the parents' marital status if this is pertinent:

> Child lives with his biological parents and a younger sister, age 7.
> Child's parents are separated, and child lives with her mother.

If the child lives with a parent's lover or partner, indicate this as well; if pertinent to the referral question, indicate the duration of this relationship and the degree of stability within the home:

> Child lives with his older sister, his mother, and the mother's boyfriend of 5 years, whom he refers to as his stepfather. The boyfriend plays a positive parental role with both children, and the home appears stable.

If the parents are separated or divorced, indicate the visitation schedule and, when germane, the type of visitation:

> Child lives with her mother and sees her father during supervised visitation one night per week.

If the child lives at a location other than either parent's home, describe the living arrangements/location.

Referral Reason   *See Chapter 8, "Reasons for Referral."*

7.3. Arriving for the Evaluation

Child arrived for the appointment with mother/father and readily/reluctantly separated from her/him at beginning of evaluation.

Child arrived for the appointment _____ minutes late, with parent(s).

Child arrived for the initial interview on time and in the company of his/her father/mother/guardian.

Child initially had difficulty/no difficulty separating from his parent/relative/caregiver/classroom and accompanying evaluator to the assessment room.

If the child is brought to the evaluation by someone other than a parent or legal guardian, indicate the reasons, as in this example:

Jason was brought to the appointment by his maternal aunt, Ms. Z., who is taking care of him while his mother (his legal guardian) is hospitalized for cancer treatment.

7.4. Other Sources of Information for the Report

Begin to describe the information sources consulted for the report with one or more statements such as the following:

In preparation for/In advance of the interview/evaluation, I received and reviewed the following records . . .

Sources of information may include the following:

Interview with parent/teacher/child/day care provider/foster mother/caseworker, other (specify): Indicate whether a structured interview format was used, and indicate dates if these are different from the date of the report, as described above.

Review of previous test results/school records/individualized education plan (IEP)/medical records/other (specify).

Standardized tests/rating scales: List each test/scale, along with its acronym/abbreviation. (*See Chapters 21–28 for test/scale names and common abbreviations.*) Include total testing time and/or duration of each testing session, as in these examples:

Met with child for two testing sessions of 3 hours each.

Met for one 30-minute interview with parent and one 2-hour testing session with child.

Group behavior rating scales by who completed each scale:

Mrs. Brown, John's mother, completed the following behavior checklists . . .

Mrs. Bagwell, John's teacher, completed the following behavior checklists . . .

Home observation: Indicate date and duration of observation, and names of family members observed.

School observation: Include date and duration of observation, and subject(s) or other activities observed.

Observation of the child during a clinical interview.

Observation of the child by other professionals.

Consultation with teacher(s) and/or other professional(s).

Results from team meeting/school conference/IEP meeting: Indicate who was present for meeting (parents, teachers, therapists, principal, etc.).

7.5. Consent and Confidentiality Statements

Please consult your agency and state guidelines for information regarding the type of information that needs to be conveyed, as well as the age at which the information needs to be explained to the child or adolescent. (*See Section 1.4 for more information on this topic.*)

> The limits of confidentiality were explained to the child and/or parents. Child/parents was/were informed that information regarding danger to the child or to others would be shared with outside agencies.
>
> We discussed the evaluation/treatment procedures; what was expected from the child, the parents, and the evaluator/therapist; who else would be involved or affected; the treatment's risks and benefits; and alternative methods' sources, costs, and benefits.
>
> The child and/or parent(s) understand the procedures that he/she is being asked to consent to and their likely consequences/effects, as well as alternative procedures and their consequences.
>
> I have advised the parents that I am not their child's treating psychologist and that we will not have a continuing professional relationship.
>
> The parents know that the results of this evaluation will be sent to _____ and used for _____.
>
> The child understands and willingly agrees to participate fully in the evaluation process.

7.6. Reliability Statements

Basis of Data

> The data/history are/is felt to be completely/quite/reasonably/rather/minimally/questionably reliable.
>
> I consider the child/parent to be an adequately/inadequately reliable informant.
>
> I have relied on the parents' report of their child's history and assumed that it was accurate (except as noted); thus I cannot assume any responsibility for any errors of fact in this report.
>
> The opinions offered in this report have not been influenced by the referrer/referring agency.
>
> The diagnoses and opinions in this report are offered with a reasonable degree of psychological certainty.

Accuracy

> The parents' description of their child was credible, forthright, and informed.
>
> Although somewhat dramatized, the core information appears to be accurate and valid for diagnostic/evaluative purposes.
>
> The child's parents are/are not astute observers of their child's behavior.

Consistency

> His/her appraisals tended to be supported/corroborated by my observations/others' records.
>
> The child's parents were poor/adequate/good/excellent historians.

Representativeness

> Results are believed to be a valid sample of/accurate representation of this child's current level of functioning/typical behavioral patterns/behaviors outside the examination setting.
>
> Because this child refused no test items/questions, worked persistently/was most cooperative

and helpful, and had no interfering emotions such as anxiety or depression, test findings/results of this evaluation are felt to be representative of her/his minimal/usual/optimal level of functioning.

Trustworthiness/Honesty/Malingering

The parents/child appeared to be honest in their/his/her descriptions of the child's strengths and weaknesses.

The parents made no special efforts to convince me of the gravity or authenticity of their child's problems.

The history offered should be taken with a grain of salt/was fabricated/grandiose.

The mother's/father's description of the child's complaints were vague, self-contradictory, and not completely consistent with any recognized clinical pattern.

The mother/father offered an exaggerated/minimized description of the child's behaviors.

The mother/father was a willfully poor historian.

Validity

Given this child's high level of motivation and cooperation, results of this evaluation are felt to be a valid indicator of her/his abilities.

Given the child's strong motivation, concentration, and cooperation, it is likely that the present results provide an accurate estimate of his/her current cognitive and psychological functioning.

In spite of the child's difficulties with impulsivity, her/his attention and effort were quite adequate on all tasks. Consequently, the results are considered valid.

In general, the following results are judged to provide a valid estimate of the child's current cognitive functioning as assessed under structured conditions.

This assessment is thought to accurately reflect his/her current level of academic/cognitive/psychological functioning.

Child was able to focus when presented with firm limits, and thus results appear to be valid.

Overall, the child was cooperative, and the results appear to be a valid representation of her/his current functioning.

Child put forth very good effort on all tasks. Although he/she was candid about disliking some tasks, he/she performed all of them attentively and often enthusiastically. Thus this evaluation appears to be a valid assessment of the child's abilities.

Questionable Validity

The following results are considered valid but may slightly underestimate the child's abilities, given his/her limited attention span.

Overall, the child was uncooperative for the evaluation. Although the results appear to be a valid representation of her/his current performance, they probably do not reflect her/his true abilities.

Child was extremely uncooperative for this evaluation, and thus the evaluation is rendered of questionable validity.

Child's limited attention had a severe impact on his/her ability to perform, and thus the evaluation is deemed invalid.

8

Reasons for Referral

This chapter covers referral reasons only. Everything else that should be included in the introduction to the report is covered in Chapter 7.

8.1. Statement of Referral Reason

In general, the statement of the referral reason should include the most pertinent identifying information, the type of evaluation, and the referral source, as well as the referral reason itself. The following are some commonly used expressions.

Patient/client is a _____-year old _____ grader, seen for _____ evaluation (indicate type of evaluation or service) **on referral of** _____ (indicate referral source/person) **to** _____ (indicate purpose of referral).

Client/patient, a _____-handed, ____-year-old male/female from _____, was referred for a _____ evaluation **by his/her psychologist/neurologist/psychiatrist,** _____, **given concerns about** _____ **and** _____ (specify nature of concerns).

Patient/client is referred by _____ (indicate referral person) **of** _____ (indicate person's affiliation/place of work) **for** _____ (indicate type of evaluation) **to obtain further information regarding** _____.

The child/family was referred by _____ (referral source/person and agency) **on** _____ (date of referral), **for** _____ (type of evaluation or other service), **to** _____ (rationale/purpose) **in regard to** _____ (referral reason).

Types of Evaluations/Reports

Classroom observation/consultation.
Clinical interview.
Cognitive evaluation.
Custody evaluation.
Diagnostic determination.
Discharge summary.
Educational placement.
Forensic evaluation.
Neuropsychological.
Mental status evaluation.
Psychological.
Psychological testing report.

Psychosocial evaluation.
Reevaluation.
Termination report or treatment termination report.
Treatment summary.

Common Referral Sources

Neurologist/pediatric neurologist.
Occupational therapist.
Nurse/clinical nurse specialist/pediatric nurse practitioner.
Parent/mother/father/guardian.
Pediatrician.
Psychologist/psychiatrist/psychotherapist.
School counselor/school psychologist.
Speech therapist.
Teacher/special education teacher.

Purposes of Evaluations

Assess academic/cognitive performance now that child has discontinued/begun _____ medication.
Assess bilingual/second-language issues.
Assess for presence of learning disorder.
Assess readiness for kindergarten/first grade/etc.
Assess social skills.
Assess treatment progress.
Assess current psychological functioning and eligibility for permanent placement versus independent living.
Better understand the origin of the child's difficulties.
Better understand the child's learning strengths and weaknesses.
Clarify diagnostic impression.
Clarify discrepancies in previous test results.
Clarify nature of the child's reading/writing/math difficulties, as well as educational needs.
Collect a baseline of psychoeducational data to measure the child's progress in the next ____ months.
Determine eligibility for special education services.
Determine whether there is a specific cause for the child's difficulties.
Determine whether behavior problems are due to a psychiatric disorder (if a specific disorder is suspected, name it).
Formulate an accurate diagnosis and translate it into a corresponding educational classification.
Help with school placement decisions.
Identify factors underlying problem behaviors.
Inform future educational plans.
Provide updated information as to the child's performance.
Suggest the most appropriate educational setting and supportive services for the child at this time, as well as any remedial and therapeutic options needed outside of school.

In the remainder of this chapter, common referral reasons are categorized by referral category.

8.2. Behavioral and Conduct Concerns

Aggressive behavior: Pushes others, grabs toys, hits/kicks/bites parents/siblings/teacher/others, throws food or objects, overturns furniture, screams/yells, violent behavior/outbursts, homicidal tendencies, threats of hurting others, expressed hatred of/desire to kill sibling/teacher/friend, talks a lot about killing and fighting, physical aggression, participates in physical fights, destructive of own/school/family's/others' property.

Attention-seeking behaviors: "Tattling," baiting, provoking others, overly demanding of attention from siblings/peers/adults, craves _____'s attention, manipulates, commits pranks, "clowns around," "class clown."

Attention span/concentration difficulties: Inadequate attention span, concerns about attention span, difficulty paying attention, difficulty following directions, difficulty staying/concentrating on task, distractible/easily distracted, difficulty focusing/lack of attentional focus, inattentiveness/inattention, inconsistent attention/behavior, insufficient attention, problems focusing/listening/concentrating, relies heavily on structured support from teachers and parents in order to remain on task and complete work, poor listening skills, often needs information repeated.

Alcohol/drug abuse: drinking/underage drinking, drug use, drug selling, smoking.

Dawdles/lingers/starts late in dressing/eating/bedtime/homework, procrastinates, wastes time.

Devaluing behavior toward others, "put-downs," insults others.

Difficulty with transitions, dislikes changes, inflexible/rigid.

Disruptive behaviors at home/school, agitates/disrupts/disturbs other children, provokes others.

Expresses emotions forcefully, intense in expression of anger/sadness, difficulty modulating emotions.

Firesetting.

Frustration: Easily frustrated, low frustration tolerance, difficulty handling new situations, becomes easily frustrated if she/he is not successful from the beginning of the task presented.

Hyperactivity/overactive/restless/fidgety, problems sitting still, problems maintaining focus in groups, excessive or inappropriate talking.

Impulsivity: Difficulty regulating impulse toward activity, impulse control problems, runs out of classroom/school, reckless behavior/activities, interrupts others, unpredictable behavior/outbursts at home/school.

Legal difficulties: Truancy, loitering, panhandling, underage drinking, vandalism, drug sales, "joy riding," auto theft, extortion, stealing, shoplifting, burglary.

Lying: Lying about homework assignments/school grades/school performance, "covers up" misdeeds.

Noncompliant/oppositional/insolent behavior toward teachers/caregivers, disregard for authority/rules, willfulness, stubbornness, headstrong.

Obsessions/hyperfocusing on certain topics, compulsions/rituals.

Regressive behavior, thumb sucking, rocking, stereotyped movements.

Self-destructive/self-injurious acts/behaviors/wishes: Cutting of wrists/arms, expressed desires/urges to harm self (e.g., jump out of moving car), etc.

Sexual behaviors: Sexual acting out/preoccupation, public/frequent masturbation, increased interest in sexual matters, initiates sexual conversations inappropriate for children his/her age, molests/molestation/molested, touched/fondled, actual intercourse/entry (oral/vaginal/anal/femoral), repeated/single-episode/recurrent, assault/rape, force used/damage/threats.

Slow-moving/lethargic.

Swearing, abusive speech, "backtalk."

Temper tantrums: Difficulty managing her/his temper, trouble calming her-/himself, "melts down" frequently, explosive behavior, prone to tantrums/severe tantrums, head banging, holds breath to point of fainting.

✓ For each behavior indicated, note duration and how it has been handled by parents/caregivers/teachers.

8.3. Cognitive Concerns

Possible cognitive impairment underlying the child's difficulties.

Developmental delays/developmentally delayed, seems behind other children his/her age with regard to cognitive skills.

Disordered thinking.

Difficulty understanding new concepts, difficulty distinguishing movies/cartoons from reality.

Forgets/forgetful.

Inability to connect cause and effect.

Memory problems.

Overwhelmed by large quantities of information.

Poor judgment.

Problems learning letter names/colors/numbers.

Processing speed difficulties.

✓ When any cognitive concerns are present, assess for/rule out mental retardation.

8.4. Emotional Concerns

Abuse (physical/sexual), consequences: Fear/anxiety, depression, dissociation, etc.

✓ Whenever abuse is suspected/reported, note source of allegations, relationship of child to alleged perpetrator, duration, etc. If allegations are not yet being investigated, notify appropriate authorities.

Anger: Angry feelings, impulsive expression of angry feelings, expresses particular anger toward mother/father/sister/brother/other; severe rage.

Anxiety: Anxiety that affects ability to perform in school/take tests, "freezing up"/experiencing a mental block, fears, phobias, nervous habits, becomes terrified for no apparent reason, panic symptoms (sweating, rapid heartbeat, etc.).

Autistic withdrawal: Lack of responsiveness to people, resistance to change in the environment.

Depression: Suicidality/suicidal ideation, sadness, anhedonia, lethargy/dysphoric mood/loss of interest in pleasurable activities, insomnia or other physical symptoms, self-harm (cutting/razor cuts, etc.), unhappy, problems with self-esteem/low self-esteem, wishes to die, feels unloved, perceives lack of friends, hates him-/herself; cries easily/chronically, cries over everything/any little thing.

Feels inadequate.

Frustrates easily, low frustration tolerance.

Guilty feelings.

Inadequate emotional reactions.

Immature emotional self-regulation, seems less emotionally mature than peers.

Imaginary playmates/fantasy.

Irritability: Irritable in a demanding/bossy way, irritable in a sad/discouraged way.

Lack of remorse for aggressive behavior.
Lethargy.
Mood: Labile/volatile mood, mood swings, moodiness, bipolar mood cycles.
Obsessive–compulsive symptoms.
Perfectionism.
Perseverative thinking.
Poor coping skills.
Posttraumatic stress disorder (PTSD) symptoms.
Psychotic symptoms.
Restricted/limited range of emotions, emotional constriction.
Shyness.

8.5. Family Concerns

Abuse (physical/sexual) by family members. *(See Section 8.4, above.)*
Argumentative with family members.
Death of mother/father/sister/brother/other family member.
Difficulty coping with recent/impending parental divorce.
Distress regarding biological father's/mother's unreliable visits.
Lies to parents.
Neglected, berated, belittled, humiliated.
Noncompliant, disobedient.
Oppositional home behaviors, talks back to parents, defies parents' authority, refuses to do chores/jobs at home, will seldom do what is asked, refuses to comply with house rules.

8.6. Learning and Academic Concerns

Academic performance below grade level, academic problems in reading/math/writing.
Attendance: Misses excessive days, absenteeism, tardiness, cuts classes, truancy.
Careless/sloppy work, problems with neatness.
Cheats, copies from peers, does not do own work.
Concerns about child's rate of progress in school, despite special education services.
Concerns relating to change in schools/move to new school district.
Deteriorating school performance.
Difficulty completing assignments, cannot work independently, does not finish things once started, difficulty organizing work.
Dropped out of school.
Effort: Insufficient effort, careless work, does not spend enough time on work.
Experiences anxiety and frustration regarding school.
Failing to seek help when appropriate.
Failure in subjects (specify).
Fatigued, too tired during the school day to put forth best effort.
Homework: Does not complete homework/in-class assignments, fails to turn in homework, turns in assignments late.
Inconsistent performance, learns something one day and forgets it the next.
Learning: Difficulty learning even simple information, trouble comprehending schoolwork.
Math: Problems learning math facts/concepts, problems retaining math concepts/rules/facts.
Motivation: Decreased motivation regarding school tasks, lack of motivation in school, does not try, makes little effort.
Organization difficulties/disorganized.

Poor attitude toward school, hates school, does not persevere, needs much encouragement, gives up easily.

Possible underlying learning disorder.

Processing problems/slow processing speed.

Procrastinates.

Refuses to do schoolwork.

Reading: Concerns about dyslexia/reading disability, failure to make progress in reading, problems with reading comprehension/decoding, difficulties acquiring reading skills, avoids reading, confuses similar words/letters, loses place while reading, forgets previously known words, trouble following written directions.

School phobia/avoidance.

Spelling difficulties: Cannot spell, can spell out loud but not as well in writing, unable to spell name.

Underachievement in school, academic underachievement.

Visual processing problems, difficulty with visual tracking.

Writing: Dysgraphia, difficulties with written output, slow writing, difficulty organizing written output, trouble copying from the board, difficulty expressing him-/herself in writing, problems with note taking.

8.7. Motor and Physical Concerns

Ambidextrous, alternates right–left, nonestablished hand dominance.

Delays in acquisition of fine motor/gross motor skills.

Eating: Poor feeding habits, poor manners, refuses food, appetite changes, odd combinations, pica.

Enuresis/bedwetting.

Fine motor difficulties: Problems with drawing/coloring/copying/cutting/staying on the line when writing, problems reversing letters and numbers.

Gross motor problems: Problems with crawling/walking/running, difficulties with skipping/climbing, unable to learn to ride a tricycle/bicycle, etc.

Hypotonia/hypertonia.

Hearing problems.

Motor coordination delays, motor control difficulties.

Motor tics.

Physically overactive.

Repetitive motor activities.

Sensory integration difficulties: Extremely sensitive to odors/clothing/textures/loud noises/particular noises/bright light/tastes, extreme sensitivity to environmental stimuli, tactile defensiveness.

Sleep: Poor sleep habits, refuses to go to bed, nightmares/night terrors, sleepwalking, excessive daytime drowsiness, parasomnias, refuses to get out of bed.

Toileting problems, unable to be toilet-trained at appropriate age.

Visual–motor integration difficulties.

Vocal tics.

8.8. Social Concerns

Attachment/bonding problems, inability to form an attachment or close relationship with others.

Clique membership/exclusion of other children.

Conversational inappropriateness: Makes rude comments, makes sexualized or grandiose statements, makes comments that have no relevance to current situation.

Difficult relationship with parents/siblings, noncompliant, fights.

Difficulty cooperating with others, trouble tolerating group situations, does not participate in group activities.

Difficulty discriminating known from unknown people.

Difficulty engaging in reciprocal conversation, problems interpreting social cues.

Difficulty interacting with peers, fights/argues frequently with playmates/peers, bossy, bullies others, deficits in interpersonal skills.

Difficulty making friends, has no friends, does not fit into peer group, is not accepted by peers, difficulty sustaining friendships, becomes obsessed with certain friends, continuing difficulties with social interactions.

Does not respect the rights and/or property of others.

Eye contact: minimal eye contact, lack of eye contact.

Immature social skills, social immaturity.

Is easily influenced/led, suggestible.

Lack of responsiveness to others.

Loner, isolates self, doesn't belong/fit in, socially isolated from peers, withdrawn, tendency to withdrawal.

Passive or uncomfortable in multipeer interactions.

Selective responses to people.

Sexual inappropriateness.

Teased or picked on in school/neighborhood by peers.

✓ For various problems in the development of social skills, assess for/rule out autism/Asperger's disorder/nonverbal learning disability; determine whether child demonstrates characteristics consistent with those found in people with autism/autistic withdrawal.

8.9. Speech and Language Concerns

Auditory discrimination weakness.

Concerns about communication skills.

Difficulty in the areas of pragmatics and verbal problem solving.

Expressive language difficulties, problems with verbal output, concerns about spoken language ability.

Failure to acquire normal speech.

Impaired language, language delays.

Mutism (elective/selective).

Poor articulation, specific speech misarticulations.

Problems understanding spoken language.

Problems comprehending and retaining information.

Word retrieval problems.

B. Background and History

9

History of Current Symptoms

The "Background Information" section of a report generally includes information provided by parents, teacher(s), and the child, as well as information from previous evaluations and records. There are two reasons to mention particular areas of a child's background and history. The first is to describe historical events that are or may be connected with the child's current problems. The second is to state that particular areas or topics were checked and reported as normal.

This chapter covers the child's history as it relates specifically to the referral question. Reasons for referral are covered in Chapter 8. Other aspects of history, such as medical/psychiatric background, developmental/family history, and academic history, are covered in Chapters 10–12. More information about psychiatric disorders can be found in Chapters 15 and 16.

✓ In child reports, the history is usually presented from the viewpoint of one or both parents. Teacher input is important in many cases as well, and, depending on the age of the child, it is helpful to provide the child's view of problem areas.

9.1. Onset of Symptoms

A formal statement of the parents'/teachers'/other authority's perception of the chief concern/problem usually starts with age of onset and perceived precipitating factors.

Age of Onset

State the child's age or grade at the time when problems were first noted. If they were only retroactively noted, indicate your conclusions about the actual onset. Different symptoms or changes in severity may have different onset dates and different precipitants.

Precipitating Factors

Indicate whether/if onset of symptoms was preceded by a particular incident or stressful event. In children, common precipitating factors include the following:

Abuse (physical/sexual).
Beginning or changing schools.
Death of parent/grandparent/sibling.
Divorce or separation of parents.
Illness, either in child or in another family member.
Move to a new home or location.

Parent's marriage/remarriage.
Separation from parents.

State the reason for seeking treatment/evaluation at the current time, and the goal(s) of treatment/evaluation.

Summary Statements

_____ (child's name) is a _____-year, _____-month-old boy/girl/male/female referred for a _____ evaluation (specify type of evaluation) by _____ (specify referral source) to address concerns regarding _____ difficulties (indicate nature of difficulties).

The current testing was requested to help characterize _____'s strengths and weaknesses in order to aid in academic planning.

This child is referred for _____ (specify type of evaluation) to obtain updated information about his/her skill levels and learning/emotional/behavioral profile. The evaluation will be used to plan educational/treatment interventions.

_____ (child's name) was described as a happy/outgoing/normal/quiet/etc. child until _____ (date), when she/he began exhibiting _____ (specify symptoms/behavior changes).

This is the first psychiatric hospitalization for _____ (child's name), who was admitted on _____ (date) due to _____ (indicate problem).

This child began exhibiting behavior/academic/attention/etc. problems at age ____.

9.2. Course

Structuring the History of the Current Problem in the Report

Provide a chronological account of the reason(s) the child has been brought for evaluation or treatment, beginning with when symptoms were first seen. This may have been at birth (e.g., in cases involving prematurity or a genetic defect); in early childhood; or in elementary, middle, or high school.

As Morrison and Anders (2001) note, children's histories often contain multiple threads, such as behavior problems, learning disabilities, and mood dysregulation. It is helpful to disentangle these strands within the report, with one paragraph devoted to each strand. Information highlighted in this area should help build a case for the diagnosis that comes later; it should particularly include aspects of the history that confirm the diagnosis, as well as aspects that refute, or perhaps weaken, the diagnosis.

Describe premorbid functioning: personality, behavioral, emotional, academic, and social.
Describe development/chronology of signs/symptoms/behavior changes. Include duration, progression, and severity of symptoms.
Single episode or multiple episodes? If the latter, describe as:

Recurrences, relapses, exacerbations, worsenings, flare-ups, fluctuating course.

Any remissions? If so, describe these as **partial** or **full/complete**. Also, indicate duration and possible reasons.
Any previous diagnoses of current problem? If so, indicate age at diagnosis, type/name of diagnosis, and validity of diagnosis; also, explain any changes of diagnosis.

Impact of Previous Treatments on Any Past Symptoms

See Section 10.7, "Psychiatric History."

Effects of Current Symptoms on Functioning

Behavioral: Indicate whether symptoms have caused increased behavior problems in other areas (e.g., whether symptoms of depression have caused aggressive behaviors toward family members).

Family: Describe effects of symptoms on family functioning and dynamics (*see Chapter 17 for descriptors*).

School: Describe impact of symptoms on school performance, grades, ability to complete homework, interest in school, and/or achievement motivation (*see Chapter 18 for descriptors*).

Social: Describe impact of symptoms on child's friendships and ability to interact with others (*see Chapter 19 for descriptors*).

10

Medical and Psychiatric Background Information

This chapter first covers a child's prenatal, birth, and early infancy histories, as well as topics relevant to adopted children. It then covers the child's medical history, use of medications, and history of previous psychiatric symptoms and treatment. Keep in mind the two reasons to mention any of these particular areas in a report, as noted at the start of Chapter 9. The first is to describe historical events that are or may be connected with the current problems; the second is to state that particular areas or topics were checked and reported as normal.

10.1. Prenatal and Maternal Health

Alcohol and Tobacco Exposure

Describe any reported alcohol or tobacco use during pregnancy, along with any possible effects of prenatal exposure, such as a child born with fetal alcohol syndrome (FAS).

> Mother denied a history of tobacco and alcohol use during pregnancy.
> Mother denied smoking during pregnancy/smoked tobacco for ____ months during pregnancy/ throughout pregnancy.
> Mother denied using alcohol during pregnancy/admitted having approximately ____ drinks a day for ____ months during pregnancy/throughout pregnancy.
> Father/child protective services worker/other (specify) reported maternal alcohol use during pregnancy.
> Child's medical record reports signs/symptoms of FAS.

Illegal Drug Exposure

Describe any reported illicit drug use; indicate the specific drug if known (e.g., cocaine, crack, heroin, marijuana); and note any possible effects of prenatal exposure, such as drug addiction at birth.

> Mother denied using illegal drugs during pregnancy/admitted using _____ (specify amount) of _____ (specify illegal drug/drugs) for ____ months during pregnancy/ throughout pregnancy.

Father/child protective services worker/other (specify) reported maternal illicit drug use during pregnancy.

The child's medical record reports he/she was born positive for/addicted to _____ (specify illegal drug/drugs).

Use of Prescription Drugs and Vitamins

Describe any drugs prescribed, reason for use, and timing of use during pregnancy. In addition, note use of prenatal vitamins.

The child's mother was prescribed and took _____ (specify prescription drug/drugs) during _____ (trimester) of pregnancy/throughout pregnancy for _____ (indicate condition).

The child's mother used prenatal vitamins during ____ months of pregnancy.

Pregnancy Course

Report the mother's previous pregnancies and miscarriages (and any complications), hospitalizations, prescribed bedrest, abnormal fetal activity, lack of medical care, preterm labor, and associated medications.

The pregnancy was normal/uneventful/uncomplicated/complicated.

The pregnancy was planned/unplanned.

The child is the product of the mother's first/second/third/etc. pregnancy.

Mother had ____ previous miscarriage(s).

Mother required bedrest for ____ months of pregnancy.

Mother was placed on partial/complete bedrest beginning at ____ weeks'/months' gestation.

The pregnancy was complicated by _____ (see the list of common complications below).

Fetal activity was very high/low throughout pregnancy.

Mother was hospitalized for _____ (see the list of common complications).

Mother received no/little/regular medical care during pregnancy.

Preterm labor was reported at ____ weeks gestation.

Preterm labor was treated with _____ (see the list of medications below).

Common Medical Complications during Pregnancy

Anemia.

Hypertension/elevated blood pressure.

Infections: Staph, sinus. (Indicate whether infections needed to be treated with antibiotics, and when during the pregnancy the infections occurred.)

Intrauterine tumors.

Morning sickness: Mild/severe; treated with _____ (specify drug, if any).

Preeclampsia.

Radiation/X-ray exposure.

Rh incompatibility.

Spotting/bleeding/threatened miscarriage.

Toxemia.

Weight gain: Abnormally low/high.

Common Medications Used to Treat Preterm Labor

Terbutaline, ritodrine, magnesium; indomethacin, nifedipine (less frequently).

Psychosocial Stressors during Pregnancy and Birth

The child's mother and father separated when the mother was _____ months pregnant.
The mother experienced mild/moderate/severe emotional stress before/during/after pregnancy.
The family was under severe stress due to parental unemployment/illness/death in family/move/divorce/separation.

10.2. Birth History

General Statements

Pregnancy and birth histories were insignificant/unremarkable/essentially normal.
Prenatal and delivery histories were reported to be free of complications.
The child was the product of a full-term, uncomplicated gestation and delivery.
Prenatal and delivery histories were significant for _____ (specify).

Labor and Delivery

Time in labor was brief/lengthy.
Birth was preceded by _____ hours in labor.
Labor was intense/difficult/induced/spontaneous.
Birth was attended by doctor/midwife.

Describe the delivery in any of the following terms that apply. In particular, report any unusual or complicating aspects of the labor and delivery that might be related to the child's current difficulties.

Normal/uncomplicated/vaginal, normal vaginal, vaginal breech, vaginal presentation under/without spinal/general anesthesia, natural delivery
Emergency Cesarean section/C-section due to fetal distress/fetal aspiration of meconium/failure to progress/maternal distress.
Scheduled C-section due to breech position/narrow maternal pelvis/other (specify).
Forceps birth/forceps were used during birth.
Meconium staining.
Vertex presentation.

Birth Weight and Gestation

The child was born full-term/born on time/at term, weighing _____ lbs. _____ oz.
The child was born at _____ weeks gestation.
The child was born _____ days late.
The child was born prematurely at _____ weeks.

Apgar Rating

The Apgar scale (Apgar, 1953) is used to evaluate the vital signs of newborns in the delivery room. The scale is administered within the first 60 seconds after birth and again at 5 minutes after birth to check a baby's appearance (color), pulse (heart rate), grimace (reflex irritability), activity (muscle tone), and respiration (breathing); note that the first letters of these five words spell the name "Apgar." Each vital sign is scored 0, 1, or 2, based on criteria described in the table below. Most infants score in the 7–10 range. Scores between 5 and 7 indicate that a baby is in need of careful observation, while scores below 4 indicate significant risk.

Apgar scores were ____ at 1 minute and ____ at 5 minutes.
Apgar scores were reportedly low/normal/good.
Child's initial Apgar score was 1, but he/she recovered quickly and 10-minute Apgar was 10.

Vital sign	0	1	2
Appearance	Blue, pale	Body pink, extremities blue	Completely pink
Pulse	Absent	Slow (below 100)	Over 100
Grimace	No response	Grimace	Vigorous cry
Activity	Limp	Some flexion of extremities	Active motion
Respiration	Absent	Slow, irregular	Good strong cry

10.3. Neonatal Health and Behavior

General Statements

Neonatal course was unremarkable.
Child was discharged home with her/his mother at the appropriate time.
Infant was hospitalized for ____ days after birth for _____ (specify).
Child had jaundice as an infant.
Infant required oxygen for ____ hours/days.
Infant had breathing difficulties due to hyaline membrane disease.
As an infant, child spent ____ hours/days/months in an incubator.
As an infant, child spent ____ days in the neonatal intensive care unit.

Reflexes

Snow (1998) describes the reflexes present in newborns as follows:

Rooting and sucking (rooting reflex should disappear by 3 months).
Grasp (replaced by voluntary grasp by 3 or 4 months).
Moro (begins to disappear by 3 months).
Babinski (disappears between 12 and 16 months of age).
Tonic neck (disappears by 4 to 6 months).
Stepping (disappears by 5 months).

General Temperament and Behaviors

Describe activity level, crying behavior, social interest, and general disposition.

The following descriptors for sensitive temperament are sequenced by degree of difficulty:

(↔ by degree) Sensitive, highly reactive to external stimuli such as clothes/sounds/touch/light/noise, pulled away from affection, unresponsive.
Moods are generally positive, is somewhat negative, tends to react negatively and cry a lot.
Adapts quickly to new experiences, is reluctant to adapt, has significant difficulties accepting new experiences.

Eating Behavior

Nursed/ate well, good eater/normal eating patterns, breast-fed well, feeding patterns were unremarkable.
Breast-fed/bottle-fed until ____ months/years of age, weaned at age ____.
Difficulty learning to suck.

Lactose-intolerant.
Reflux/problems with gastroesophageal reflux; spit up frequently.

Sleeping Behaviors

Slept well, good sleeper, normal/unremarkable sleeping patterns.
Difficulty falling asleep/had trouble falling asleep, poor/light sleeper, awoke frequently during the night.
Slept through the night at _____ weeks/months.

10.4. Adopted Children

Report the child's age at adoption, and describe what is known about the home prior to adoption (or, if appropriate, indicate the country from which he/she was adopted).

The child was adopted at birth/_____ months/years of age.
The child was fostered by the _____ center/foster mother for _____ days/weeks/months.
Records indicate that the child lived with her/his biological mother until age _____.
The child was adopted from an orphanage in _____ (specify nation).

✓ Often little is known about an adopted child's prenatal and birth histories. In these cases, report what is known, as in these examples:

Little is known about the child's birth parents, except that his/her mother was a young teenager and the father was employed as a _____.
Little is known about the child's prenatal or birth history.
The child was adopted from Korea, and there is no information regarding prenatal history.

10.5. Medical History

As relevant, note the following:

Current/recent illnesses.
Symptoms.
Surgeries and other treatment.
Injuries and accidents—especially traumatic brain injury, closed head injury, and all other traumatic incidents resulting in loss of consciousness.
Drug treatment, use, and abuse. Note especially use of illegal/illicit drugs, as well as of nonprescription drugs, over-the-counter medicines, vitamins, herbal remedies, supplements, etc.
Exposure to toxins: Duration, amount, type, source, and treatments.

Medical Problems Frequently Observed in Children

Allergies. Descriptors:

The child is allergic to _____/has seasonal allergies/hay fever.

Asthma. Descriptors:

The child has asthma treated with _____ (specify medication).
Asthma is allergenic/seasonal/exercise induced.
Asthma resulted in _____ (specify number) hospitalizations/emergency room visits.

Bowel disorders: Colitis, Crohn's disease, irritable bowel syndrome, frequent diarrhea.

Brain tumors: Meningiomas, primary neoplasms, gliomas, secondary neoplasms.

Cerebral palsy. Hallahan and Kauffman (1994) describe two approaches to classifying cerebral palsy. The first classification is according to the parts of the body involved:

Hemiplegia (condition where one side of body—right or left—is paralyzed).
Diplegia (condition where legs are paralyzed to a greater extent than arms).
Quadriplegia (condition where all four limbs are paralyzed).
Paraplegia (condition where both legs are paralyzed).

The second classification is according to type of brain damage and consequent motor disability:

Pyramidal (spastic). Brain damage is to the pyramidal cells in the cerebral cortex, resulting in spasticity.
Extrapyramidal (choreoathetoid, rigid, and atonic). Damage to brain is outside of pyramidal tracts and results in involuntary movements, stiffness, or floppiness.
Mixed.

Childhood illnesses: Anemia, chicken pox, diphtheria, encephalitis, German measles, measles, meningitis, mumps, rheumatic fever, scarlet fever, sustained high fever, tuberculosis, whooping cough.

Congenital infections: Human immunodeficiency virus (HIV), herpes virus, syphilis, toxoplasmosis.

Cystic fibrosis (a fatal disease affecting the lungs and intestinal tract).

Ear infections/otitis media: Indicate frequency of the infections, timing of ear infections (e.g., first year of life), severity, and impact on development, if any; indicate also whether child received tympanostomy tubes to treat condition, and, if so, age at operation. General statement about ear infections:

The child's medical history is remarkable for frequent otitis media during critical language periods.

Ehlers–Danlos syndrome: Include what effect disorder has had on psychological/physical functioning, and whether surgery (e.g., skin grafts) was needed.

Epilepsy/seizure disorder. Indicate type of seizure disorder, age at diagnosis, frequency and length of seizures, and medication used to control seizures. Lezak (1995) provides the following clinical classification of epilepsy:

Partial seizures: Can be simple, complex, or partial evolving to generalized seizures.
Generalized seizures: Can be nonconvulsive/absence/petit mal, or convulsive.
Unclassified: Includes seizures that are poorly documented or don't fit into previous categories.

Enuresis/bladder incontinence, encopresis/bowel incontinence: Indicate whether it occurs during daytime/nighttime/both day and night; also indicate age of onset and whether condition is secondary to a medical condition.

Eczema/other skin problems.

Febrile seizures: Indicate number of seizures, age(s) at occurrence, and cause(s).

Fibromyalgia: More commonly diagnosed in adolescence than in childhood. Symptoms that commonly occur with fibromyalgia include unrestful sleep, fatigue, morning stiffness; less common symptoms include headache, Raynaud's syndrome, irritable bowel syndrome, and depression.

Head injury/concussion: Indicate age at injury; whether loss of consciousness was observed; circumstances (car accident, fall, etc.); whether stitches were needed; whether skull was fractured; and impact on child's functioning, both immediately following injury and later.

Hearing loss/impairment: Indicate severity and whether problem is bilateral/unilateral.

Heart murmur: Indicate whether problem was resolved without/with intervention (and age at surgery, if applicable) or remains unresolved.

Hemophilia.

Hernia: Report age at operation.

Hydrocephalus: Report whether hydrocephalus was congenital or developed later (if later, age of onset); whether ventriculoperitoneal shunt was placed and at what age; and sequelae (e.g., seizure activity).

Juvenile rheumatoid arthritis or **osteoarthritis**.

Musculoskeletal conditions: Clubfoot, scoliosis, Legg–Calvé–Perthes syndrome, osteomyelitis.

Respiratory problems: Pneumonia, bronchitis, croup, asthma (see above), other pulmonary problems, seasonal wheezing; indicate frequent hospitalizations or emergency room visits.

Sinusitis: Report age of onset, and note whether it affects ability to concentrate or results in frequent headaches.

Spina bifida (deficit resulting from failure of bony spinal column to close during prenatal period).

Stomach disorders: Acid reflux, gastroesophageal reflux, esophageal strictures (indicate whether and when surgery was performed to treat condition), lactose intolerance.

Tonsillitis: Report whether tonsillectomy was performed (at what age) and whether adenoids were removed.

Undescended testes: Indicate whether child received surgery for this and age at surgery.

Vision loss/impairment: Indicate severity, whether corrective glasses are effective in treating condition, and whether problem is bilateral/unilateral. Also report color blindness, if present.

Summary Statements

Unremarkable Medical History

The child's health history is essentially benign.

Her/his medical history is unremarkable, and immunizations are up-to-date/complete.

Child's medical history has included no significant medical illness, head trauma, loss of consciousness, or seizure disorder.

Medical history is noncontributory.

Remarkable Medical History

Medical history is remarkable for _____. (Include information about current/past illnesses, past/current surgeries, injuries, exposures to toxins, etc.)

10.6. Medication History   *See Chapter 38, "Medications."*

Indicate any medications that the child is currently taking or has ever taken for longer than 6 months; in each case, include the type of medication, the reason for taking it, and the duration for which it has been or was taken.

Summary Statements

_____ (child's name) is not currently taking medications.

The child has not received any medication, either currently or in the past, for his/her symptoms.

_____ (child's name) currently takes _____ (name of medication) for _____ (name of disorder/symptoms). In the past, she/he has taken _____ (name of medication) **during** _____ (grades/years) **to help with** _____ (name of disorder/symptoms).

The child takes _____ (name of medication) **to help him/her manage problems with** _____ **and** _____ (name of disorder/symptoms).

10.7. Psychiatric History

See Chapter 9, "History of Current Symptoms," for guidance in describing the history of the present concern.

Describe psychological difficulties in the past, as well as any treatment(s) and professional help sought.

Hospitalization: Report number of previous psychiatric admissions; reason for psychiatric admissions; length of hospital stays; therapies instituted during hospitalization, and responses to these treatments; condition on discharge from inpatient treatment; involvement with other agencies/treaters.

Previous diagnoses: Indicate whether child was ever previously diagnosed with a psychiatric disorder:

Child was diagnosed with _____ (name of disorder) **in** _____ (date) **by Dr.** _____ (name).

Past psychiatric medications: Report all medications previously prescribed, as well as their effects, the child's response, and the side effects.

Previous outpatient therapies: State the history of previous interventions; for each intervention, note the type of therapy, reason for therapy, dates of therapy, name of therapist, and outcome. Types of outpatient therapy may include the following:

Psychiatry, psychotherapy, occupational therapy, physical therapy, speech/language therapy, special education services.

Previous testing: Report any previous evaluations by type:

Neuropsychological, psychological, intellectual, emotional, projective, speech/language, occupational, physical, neurological, vocational.

Postdischarge history: Report any follow-up treatments or referrals and compliance with these, or report as lost to follow-up.

Summary Statements

The child has never been treated for any psychiatric disorder.

The child previously received _____ (indicate type of therapy) **to treat** _____ (name of disorder/symptoms) **symptoms from** _____ **to** _____ (dates).

No significant mental health problems were reported, except for _____ **at age** ____.

11

Developmental
and Family History

This chapter covers pertinent aspects of a child's developmental and family history, as well as providing listings of age-appropriate developmental milestones in various areas.

11.1. General Statements

Developmental milestones were all generally considered to be within normal limits.
Developmental milestones were acquired within age expectations.
Developmental milestones were within normal limits, with the exception of _____ (specify).
Developmental milestones were reportedly delayed.
Parents report that certain developmental milestones were late (specify).
Parents report delayed acquisition of both motor and communication developmental milestones.
The child was described by her/his mother as acquiring developmental milestones early.

11.2. Adaptive Skill Development

Statements about Specific Skills/Problems

Bedwetting	Daytime/nighttime bedwetting occurred at age ____. History of enuresis at age ____.
Bottle	Gave up bottle at age ____.
Dressing	Dressing skills were mastered at age ____.
Eating	Became a picky eater at age ____. Fed him-/herself finger food at age ____ months. Ate with spoon/fork at age ____. Was a good/poor eater as an infant/toddler/child/adolescent.
Nightmares	Nightmares began at age ____. The onset of nightmares at age ____ coincided with _____ (specify event).

Separation	No problems with separation.
	At age ____, child exhibited difficulty tolerating separations from parents.
Sleep	Took time to settle into a sleep routine.
	Began sleeping more at age ____.
	History of increased sleeping/delayed sleep onset since age ____.
Toilet training	Was toilet-trained at age ____.
	Was bladder-trained at age ____ and bowel-trained at age ____.

Adaptive Skills Milestones

Average ages at which important adaptive skills milestones appear are as follows (Santrock, 1997; Snow, 1998):

30–36 months	Dresses self with supervision.
48 months	Uses toilet alone.
5 years	Ties shoes.
7 years	Can brush and comb hair in an acceptable manner.
	Can use a knife for cutting meat.
8 years	Can help with routine household tasks, such as dusting and sweeping.
10 years	Can wash and dry own hair without difficulty.

11.3. Language Development

General Statements

Articulation difficulties (mild/severe, specific/multiple) noted at age ____.
Began speaking at age ____, began using single words at age ____, began combining words at age ____.
Experienced difficulties with speech.
Expressive language was delayed/average/above average.
Did not use words until age of ____.
Has history of expressive/receptive language difficulties.
Idiosyncratic speech patterns developed at age ____.
Receptive language was delayed/average/above average.
Slow to speak/talk.
Speech therapy was prescribed/used to treat problems with _____ at age(s) ____.
Spoke in sentences at ____ months.
Stuttering began at age ____/was noted briefly at the age of ____.

Language Milestones

Average ages at which important language milestones appear are as follows (Bee, 1997; Sattler, 2002):

1 month	Responds to voice.
2 months	Coos.
4 months	Turns head to sound.
5–6 months	Babbles.

8 months	Vocalizes three different vowel sounds.
12 months	Jabbers expressively.
13 months	First words.
18 months	First two-word combinations.
22 months	Combines words and gestures.
2 years	Mean sentence length of two words.
34 months	Poses questions.
3 years	Mean sentence length of three words.
42 months	Understands two prepositions.
4 years	Mean sentence length of four words. Follows three commands.

11.4. Motor Development

General Statements

Gross/fine motor skills are described as being within the normal range.
Mild/moderate/severe difficulties with fine/gross motor skills.
Motor skills were age-appropriate/well developed/good/fair/delayed.

Statements about Fine Motor Skills

Avoided fine motor tasks.
Child had difficulty in/was adept in buttoning pants/coat, tying shoes, drawing/coloring/writing/copying/staying on line when writing, cutting with scissors, fastening clothes, putting puzzles together, snapping/zippering garments (pants, jacket, etc.).

Statements about Gross Motor Skills

Activity level	Preferred being active/inactive. Did not like sitting in a stroller.
Balance	Shows good/normal/poor balance. Described by parents as "clumsy"/"accident prone."
Bike riding	Rode a bike at age ____. Had difficulty/became easily frustrated learning to ride a bike.
Catching/throwing	Catching/throwing a ball was difficult.
Climbing	Was a fearless/fearful climber.
Crawling	Crawled at age ____. Never crawled.
Running	Ran at age ____. Has an awkward run. Was a "floppy" runner.
Stair use	Walked up/down stairs at age ____. Had difficulty learning to walk up/down stairs.
Walking	Walked at ____ months. Took first steps at ____ months and began to walk shortly thereafter. Walked within normal limits.

Motor Milestones

Average ages at which important motor milestones appear are as follows (Bayley, 1969; Bee, 1997; Santrock, 1997):

1 month	Thrusts arms or legs in play.
	Makes fists.
2 months	Holds rattle briefly.
	Rolls from side to back.
3 months	Attempts to bring hand to mouth.
4½ months	Rolls from back to side.
5 months	Uses eye–hand coordination in reaching.
	Picks up cube.
7 months	Sits alone.
	Transfers objects from hand to hand.
	Makes early stepping movements when standing.
7–10 months	Crawls.
	Pulls self to standing position.
11 months	Stands alone.
	Pincer grasp.
	Walks sideways while holding onto furniture.
	Sits from standing position.
12 months	Walks alone.
12–18 months	Scribbles with crayon on paper.
	Builds four-block tower with 2-inch cubes.
	Throws ball while standing.
18–24 months	Unscrews a lid put loosely on a jar.
	Zips and unzips large-sized zipper.
23 months	Jumps in place.
25 months	Runs with coordination.
31 months	Builds tower of eight cubes.
	Swings leg to kick ball.
37–48 months	Catches large ball.
	Cuts paper with scissors.
	Draws circle and plus sign.
	Hops three hops with both feet.
	Walks up stairs, alternating feet.
	Throws ball overhand.
49–60 months	Bounces and catches ball.
	Copies figure X.
	Cuts following line.
	Kicks 10-inch ball toward target.
	Hops on one foot.
	Prints first name.
	Skips.

61–72 months	Draws rectangle, circle, square, and triangle.
	Skips.
	Reproduces letters.
	Rides bicycle with training wheels.
	Jumps rope.
7 years	Can balance on one foot without looking.
7–8 years	Rides bicycle without training wheels.

11.5. Social Development

General Statements

Extremely social baby/toddler/child.
Social skills were age-appropriate at all stages of development.
Social skills were reportedly delayed.
History of difficulty in social situations with peers.
Difficulties in social interactions beginning at age ____.
Social situations more/less difficult than academic pursuits.

Statements about Specific Skills/Problems

Affection	Always/never showed affection to others.
	Constantly pulled away from others.
	Affectionate at an early age.
Being bullied	Was bullied at age ____ by _____.
Eye contact	Avoided eye contact as an infant.
	Did not engage in eye contact until age ____.
Fears	Became fearful of _____ at age ____.
Friends	Had few friends in preschool/elementary/middle/high school.
	Isolated him-/herself in preschool/kindergarten/etc.
Play	Play skills were excellent/awkward.
	Engaged in imaginary play until age ____.
	Had trouble playing with other children from an early age because she/he was bossy/withdrawn/rigid/insensitive/argumentative/etc.
	Preferred individual activities to playing with other children in the neighborhood/at school.
	Preferred playing with younger children at an early age.
	Preferred playing with boys/girls.
Shyness	Was shy/uncomfortable meeting new people at age ____.
	Was very quiet in ____ grade/at ____ age.
	Socially introverted when younger.

Social Milestones

Average ages at which important social milestones appear are as follows (Berk, 1994; Santrock, 1997; Snow, 1998):

1–2 months	Social smile emerges.
	Adjusts in anticipation of being held.
3–4 months	Laughter appears.
5–8 months	Plays peek-a-boo.
6 months	Smiles at mirror image.
7–12 months	Attachment to caregiver as a secure base emerges.
10 months	Cooperates in game.
2–3 years	Parallel play appears.
3–5 years	Friendships are concretely viewed in terms of play and exchange of material goods.
	Limited ability to take perspective of others.
6–10 years	Friendship emphasizes mutual trust and assistance.

11.6. Living Arrangements/Home Environment

Report the child and family's cultural/ethnic background as appropriate, country of birth, and language(s) spoken in the home. If doing so is pertinent to the history and referral reason, chronicle the child's home locations and relocations, and with whom the child was living with at each location (e.g., parents, foster homes, grandparents, extended family, etc.). For foster home/group home placements, report age of child at time of each placement, circumstances regarding the placement, and length of time in the placement.

General Statements about Living Arrangements

The child lives with his/her parent(s)/mother/father/mother's boyfriend/father's girlfriend and with _____ older/younger sister(s)/brother(s).

The child lives with his/her legal guardian, _____ (name). (Indicate when guardianship was awarded, to whom it was awarded, relationship of guardian to child, and reasons for transfer of guardianship.)

The child lives with his/her grandmother/grandfather/aunt/uncle/etc., who is her/his legal guardian.

The family resides in _____, _____ (city, state), a metropolitan/urban/suburban/rural/military location.

The child lives at home with her/his mother, father, and _____ siblings ages _____, _____, and _____.

The child is one of _____ (number) children born to _____ (names of parents). The family is intact and lives in _____.

Family is originally from _____ and has been residing in _____ for the past _____ years/months.

For a Young Adult/Adolescent Living Independently

If a young adult/adolescent client is living independently of the family of origin, report the following:

Living circumstances:

Client is living alone/with relatives/friends/boyfriend/girlfriend.

Reasons for move from family of origin.

If client is married: Age at marriage, date of marriage.

If client has child(ren): Age at birth(s) of child(ren), circumstances surrounding birth(s), effects of birth(s) on client, client's relationship with child(ren)'s other parent.

Aspects of the Home Environment

Type of home:

> Apartment/flat, house/single-family home, public housing, motel/shelter, homeless.

Language(s) spoken:

> Language(s) spoken in home is/are _____ (English, Spanish, etc.).
> (For a bilingual home:) **Child's primary language is** _____ **, while parent's primary language is** _____ **.**

Socioeconomic status:

> **Lower/middle/upper income level, impoverished/destitute, "working poor," modest means, prosperous/well-to-do.**

Quality of home environment:

> **Enriched environment/environment was lacking in enrichment/unstimulating.**
> **Home is overly structured/rigid/unstructured, stable/unstable.**
> **Parents describe immediate family members as very close to/distant from one another.**
> **Family atmosphere was described as positive/close/distant/isolated/volatile/violent.**
>
> ✓ If violence in the home is reported, note type of violence (physical, emotional); target of violence (e.g., mother, child); and whether and how frequently the child witnessed violence.

Extended family relationships:

> **Grandparents live with/near parents.**
> **Child has positive/negative relationship with grandparents/uncles/aunts/other extended family members** (specify).
> **Family does not do things with extended family members or with other families.**
> **Family is estranged/cut off from extended family.**

11.7. Parents

General Information about Parents

Age(s)/year(s) of birth; age(s) at birth of child.

If applicable, date of a parent's death; cause of death; child's age and reaction to death and its consequences.

> General physical and mental health; present health; chronic or severe illnesses, disabilities.
> Years of education/degrees.
> Ethnicity/nationality.
> Discipline style:
>
> > **Authoritarian/authoritative/controlling, lenient/laissez-faire/hands-off/permissive, strict/ firm/harsh/stern.**

Parents' Work History

Report the parents' occupations; indicate whether neither parent, one parent, or both parents work; and indicate place(s) of employment (outside or inside home, and location[s] if outside home).

> Mother/father/both parents worked outside of home when child was age ____/until child was age ____.
> Parent's job hours are flexible/inflexible.
> Parent's job requires much travel.
> Parent's job requires him/her to work away from home indefinitely/for extended periods of time.

Parents' Legal History

Report the parents' legal history *only* if it is relevant to the child's diagnosis or treatment.

> Arrests: Number, reason(s), whether child was a witness to arrest(s).
> Incarcerations: Number, reason(s), age of child at incarceration(s), effect on child.
> Other legal history: Indictments, prosecutions, convictions, probations, parole, bankruptcy.

Parents' Medical and Psychiatric History

> **Family medical/psychiatric history is significant for _____.** (Try to avoid identifying the particular family member by name in the report, unless absolutely necessary. This is particularly true for psychiatric disorders.)

> Alcohol and drug use histories: Note any history of alcohol/drug use/abuse/addiction, as well as any treatment history for alcohol or drug use.
> Learning disabilities: Note name of disability/disabilities; if not formally diagnosed but suspected, list symptoms reported by parent.
> Medical history: Note good health; for any health problems, record name(s) of disorder(s), age(s) at which disorder(s) was/were diagnosed, and impact of parent's medical problems on child's development.
> Psychiatric history: Note whether any psychiatric disorders were reported; for any psychiatric problems, record name(s) of disorder(s), age at which disorder(s) was/were diagnosed, hospitalization of parent during child's lifetime, and impact of disorder(s) on child.

Absence/Death of a Parent

> Absence:

> > Child's father/mother is not involved in her/his care.
> > Child sees his/her father/mother very infrequently; his/her last contact was ____ months/ years ago.

> Death: Indicate ages of parent and child at time of parent's death and circumstances surrounding death.

> > Child's father/mother died of _____ when child was ____ years old.
> > Parent died unexpectedly/after a long illness/violently.
> > Child witnessed death/found parent.

Parents' Marital/Couple Relationship

If married: Note year of marriage.

If separated: Note status of separation (legal vs. informal), time of separation, age of child at separation, and effect of separation on child's behavior.

If divorced: Note year of divorce, age of child at divorce, and effect of divorce on child's behavior.

Quality of parental relationship (↔ *by degree*):

Close/secure/warm/cordial, functional, unsettled/"up and down," distant, dysfunctional, tempestuous/violent/stormy/abusive.

Summary statement:

_____ (child's name) **is the oldest/youngest/etc. child in an intact family.**

The child's parents separated/divorced when she/he was ____ years old, and the child lives with her/his mother/father.

The child's parents divorced when he/she was ____ years old, and his/her father/mother is remarried.

Parents' Relationship(s) with Other Partners

Dating:

Parent has a boyfriend/girlfriend who has poor/good relationship with child.

Parent's boyfriend/girlfriend lives with parent and child.

Remarriage(s): Note age of child at remarriage(s) and child's relationship with stepparent(s).

Visitation and Contact with Noncustodial Parent

Visitation: Note frequency, schedule (including holidays), length of visits, and supervision status, as well as the effects of visitation on the child's functioning.

The child sees her/his father/mother weekly/monthly/etc.

Child saw his/her father/mother for 1/2/etc. days every/every other/etc. week from ages ____ to ____.

Child spends holidays with mother/father every/every other/etc. year.

Visitation takes place for ____ hours per week/____ weekends per month.

Visitation is unsupervised/supervised.

Other contact with noncustodial parent: phone calls (indicate frequency of phone contact); letters to/from parent/child (indicate frequency).

11.8. Siblings

_____ (child's name) **is an only child.**

Child reportedly gets along well/poorly with his/her brother(s)/sister(s)/sibling(s).

Child has normal relationship with siblings.

Quality of Sibling Relationships

Close/protective, good, average/fair, poor, "love–hate," volatile/explosive.

Sibling Rivalry

Sibling rivalry is nonexistent/typical/intense.
Rivalry increased with onset of birth of sibling/divorce of parents/other event (specify).
The child had difficulty adjusting to birth of sister/brother, but now has good relationship with her/him.
The child responded positively to birth of new brother/sister.

Information about Siblings

Age of siblings (if parents are expecting another child, note the due date). Birth order of siblings, and patient's location in birth order.
Living arrangement of siblings: Note whether living at family home or not; if not, note year sibling left home, reasons for living outside of family situation.
Medical history of siblings: Note important medical diagnoses, years of diagnoses, effect on child's development.
Psychiatric history of siblings: Note psychiatric diagnoses, psychiatric care (including hospitalizations), effect on child's development.

11.9. Family Genogram

A "genogram" is a diagram that maps family patterns and relationships across generations. It is more comprehensive than a family tree, because it provides information about the quality of the relationships, communication, and other behaviors. The figure below offers a key to the conventions of constructing genograms. It is reprinted with permission from Zuckerman (2005). For more information, consult Bowen (1980), Kramer (1985), or McGoldrick, Gerson, and Shellenberger (1999).

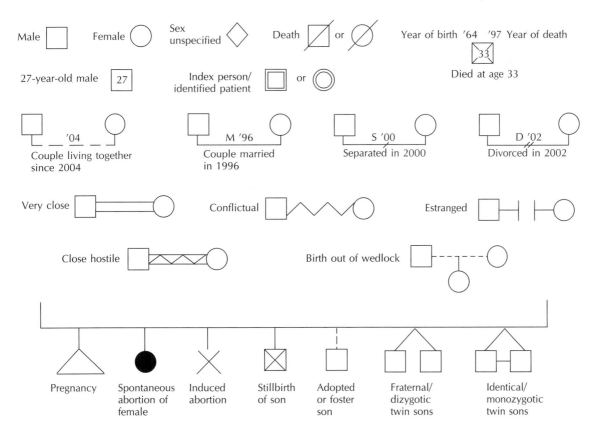

12

Academic and School History

This chapter describes general issues related to school and academics. For more information about intellectual functioning and academic achievement, see Chapters 21 and 22. For more information about current school functioning, see Chapter 18.

What follow are some of the more common issues that are encountered at different points in a child's school history. Although these issues are categorized, there is much overlap between categories.

✓ It is often helpful to construct an outline, using each academic year or time period as a guideline. For each year or time period (e.g., preschool, elementary, middle school), record significant school experiences: any change in school or grade retention; problems in specific academic areas (e.g., reading, spelling, math); grades received; special education services; evaluations; frequent absences; school behavior problems; and concerns about particular teachers.

12.1. Educational Situation

Highest grade completed:

> Preschool/kindergarten/first/second/etc., elementary school, middle/junior high school, high school, technical school, college, dropped out of school in grade ____.

Nature of enrollment:

> Day, full-time, part-time, boarding, summer school.

Special education: *See Section 12.16, "Special Education."*

Types of classrooms:

> Traditional/regular, language-based, mixed-age/open classroom, structured/unstructured/ rigid/loose, lacked a sense of control/seemed overcontrolled.

Age at school entry:

> Began preschool/nursery school/kindergarten/elementary school at age ____.

Types of schools:
Preschools:

> Montessori, play-based, parent cooperative, integrated/inclusion program, special-needs program, early intervention program, Head Start.

Kindergartens:

Traditional, Montessori/Waldorf, full-day/half-day, public/private/parochial, integrated/inclusion program, special-needs program.

Elementary and high schools:

Public/private/preparatory/parochial/vocational/religious/sectarian, residential boarding school, traditional/regular/special, Montessori/Waldorf, bilingual, charter school, home school/cyberschool.

Location(s) of school(s):

Rural, suburban, metropolitan/urban/inner-city.

Name(s) of teacher(s), relationship(s) with teacher(s), teacher report/description of problems.

Class assignment/level (specify), age–grade discrepancy (if any).

Educational program:

Academic, technical/vocational, college preparatory, etc.

Extracurricular activities:

Athletics, social service, music, scholarly, religious, political, special interests (specify), other (specify).

Other aspects: Favorite subjects, peer and teacher relationships, position in peer group, aspirations.

12.2. General School Issues

Overall level/quality of academic achievement/performance/grades, grade point average, standing in class.

Grades:

Consistently good/poor/mediocre, should be higher.
Received mostly A's/B's/C's/etc. in grade(s) ____.
Typical grades in elementary school/middle school/high school were described as A's/B's/C's/etc.
Uneven/variable grades.
Grades got worse/better in middle school/high school.

Summer school:

Attended summer school in _____ (indicate years) to help with _____ (specify difficulties).

Child–teacher interactions:

Child enjoyed his/her ____th-grade teacher.
Child had a strong bond with teacher.
Child was not comfortable with her/his classroom teacher.
In grade ____ there was a bad match between child and teacher.

Teacher behaviors:

Warm/caring, strict/rigid, became easily angered with child.

Standardized testing:

> The child earned scores on the Iowa Tests of Basic Skills/Stanford Achievement Tests/etc. of _____ in grade(s) ____.

Summary Statements

The child has always been a good/poor/average student.
The child was always a good student until grade/age ____.

12.3. Early Care/School Experiences

Day Care

Age at entry:

> Began day care at age ____.

Types of daycare and day care providers:

> Family day care, in-home care (includes nannies, au pairs), center-based day care.

Time spent in day care:

> ____ days a week for ____ hours a day beginning at age ____, for ____ months/years.
> An average of ____ hours a week in outside-the-home day care.

Day care provider behaviors:

> Caring/loving, mean, unkind, aggressive/abusive.

Positive child behaviors:

> No significant difficulties were noted.
> Was attached to day care provider.

Child behavior difficulties (see also Section 12.8, "Behavior Difficulties"):

> Aggression/was extremely aggressive, bit/hit/pushed other children.

Preschool/Nursery School/Kindergarten

Preschool/nursery school experience:

> Attended preschool/nursery school at age ____/from ages ____ to ____ and reportedly did well/poorly.
> Experienced difficulties in _____ (specify).

Kindergarten readiness:

> No problems/difficulties were seen in kindergarten readiness screening.
> Was below/at/above age level on tests of academic skills/perceptual development/social-emotional development/cognitive functioning in kindergarten screening.
> Failed kindergarten screening.

Transition to kindergarten:

> Uneventful/difficult/very traumatic.

Reasons for repeating kindergarten:

"Young" for age/grade, more interested in playing than working, socially immature, lacked appropriate academic skills, lacked attention skills necessary for kindergarten environment.

12.4. Academic Difficulties

Preschool/Nursery School

Had no interest in prereading activities/demonstrated difficulties with prereading skills, problems with fine motor tasks (cutting/holding crayon/etc.), problems learning letter names/colors/shapes, was reluctant to engage in language/fine motor/gross motor activities, had trouble writing, was slow to learn the alphabet.

Kindergarten

Was identified as a child at risk, had difficulty finishing work and organizing her-/himself, problems with fine motor/gross motor tasks, had difficulty acquiring prereading/premath/writing skills, did not perform at a level expected for a typical kindergarten student, had difficulty attending.

Elementary School

Trouble with task completion/difficulty completing assignments/took longer than other children to complete assignments, difficulty with handwriting/math/reading, needed help expressing ideas clearly, visual–spatial difficulties, did not meet grade expectations for reading/math/etc., could not keep up with class, had difficulty acquiring core academic skills, had a dependent learning style, had poor penmanship, had difficulty putting ideas in writing.

Middle School

Problems changing classes/dealing with more than one teacher, long-standing difficulties with reading/math/written expression/etc. continued in middle school, problems completing homework, problems organizing written work, could not complete grade-level work without considerable tutorial support.

High School

Often got lost getting from one class to another, had difficulty with increased course load and amount of homework, failed to do homework conscientiously, did not know how to study.

Summary Statement

The child had difficulty in the acquisition of age-appropriate academic skills.

12.5. Academic Progress

Elementary School

Good/much progress, performed well academically with exception of math/reading/spelling/writing, good progress in _____ (specify), satisfactory marks were noted in all/some subjects, was above grade level in all/some subjects, was noted by teachers to be working hard to develop math/reading/etc. skills, made good progress in all academic areas, was an early reader, had a knack for numbers.

Middle School/High School

Has made much/little academic progress during middle and high school years, was able to keep up with classmates in all academic areas except for _____ (specify).

12.6. Anxiety and Separation Difficulties

Separation anxiety/difficulties, had initial separation difficulties that resolved quickly, had difficulty tolerating separations from parents, was shy.

12.7. Attention Difficulties

Had attention problems/was inattentive, was easily distracted, problems following directions/ processing information, had a short attention span, was frequently unresponsive when teachers called his/her name; seemed to "fade out," often "spaced out."

Had great difficulty attending/paying attention/focusing, appeared not focused enough to complete all tasks in class, difficulty with listening tasks/listening comprehension, problems staying on task, had difficulty retaining information.

12.8. Behavior Difficulties

Preschool/Nursery School

Aggression/aggressive behavior, bit other children, expelled from preschool due to biting/hitting/lack of toilet training, impulsivity, refused to participate in structured activities, was always "on the go," had a difficult time sitting still, was easily overstimulated, had severe temper tantrums, bossy/uncooperative.

Kindergarten

Engaged in significant acting-out behavior that interfered with classroom functioning, was defiant/oppositional, demonstrated lack of response to reward systems, problems with mood regulation, violent outbursts, was disruptive, walked out of class on ____ occasions, had a propensity to fidget and move about, had difficulty remaining in his/her seat, was very impulsive.

Elementary School

Got into fights with other students, had trouble delaying gratification, demonstrated increased behavior problems in grade(s) ____, stole from classmates, was argumentative, did not complete work on time/did not use time wisely, could not work without disturbing others, poor self-control, difficulty with classroom compliance/problems following directions, fighting in the schoolyard, demonstrated disobedience toward teacher(s)/substitute teacher(s), hyperactive, unable to stay in seat.

Middle School/High School

Truant from school on a number of occasions, disruptive, unmotivated, brought gun/knife/drugs to school.

Was defiant, showed problems with mood regulation, fought with teachers/other students, stole items from other students/teachers/school property.

12.9. Language Difficulties

Preschool/Nursery School/Kindergarten

Problems with expressive/receptive language observed by teacher, had difficulties engaging appropriately in conversation, problems with auditory comprehension/processing, poor articulation, problems with self-expression.

Elementary School

Had difficulty with pronunciation of vowels/consonants/etc. in first/second/third/etc. grades, problems with verbal comprehension/articulation/word retrieval/written language/spoken language.

12.10. Math Difficulties

Difficulty learning basic math facts, had trouble learning multiplication tables, difficulty comprehending high-level problem solving.

12.11. Medication

The following statements relate specifically to the impact of medication on a child's educational progress and history. Medication history is covered in detail in Chapter 10.

Medication has helped with _____'s behavior and her/his academic performance in school.

He/she has been medicated with _____ since _____, and his/her teachers have indicated that this is very helpful.

Although medication was effective in school, in the evenings the medication wore off, and _____ had a great deal of difficulty focusing on homework and coping.

Medication had significant/little/no impact on school performance.

Parents tried medication for ____ weeks/months, but school personnel did not see a difference.

12.12. Positive Behaviors

Preschool/Nursery School

Did well, no academic difficulties, parents described preschool as a positive experience, _____ was a great student, was actively interested in classroom materials.

Kindergarten

Solid academic skill development, maturity, contributed a great deal to class discussions, kindergarten year was successful, _____ was an early reader.

Elementary School

Was able to follow directions/listened well, cooperated with others, accepted responsibility, was courteous and well mannered, displayed self-control, had a positive attitude, demonstrated strong effort, demonstrated good behavior and academic performance at school.

Middle School/High School

Did not have to study to get good grades, was a quick student who rarely needed to study, enjoyed sports/other extracurricular activities, demonstrated positive behavior/leadership.

12.13. Reading Difficulties

Kindergarten

Was not interested in reading activities, had trouble blending sounds, difficulties learning to read, problems learning letter names, difficulty rhyming words, problems learning sound–symbol associations, trouble learning the alphabet.

Elementary School

Difficulty learning to read, problems learning letter names/sounds, difficulty comprehending what she/he read.

Middle School/High School

Did not read for pleasure, problems with reading comprehension, continued to struggle with reading difficulties in middle school/high school.

12.14. Social Difficulties

Preschool/Nursery School/Kindergarten

Poor peer interactions, often isolated him-/herself, had difficulty connecting with others/did not connect with children in her/his class, did not engage in cooperative play, didn't participate in circle time, was socially immature, did not initiate peer interactions, had high levels of solitary or parallel play, appeared emotionally vulnerable.

Elementary School

Problems with peers/peer relationships, often teased by others, was a "loner"/avoidant/withdrawn, would react to teasing with verbal or physical aggression, often dominated classroom discussions, had difficulty picking up on verbal cues, had difficulty keeping friends, often angry at peers, had difficulty letting an argument go.

12.15. Social Skills

Elementary School

Was able to make friends at school, demonstrated extremely good social skills, made friends easily, was good-humoredly teased by peers, had many friends, child's sense of humor and likeability kept him/her out of trouble.

Middle School

Began to make friends, in contrast to elementary school history.

High School

Had many friends/several close friends, was very involved in extracurricular activities, played sports such as _____, was involved in drama/band/chorus/music/etc.

12.16. Special Education

Special education services are services designed to meet the needs of a child whose needs cannot be met within the general educational program (i.e., the regular classroom). Special education services can include special materials, teaching techniques, or equipment; special transportation; physical, occupational, or speech/language therapy; consultation services; and counseling. The brief listings below of possible services are by no means exhaustive.

✓ It is important to document a child's history of special education services at each grade level. For each type of service provided, note the frequency and duration of delivery.

Math Services

Had remedial math help, received specialized math tutoring focusing on _____ (specify).

Peer Relationships and Special Education

Was teased by peers about going to the learning center, is frequently ridiculed by classmates for being "dumb."

Reading Services

Participated in small-group reading instruction, received Chapter 1 reading resource assistance, took part in Reading Recovery/Project Read/Orton–Gillingham program/Wilson program/Lindamood Bell program/other (specify).

Writing Services

Writing workshop, help with organizing written work, occupational therapy.

Specialized Services

Occupational therapy, physical therapy, speech/language therapy, sensory integration therapy, music therapy, counseling, other (specify).

Other Special Education or Support Services

Mild/moderate/significant support from learning disability specialists, special help from teacher out of class, private tutoring, Lunch Bunch/other lunchtime activities, other (specify).

Types of Classroom Settings

Regular classroom setting with support, classroom for emotional and learning difficulties, inclusion language arts classroom, integrated classroom with remedial services, mainstreamed classroom, resource room/learning center.

Individualized Education Plans

See Section 35.9 for a sample individualized education plan (IEP).

It is useful to review the child's history of services as outlined in current and past IEPs. An IEP, by law, must include the following information: statement of present educational performance; instructional goals; educational services to be provided; and criteria and procedures for determining that the instructional objectives are being met.

Summary Statements about Special Education Services

The child has not received special education services and has done well academically.
The child never received special services during elementary or middle school.
The child has never needed special services or accommodations.
The child has received special education services throughout his/her school history.
The child receives resource room support/speech and language therapy/occupational therapy/ counseling/etc. for ____ minutes/hours a day/week.

C. The Child or Adolescent in the Evaluation

13

Behavioral Observations

This chapter covers the following areas: physical appearance, clothing, activity level, speech and language skills, and motor skills. How the child responded to the evaluation and presented him-/ herself in the evaluation is covered in Chapter 14.

13.1. Physical Appearance

✓ Use behavioral observations of the child's appearance to consider or rule out certain syndromes. For example, head shape and facial appearance are important in diagnosing disorders such as fetal alcohol syndrome (FAS), Sotos syndrome, and fragile X syndrome, while eye and hair colors are important in diagnosing Waardenburg syndrome.

Overall Physical Appearance

Child/adolescent presented as an attractive/handsome/pretty, well-groomed girl/boy/young woman/young man who appeared her/his stated age.
Child appeared to be well cared for/neglected.
The child seems to be well kept, well nourished, and in no apparent distress.
Hygiene is managed independently, effectively, and appropriately.
Clean, well groomed, and well dressed.
The child and/or his/her parents took good care of his/her appearance in regard to dress, hygiene, and grooming.

Child's appearance was appropriate for age.
At the time of this assessment, hygiene, grooming, and attire were appropriate for sex, age, and social norms.
_____'s appearance is not unusual.
No unusual visible features/deformities/dysmorphic features.
Nothing unusual/remarkable/noticeable about her/his posture, bearing, manner, or hygiene.

Child arrived for appointment poorly groomed.
This child showed some signs of neglect, specifically _____ (indicate).
Haggard, weak, pale and wan, frail, sickly, sleepy/tired. (Note time of day; ask about sleep.)

Height and Weight

It is best to describe height and weight by using the actual numbers. It is also helpful to note at which percentiles height and weight fall for the child's age. Current stature-for-age and weight-for-age percentiles can be found at a U.S. government website (www.cdc.gov.growthcharts).

Build

As explained in the Introduction to this book, the following table and similar tables in this and later chapters are ↔ *by degree across columns only* (i.e., individual entries that happen to fall within the same row in a table do not necessarily represent points on a mini-continuum).

Gaunt	Small for age	Average for age	Large for age
Emaciated	Thin	Well-nourished	Obese
Frail	Petite	Healthy	Tall
Malnourished	Underweight	Trim	Large Frame
Skinny	Slender	Robust	Plump
Lean	Little	Well-developed/	Fat
Bony	Short	well-built	Lanky
Scrawny	Diminutive	Weight proportionate	Long-limbed
Too thin	Slim	to height	Leggy
Underfed	Willowy	Within usual range	Tall and thin
"Skin and bones"	Tiny		Rotund
Undernourished	Undersized		Stout
Skeletal	Short-statured		Overweight
Gaunt	Bony		Heavy
Cachectic	Wiry		Corpulent
	Lanky		Chubby
	Skinny		Big for age
	Small-boned		Heavy-set
			Stocky
			Pudgy

Summary Statements for Build

Appeared smaller/larger than her/his stated age.
Appeared his/her given/stated age of _____ years.
Stature in relation to age is short/normal/tall.
Child is quite tall/large/small for her/his age and looks older/younger than her/his _____ years would indicate.
Child is at the _____, and _____ percentiles (respectively) of the standard table for height, weight, and head circumference for children.
Height/weight is average/below average/above average for age, at the _____ percentile for height/weight.
Child is not obese but appears to be tall and heavy-set.
Child is at _____ Tanner stage of sexual development (Tanner, 1978).

Eyes

Appearance/size/shape:

Large, small, squinty, sunken, hollow, deep-set, bulging, close-set, wide-set, cross-eyed, bloodshot, wide-eyed, hooded, almond-shaped, reddened, bleary-eyed.

Brows:

Light/heavy, raised, pulled together, pulled down, shaven, plucked.

Color:

Blue, gray, green, brown, hazel.

Eye contact:

(↔ *by degree*) No/avoided eye contact, stared into space, kept eyes downcast, poor, broken off as soon as made/passing/intermittent, wary, looked only to one side, brief, flashes/fleeting, furtive/evasive, variable, appropriate, normal, expected, good, had a frank gaze, lingering, staring, steady, glared, penetrating, piercing, confrontative, challenging, stared without bodily movements or other expressions.

Expression:

Sleepy, tired, heavy-lidded, had dark circles under his/her eyes, eyes looked red/pink, often rubbed her/his eyes, staring, unblinking, penetrating, squinting, nervous/frequent eye blinking/fluttering, vacant, glassy-eyed.

Glasses:

Wears/does not wear glasses for distance/reading, wears contact lenses, wears regular corrective lenses, wears sunglasses, glasses needed but not worn, glasses broken/poorly repaired.

Facial Complexion

Rosy, flushed, ruddy, tanned, glowing, healthy-looking, sallow, sickly, pale, jaundiced, wan, washed-out, ashen, pallid, pallorous, pasty, scarred, blemished, pocked, pimply, warty, mottled, shows negligence, birthmarks/port-wine stains, scars.

Facial Expressions   *See also Chapter 15, "Affective Symptoms and Mood/Anxiety Disorders."*

Smiling, happy, cheery/cheerful, positive, joyful, silly, delighted, elated.
Attentive, alert, vigilant, observant, interested, focused.
Calm, tranquil, peaceful, composed, serene, relaxed, dreamy, head bobbed as if nodding off.
Grimace, frown, scowl, sad, unhappy, glare, puckered brow, tense.
Crying, weeping/weepy, sobbing, sniffling, tearful/in tears, eyes watered/teared up.
Frightened, scared, terrified, startled, anxious, upset, worried, panicky, withdrawn, agitated, alarmed.
Annoyed, angry, irritated, cross, enraged, defiant, sneering, tight-lipped, disgusted.
Indifferent, uninterested, listless, droopy, lethargic, apathetic, meek, withdrawn, reserved, vacuous, blank, mask-like, flat, lifeless, unresponsive, tended to stare with little affective/emotional variability, lifeless, rigid.

Teeth

Unremarkable, crooked, wore braces, had many missing teeth (indicate if inappropriate for age), poor dental hygiene was apparent, bad breath/breath odor/halitosis.

Hair

Color:

Dark/light, brown, brunette, chestnut, black, red/red-haired/coppery/auburn, golden-brown, platinum, blond, strawberry-blond, fair-haired, streaked, albino, bleached, colored/dyed, frosted, streaks of color, different-colored roots.

Neatness:

> Clean, dirty, unkempt, messy, tousled, greasy, oily, matted, tangled, knotted, disheveled, uncombed.

Hairstyle:

> Fashionable length and style, long, short, "edgy," braided, cornrows, "relaxed, " crew/brush cut, tousled, uncombed, frizzy, curly, wavy, straight, dreadlocks, natural/Afro, ponytail, "pigtails," finger curls, "Goth/Gothic," "Mohawk," shaved head, stylish, currently popular haircut, unusual cut/style/treatment, moussed, permed, unremarkable.

Facial hair:

> Clean-shaven, beginning to get "peach fuzz," full beard, goatee, moustache, light facial hair.

13.2. Clothing

✓ What is most relevant about a child's clothing is what it says about the parents' ability to care for the child and the parents' judgment of appropriateness. Fashion, cost, or newness of a child's clothing is usually not important in itself. For an adolescent, dress is evaluated as to how appropriate it is when compared to that of the typical adolescent, as well as whether the clothing is being used to make a statement (as in the case of extreme hairstyles, dress, piercings, etc.).

Appropriateness

Dressed suitably/presentably, dressed appropriately for weather/climate, dressed in a style popular in his/her age group, school uniform.
Casually dressed, care of clothing was only fair, dressed carelessly.
Not suitably dressed for age/clothing suitable for a much younger/older child.
Inadequately dressed for the weather, lacked shoes/coat/boots.
Clothing was out-of-date/old-fashioned/unfashionable, unconventional, eccentric/odd/peculiar.
Garish/bizarre clothing, dressed to offend, attention-seeking/drawing, outlandish.

Qualities of Clothing (↔ by degree across columns only)

Dirty	Disheveled	Neat	Stylish
Unclean	Messy	Well-groomed	Smartly dressed
Filthy	Unkempt	Neatly dressed	Chic
Grimy	Tousled	Clean	Elegant
Soiled	Ill-fitting	Trim	Fashionable
Grubby	Too tight	Well-dressed	Trendy
Muddy	Sloppy	Spotless	Classy
Encrusted with food/ etc.	Tattered	Dirt-free	Hip
Caked with mud/etc.	Shabby	Unsoiled	The latest thing
Smelly	Frayed	Tasteful	Cool
Dusty	Threadbare	Well put together	Meticulous
Musty	Worn	Clothes-conscious	Immaculate
	Unzipped	Careful dresser	Overdressed
	Unbuttoned	In good taste	Seductive
	Rumpled		Revealing

Dirty	Disheveled	Neat	Stylish
	Disheveled		Flashy
	Clean but worn		
	Torn		
	Baggy		

13.3. Demeanor/Presence/Style (↔ *by degree across columns only*)

Withdrawn	Anxious	Shy	Friendly/confident	Immature or eccentric
Reserved	Threatened	Guarded	Outgoing	Silly
Neutral	Tense	Quiet	Energetic	Atypical
Unreadable	Overwhelmed	Inhibited	Polite	Bizarre
Expressionless	Apprehensive	Introverted	Engaging	Dramatic
Distant	Distrustful	Timid	Likeable	Infantile
Asocial	Nervous	Retiring	Warm	Odd
Detached	Worried	Bashful	Delightful	Peculiar
Isolated	Concerned	Reticent	Personable	Strange
Uninvolved	Uneasy	Apprehensive	Appealing	Unconventional
Uninterested	Apprehensive	Tentative	Sociable	Unusual
Impassive	Fearful	Demure	Playful	Out of the
Estranged	Frightened	Passive	Gracious	ordinary
Solitary	Hesitant	Reserved	Calm	Affected
Aloof	Suspicious	Humble	Relaxed	Histrionic
Dejected	Wary	Subdued	Open	Abnormal
	Edgy	Restrained	Pleasant	Idiosyncratic
	Jumpy	Composed	Affable	
	Panicky	Placid	Civil	
	Distraught	Mild-mannered	Well-mannered	
	Weak	Unassuming	Courteous	
	Vulnerable	Plaintive	Respectful	
	Fragile		Attractive	
	Low-resilience		Charming	
	Threat-sensitive		Agreeable	
			Amiable	
			Jolly	
			Warm	
			Extroverted	
			Chipper	

13.4. Movement/Activity Level

High Activity Level   *See also Section 16.1, "Attention-Deficit/Hyperactivity Disorder (ADHD)."*

Child had difficulty staying in seat/chair, difficult for child to sit for short periods of time, was nearly impossible for child to sit in a chair, high activity level, motorically active.

Child was very active and in constant motion, many out-of-seats, restlessness and distractible, difficult to redirect.

Child exhibited continual body movements while completing tasks.

Child often asked to get a drink/take a break/go to the bathroom/check to see whether parents were in waiting room.

Exhibited increasing motor restlessness as the day went on.

Was excited and tried to go too fast for accuracy.

Investigated all the contents of the room/desk/testing materials, intrusive, a "darter."

Child was fidgety/exhibited moderate to pronounced fidgeting, level of fidgeting increased as tasks increased in difficulty/became less challenging, child was "antsy"/wiggly.

Mild/moderate/severe impulsivity was noted in response style, child did not wait for feedback or directions and would impulsively respond, child began responding before the examiner finished explaining the task at hand.

Variable Activity Level

Movement was transient, activity level was changeable, still and pensive moments were followed by abrupt change to hyperactivity.

Although child was quite hyperactive, she/he was also easily fatigued and wanted to give up easily.

Child's level of arousal fluctuated during testing, child was sometimes highly distractible and at other times demonstrated good attention to the tasks.

Low Activity Level

Appeared tired, frequently stated that he/she was tired or did not get enough sleep, was initially tired but brightened considerably as evaluation/interview progressed.

Child frequently put her/his head on the table and complained that she/he was often tired.

Behavior was significant for slow performance speed.

Signs of fatigue were noted after a ____-minute work period.

Mannerisms/Odd Physical Behaviors

Twirling, rocking, self-stimulating, hand flapping, aimless/repetitious/unproductive/counter-productive movements, head bobbing, wriggling, hand or finger movements, bounced leg, posturing.

Played with lips, clicked tongue, stuck out tongue, bit lips, tongue chewing, lip smacking, whistling, made odd/animal/grunting sounds, belching, pulled lips into mouth.

Played with hair, picked at eyelashes/eyebrows.

Sniffled repeatedly/loudly, used/needed but did not use tissues/handkerchief, freely and frequently picked nose, repetitively "cleaned" ears with fingers.

Tapped fingers on table, tapped teeth with fingers.

Yawned frequently/excessively/regularly/elaborately, rubbed eyes.

Was often red in the face, as if straining his/her bowels.

Made audible breath sounds.

Chewed fingernails, nails were chewed down to a marked extent, bit nails down past the quick of all/some fingers.

Deliberately dropped items so she/he could retrieve them.

Sat on feet or knees, laid body on table, made faces, shook head back and forth, tried to look at examiner's test book, crawled under the table, did headstand on the chair, preferred to stand for most of the evaluation, tipped chair back and forth, twirled hair, moved arms in and out of shirt.

Kept thumb in mouth for ____ minutes of the ____-hour session, sucked fingers.

Covered face with hands and peeked out.

Walked on toes/heels/ankles.

13.5. Motor Skills

Fine Motor Skills

General Statements

Basic hand development was good.
No difficulties were noted in his/her fine motor abilities.
Fine motor skills were appropriate/delayed for age.
Difficulties with dexterity and fine motor control were evident in her/his manipulation of
   test materials.

Handedness

Right-handed/left-handed, demonstrated clear right/left-hand preference, has a well-established
   dominance of right/left hand, ambidextrous, no hand preference observed, appears unde-
   cided about hand preference.

Pencil Grip

Demonstrated appropriate/poor pencil grip, grasped crayon/pencil with pronated grip, whole-
   hand pencil grasp with no evident web space between thumb and index finger, awkward
   grasp, palmar grasp, tense grip, mature pencil grip.

Scissors Use

Unable to grasp scissors appropriately or snip without maximum assistance, snipped paper
   with scissors when maximal assistance was given for hand placement and holding the
   paper, able to cut a 2-inch line, demonstrates no difficulty with cutting skills.

Writing

Writing was graceful/neat/precise/poor/sloppy/small/large/difficult to read/illegible, child was
   able to scribble spontaneously, able to imitate crayon strokes, able to copy circle/square/
   triangle, able to write name, demonstrated poor letter formation, handwriting was labored
   and obviously difficult for him/her, could not cross midline in writing, wrote with good/
   poor speed for each task, stabilized paper with her/his right/left hand, placed excessive
   pressure on pencil.

Other Observed Skills

Child was able to build block designs for _____-cube tower, build bridge of cubes, fold paper
   with crease, unscrew cap from a bottle, complete puzzles, string small/large beads, button/
   zip/snap, draw a person.

Tests of Fine Motor and Visual–Motor Skills

See Chapter 25 for citations and more information on some of these tests.

Beery–Buktenica Developmental Test of Visual–Motor Integration, Fifth Edition (Beery VMI)
Bender Visual–Motor Gestalt Test (Bender Gestalt)
Bruininks–Oseretsky Test of Motor Proficiency, Second Edition (BOT-2)
Developmental Test of Visual Perception, Second Edition (DTVP-2)
Developmental Test of Visual Perception—Adolescent and Adult (DTVP-A)
Finger Tapping or Finger Oscillation Test

Grooved Pegboard
Rey–Osterrieth Complex Figure
Wide Range Assessment of Visual Motor Abilities (WRAVMA)

Gross Motor Skills

General Statements

Child has excellent/good/poor gross motor skills.
Gross motor planning is poor/good/age-appropriate/excellent.
Gross motor skills are notable for difficulties with balance/coordination/motor planning and output/neuromaturational delay.

Balance

Balance was good, excellent/good/poor balance reactions, balance is steady/normal/firm/solid, child could stand on one leg for _____ seconds, is able to maintain control on a playground swing without back support, complained of dizziness/lightheadedness, balance is wobbly/shaky/unstable/uneven/unsteady.

Gait

(↔ *by degree*) Astasia/abasia, ataxic, steppage, waddling, awry, shuffles, desultory, effortful, dilatory, stiff/rigid/taut, limps, drags/favors one leg, awkward, unusual, odd, abnormal, atypical, collided frequently with other children/people/furniture, walks with slight posturing, lumbering, leans, rolling, lurching, collides with objects/persons, broad-based, knock-kneed, bow-legged, normal, ambled, no visible problem/no abnormality of gait or station, fully mobile (including stairs), springy, graceful, relaxed, glides, brisk/energetic, limber.
Runs/walks in a manner mature/immature for age.
When running, child had poor to fair coordination and balance with overflow movement of his/her arms and hands (indicating neuromaturational delay).
Contact with floor is a mature heel–toe pattern/a flat-footed pattern.

Muscle Tone/Strength

Muscle tone and strength are normal/within a typical range, upper/lower extremities were found to be within functional limits, strength appeared appropriate for child's age and size, exhibited low/high muscle tone in trunk/shoulder girdle/legs/etc., presented with poor/weak strength in upper abdominal/lower leg/etc.

Posture

Postural reactions are good, posture is erect/upright/straight/rigid/stiff/"military," sat on edge of chair, posture is slouched/slumped/droopy/stooping, hunched over/curved spine, "hunkered down," round-shouldered, limp, hangs head, peculiar posturing/atypical/inappropriate (sat sideways in the chair, reversed chair to sit down), relaxed.

Proprioception

Child consistently sought out activities that provided vestibular input and proprioception through climbing/jumping/falling/swinging/etc., visual attention/sensory modulation/etc. improved when child was provided with proprioceptive input.

Other Observed Skills

Able to walk forward/backward on balance beam with/without heels and toes touching, walks up/down (ascends/descends) stairs with/without handrail, can catch and throw small tennis ball, able to kick a stationary/moving ball, able to perform long jump, can hop on one leg.

Tests of Gross Motor Abilities   *Chapter 25 provides more information about BOT-2.*

Bruininks–Oseretsky Test of Motor Proficiency, Second Edition (BOT-2)
Peabody Developmental Motor Scales–Second Edition
Test of Gross Motor Development–Second Edition (TGMD-2)

Summary Statements about Motor Skills

Child's motor planning and fine motor skills appeared age-appropriate at this time.
Motor ability appeared unremarkable.
Child demonstrated poor fine motor/handwriting skills.
Visual–motor control (eye–hand coordination) was age-appropriate/delayed.
Overall, the child's fine/gross motor skills are delayed, but many of the skills are emerging.
Graphomotor skills were awkward and laborious, and there were difficulties with motor output skills.

Glossary of Terms Frequently Used in Motor Skill Evaluations

In more specialized evaluations of motor skills, the following terms are often used; the simple definitions provided below can be used in report writing.

Bilateral coordination: Ability to use both sides of the body in a smooth and coordinated fashion.

Eye–hand coordination: Ability to use the eyes and hands together in a coordinated fashion for tasks such as writing, throwing, cutting, etc. (see also visual–motor integration, below.)

Kinesthesia: Ability to perceive the movement of individual body parts.

Motor planning skills: Ability to formulate an idea for a motor task (hitting a ball with a bat, tying shoes, etc.), as well as to organize and sequence a plan for the task.

Ocular motor control: Ability to smoothly locate and follow a moving object with one's eyes.

Postural stability: Sufficient muscle strength and control to participate in daily activities without excessive fatigue or clumsiness.

Proprioception: Ability to process and integrate information from muscles and joints to determine where, how, and with what force they are moving.

Range of motion: Amount of movement in extremities or joints.

Sensory processing: Ability to take in information from the environment and organize it into motor and social responses.

Tactile discrimination: Ability to determine, without vision, where one is being touched and with what.

Tone: Tension in a muscle at rest and/or reaction to passive stretch.

Vestibular processing: Ability to monitor the position of the head as one moves through space.

Visual–motor control: Use of visual skills in conjunction with motor skills, such as writing, drawing, and painting.

Visual–motor integration: Ability to translate with the hands what is perceived visually; this is especially important for writing.

Visual perception: Visual skills that do not necessarily involve a motor response; they are important for learning left versus right, doing matrix puzzles, etc.

13.6. Speech and Language Skills

Articulation

If articulation is unclear, indicate whether the lack of clarity is within normal limits for age.

> Good/moderate/variable/fair intelligibility, unclear/unintelligible, intelligibility was excellent/
> poor/within normal limits, was difficult to understand due to poor articulation, child's
> articulation was so poor that his/her mother/father needed to interpret his/her responses,
> stumbles over words, mumbles, whispers to self/mutters under breath, lisps, slurred/gar-
> bled, clear/precise/clipped, choppy and mechanical, poor diction/enunciation.
>
> Child's vocabulary outpaced her/his pronunciation ability.
> Child stammered/had noticeable speech impediment.

> ✓ When a child has a regional or foreign accent, note this fact only if the accent is strong
> enough to interfere with clarity. If the child's first language is not English, consult (if possi-
> ble) with a native speaker of the child's first language to determine whether the child has
> articulation difficulties in that language.

Voice Qualities

> Voice quality was unremarkable/appropriate for age.
> Soft/quiet/weak voice, speaks so softly it is difficult to hear him/her, soft-spoken, voice is frail/
> feeble/thin/"small"/barely audible, whispered/aphonic, tremulous/quivery.
> Used baby talk (including higher-pitched tone), spoke in a very high-pitched voice, sing-song,
> strident/whiny, shrill/squeaky.
> Hypernasality/nasal tones.
> Low tone of voice, flat voice tone, gravelly/hoarse/throaty/croaky/raspy, bellowed, monoto-
> nous pitch/tone, sad/low tone of voice.
> Spoke in a loud voice, screamed/squealed/shrieked/yelled/shouted, noisy, brash, harsh.

Comprehension

> Demonstrated understanding of prepositions, size differences, body parts, number concepts,
> etc.
> Frequently asked for repetition of information.
> Problems with auditory comprehension were noted.
> Has difficulty processing simple "wh-" questions (what, where, when, etc.).

Responses to Questions

> Responded appropriately to questions posed by the examiner, eagerly answered examiner's
> questions.
> Despite child's good understanding of question forms, she/he was not always responsive to
> questions when they were asked.
> Brief responses, did not initiate conversation/did not volunteer information, tended to offer
> the minimal answers to questions.
> Child echoed the last word of what he/she heard (in)consistently, often repeated part of the
> verbal question before responding.
> When asked direct questions, would frequently ask for repetition or only acknowledge half of
> the question.
> Tended to mumble when asked a question, verbal responses were vague and imprecise.
> When child was unsure of a verbal answer, she/he frequently provided a tangential re-
> sponse.

His/her answers indicated considerable failure to understand the intent of the question.
Answered questions impulsively, responses were disorganized and did not appear well
thought out.

Responses to Directions

Quickly understood directions.
Followed one-step/two-step/etc. related/unrelated commands.
Often took instructions/directions too literally.
Often had trouble understanding directions, seemed to mishear or misunderstand administered questions, often needed to have test instructions repeated and clarified.
Had difficulty consistently following oral directions, followed one- and two-step commands
but frequently needed visual cues for full compliance, was able to follow commands but
did better when a task was demonstrated and he/she was verbally instructed to attend to
the demonstration.

Speech Amount/Rate/Rhythm/Productivity *(↔ by degree across columns only)*

Slow	Normal	Pressured	Verbose
Stammered	Talkative	Fast	Hyperverbal
Reticent	Articulate	Rambling	Dramatic
Mute	Fluent	Garrulous	Effusive
Unspontaneous	Communicative	Loquacious	Long-winded
Taciturn	Spontaneous	Impulsive	Wordy
Slow response time	Natural	Forced	Long and drawn out
Uncommunicative	Chatty	Expansive	Excessively detailed
Sluggish	Smooth	Rapid	Bombastic
Unhurried	Clear	Unrestrained	Overproductive
Measured	Coherent	Excessively wordy	Nonstop
Deliberate	Lucid	Hurried	Vociferous
Unforthcoming	Expressive	Rushed	Overabundant
Restrained	Initiates	Animated	Copious
Silent	Concise	Voluble	Overresponsive
Terse	Grammatical	Blurts out	Voluminous
Brusque	Intelligible	Run-together	Flight of ideas
Curt	Well-spoken	Raucous	
Clipped	Productive		
Halting	Animated		
Incoherent			
Paucity			
Impoverished			
Laconic			
Economical			
Single-word answers			

Vocabulary and Expressive Language

Child appeared to have good verbal skills, was highly verbal, engaged in pleasant conversation
using interesting vocabulary.
Child was remarkably verbal for his/her age.
Child uses words well with good sentence structure.
_____ (child's name) is a highly articulate child, whose vocabulary and the ideas

she/he expressed were well beyond what would be expected for her/his chronological age.

Child spoke in complete sentences.

Often used colloquial language such as "That was wicked good," "This sucks."

Verbal responses were severely limited/limited to one or two words, expressive language included mostly labeling.

Expressive language was mildly/moderately/severely delayed.

Often said "uh" before speaking as if trying to find the right word.

Hesitated before speaking.

Child was unable to formulate spontaneous sentences to express his/her thoughts.

Child's sentences were out of context or inappropriate to what the examiner presented to her/him.

Conversational Style

Child used appropriate turn-taking skills in conversation.

He/she is a reciprocal conversationalist/engaged spontaneously in dialogue/is able to carry on a conversation.

Child readily engaged in conversation/initiated and maintained dialogue appropriately.

Thoughts were connected and flowed logically, child did/did not skip randomly from one topic to another.

She/he appeared quite comfortable conversing with an adult/child.

He/she was able to maintain a conversation and enjoyed asking questions to obtain information.

Child follows the conventions/social rules of communication (including appropriate phrasing and turn taking) and understands the suppositions and expectations of native speakers of American English.

Child offered no spontaneous comments during the evaluation but answered questions easily.

Child spoke in single words and short phrases (most of which were difficult to understand).

Child demonstrated marked impairment in the ability to sustain conversation/was unable to carry on a conversation.

Speech was slow/deliberate/sometimes evasive.

Child was verbal but not articulate.

Child was excessively verbal, examiner had to interrupt her/him to redirect attention to task at hand, child ran on verbally, has difficulty limiting the amount of talking she/he does.

Conversational speech was noted for a quick rate of speech and a tendency to respond tangentially to verbal questions.

When conversing with peers, tends to talk excessively on the same topic without taking other people's point of view into account.

Where one word would suffice/answer the question asked, he/she produced a paragraph.

The child's speech needed more braking than prompting.

The child attempted to be helpful by trying to tell a great deal and so created pressured speech.

Problematic Communication Behaviors

Anomia (child could describe objects but was unable to name them).

Child often asked questions at inappropriate times.

Child frequently complained.

Child subvocalized (softly whispered) as she/he worked, was observed to hum/sing/laugh/giggle throughout session.

Child exhibited significant frustration over his/her inability to express thoughts spontaneously.

Echolalia was present in some/many/most responses, echolalia was noted throughout the sessions.

Malapropisms (e.g., "reef" for "wreath," "elephant" for "elegant").

Syntactical errors. (Indicate whether errors are appropriate for developmental age.)

Commonly Used Tests of Speech and Language Ability

See Chapter 23 for citations and more information regarding most of these tests.

Expressive One-Word Picture Vocabulary Test (EOWPVT), 2000 Edition
Illinois Test of Psycholinguistic Abilities—Third Edition (ITPA-3)
Peabody Picture Vocabulary Test—Third Edition (PPVT-III)
Receptive One-Word Picture Vocabulary Test (ROWPVT), 2000 Edition
Test of Early Language Development—Third Edition (TELD-3)
Test of Language Development—Intermediate: Third Edition (TOLD-I:3)
Test of Language Development—Primary: Third Edition (TOLD-P:3)

13.7. Other Behavioral Observations

Sensory Input

Demonstrated sensory processing regulation deficits.
Displayed an oversensitivity/hypersensitivity to light touch/lights/noise/messy substances.
Threshold level for sensory input was very low.
Is irritated by certain textures and will not touch some things (lotion, shaving cream, etc.).
Certain auditory/visual/tactile input was aversive to the child.
Demonstrated a mild/moderate/severe level of tactile defensiveness, perceived light touch as threatening and noxious.
Lacked ability to regulate her/his sensory system without additional sensory input.

Attention to Detail

Lost sight of the "bigger picture" and tended to become overly focused on irrelevant details.
Excessive attention to detail slowed the child's performance considerably.

Personal Space

Examiner did/did not note difficulties with personal space.
Child would get too close to examiner (about _____ inches from face).
Child needed to be reminded that he/she was in the examiner's personal space.
Child seemed unaware of physical boundaries.

Tics

Motor tics:

Blinking, facial grimacing, twitching/jerking of specific body parts (e.g., head, shoulder, extremities), abdominal tensing.

Vocal tics:

Coughs, sneezes, grunts, snorts/sniffs, throat clearing, mutters phrases or single syllables, barks.

Miscellaneous Observations

Child often sucked her/his thumb between responses to questions.

Frequently asked for a snack or drink throughout the evaluation.

Child often placed head in his/her hands and rested it on the table as a strategy to visualize the auditory information.

There appeared to be little appreciation of danger (e.g., ran out of office onto street), safety awareness was poor.

Brought items to the examination (possessions, presents, refreshments/candy/food/gum, stuffed animals, iPod, etc.).

14

Attitude toward Testing

14.1. Response to Examination Process

Child's Interaction with Testing and Examiner

(↔ *by degree*) The following groups of descriptions are presented in order from most to least cooperative.

Very cooperative:

Seemed highly interested in the testing, exhibited an optimistic attitude, was an eager participant, appeared to be comfortable with the evaluation process, was eager to participate in all tasks presented, demonstrated test-appropriate behavior, was cooperative and willing to comply with all directives, had a good understanding of why she/he was undergoing evaluation, appeared relaxed and comfortable in the testing/therapy environment, insight appeared to be good for age, approached the testing with enthusiasm.

Dependent:

Consistently required visual/verbal modeling before attempting a task unfamiliar to him/her, did not initiate spontaneous interactions but would imitate play after visual cues were given, responded positively to organizational cues provided by therapist, would only attempt testing items after much cajoling and creative play with examiner, often asked the examiner for assistance, was able to engage in testing but was distracted by new playroom, therefore difficult to engage her/him for very long in directed activities.

Variable:

Could be quite cooperative when tasks were interesting to him/her but quite uncooperative when they weren't, cooperation and behavior depended on child's mood, was able to perform on task yet clearly did not enjoy the demands of the testing process, appeared somewhat uncomfortable with the examiner and the testing environment.

Difficulty cooperating during the evaluation:

Indicated by words/actions that she/he did not like the testing process, resisted formal attempts to administer tests, refused several test items, often complained "When will this be over?" or "I want to go home," wanted to give up easily, did not respond to limit setting.

Difficulty understanding the purposes of or completing the evaluation:

Appeared to be untestable, did not understand the significance of the evaluation, denied knowing reason for the evaluation, did not meet minimum requirements for appropriate social interaction.

Parent's Interaction with Examiner

Parent related to the examiner in an appropriate, trusting, warm/friendly/gracious, open/unguarded, sociable/pleasant/affable way.

Parent's manner of relating to examiner was arrogant/threatening, suspicious/distrustful, impatient, uncooperative, controlling/manipulative, seductive, needy/dependent, grudging/condescending, aloof/detached/cold, etc.

Parent's attitude did/did not change during the interview.

Parent took _____ role and assigned _____ role to examiner during interview (specify).

Child's Behavior with Parent

Child actively explored environment with parent/guardian present, was quite affectionate and loving toward his/her parents, appeared to have a very good relationship with parents, actively participated in the interview, elaborated on her/his mother's/father's comments and added her/his own opinions about what the problems were.

Child was seen initiating hand holding with his/her father/mother upon leaving the clinic, showed great exuberance when reunited with parents at the close of the session.

Child played easily/unwillingly/not at all in the waiting room, did/did not put away the toys used.

Child exhibited _____ level of play, used playthings appropriately/inappropriately for his/her age.

Child did not display a warm reaction to mother/father when parent entered the examination room.

Parent's relationship to child was unsupportive/unilaterally controlling/harsh/etc.

Child was noted to be curt/bossy/noncompliant/etc. to her/his mother.

Parent used control in _____ ways (specify degree, kind/methods/means, timing), over issues of _____ (specify).

Parents showed agreement/disagreement/conflict over discipline, rewards, language, attention given, etc.

Child's Separation from Parent

Child had no difficulty separating from his mother/father/parents.

Child came willingly to the testing/entered the testing environment willingly.

Separated with minimal/appropriate anxiety from his/her father/mother and quickly became engaged with the examiner.

Child was aware that her/his parents were meeting in the adjoining room, but she/he was not distracted by their presence.

Child displayed some initial separation anxiety, but quickly became comfortable with the therapist/examiner.

Child initially requested that his/her mother/father accompany him/her for testing, but accepted without difficulty that she/he needed to remain in the waiting room.

Child showed initial hesitation to engage in testing.

Preferred to play with toys in the waiting room and was reluctant to begin examination.

Child was shy at first and needed some time to warm up to the examiner.

During stressful times during the evaluation, child requested to see his/her parents in the waiting room, apparently to verify that they were still there.

Upon separation, child showed excessive/expected/limited/no anxiety, expressed as _____ (specify).

Child used appropriate/a few/no coping mechanisms upon separation (if any, specify).

Child separated easily/poorly/reluctantly from the parent/examiner.

Child's reaction upon rejoining parent was _____ (specify).

Child showed anger and distress when separated from her/his father/mother at the beginning of testing.

Child refused to be separated from parent and thus evaluation was completed with parent in the room at all times.

Observations of Child's Play

Isolates him-/herself from other children and prefers solitary play.

Play was mostly self-directed parallel play.

When invited to play, child had some difficulty initiating play.

Child initially rejected toys presented to him/her, but became increasingly cooperative.

Preferred self-directed play to examiner-directed play.

Child was able to enter into cooperative play.

Child enjoyed imaginative play.

Play was interactive.

Child was overly aggressive when playing with other children.

Child tended to want to control play activities.

Child exhibited appropriate/inappropriate play with toys.

Child played eagerly/willingly/unenthusiastically/not at all with same-age/younger/older peers.

Child showed eager/expected/limited/no approach to and interest in toys/materials.

Toys/materials actually used were _____ (specify).

Manner of play was constructive/disorganized/mutual/parallel/distractible/disruptive/other (specify).

Child was tractable/intractable to discipline, such as _____ (specify).

Child's Response to Transitions

Transitions between activities were challenging for the child.

When child was asked to change activities, she/he refused/became aggressive/began to cry/showed visible signs of anxiety/threw the materials across the room/ran from the room/became oppositional.

Child consistently became disorganized when transitioning demands were placed on him/
her.
She/he made transitions from task to task well.
Child was sensitive to changing task parameters.

Child's Separation from Teacher/Classroom

Child separated comfortably from his/her teacher to accompany the examiner to the testing
room.
Child separated from class with ease.
Child did not want to separate from class environment and very reluctantly joined the exam-
iner.
Child refused to accompany the examiner.

14.2. Rapport with Examiner

Cooperative Behaviors

(↔ *by degree across columns only*)

Friendly	Cooperative	Dependent	Indifferent
Enthusiastic	Responsive	Shy	Unresponsive
Vivacious	Attentive	Obsequious	Uninterested
Enjoyed one-to-one	Compliant	Deferential	Apathetic
contacts	Diligent	Ingratiating	Passive
Engaging	Hard-working	Tried too hard to	Careless
Solicited interaction	Curious	please	Noncommittal
Imaginative	Flexible	Needy	Blasé
Playful	Considerate	Overly reliant on	Aloof
Sweet-natured	Polite	examiner's input	Remote
Entertaining	Tactful	Sycophantic	Lazy
Amiable	Agreeable	Fawning	Bored
Upbeat	Cordial	Submissive	Curt
Chummy	Kind	Docile	Submissive
Enjoyable	Civil	Meek	Nonchalant
Amusing	Forthright	Overly obedient	Neutral
Sociable	Obliging	Help-seeking	Minimal cooperation
Good-natured	Accommodating	Eager to please	Submissive
Affable	Courteous	Accommodating	Passive
Likeable	Well-mannered	Effusive	
Good-humored	Respectful	Pleading	
Cheerful	Thoughtful	Oversolicitous	
Optimistic	Direct	Compliant	
Bubbly	Frank	Overapologetic	
Cheery	Candid		
Familiar	Open		
Tactful			
Cordial			
Solicitous			

Negative Behaviors

(↔ *by degree across columns only*)

Guarded	Brusque	Defensive	Challenging	Antagonistic	Aggressive
Unreadable	Curt	Reticent	Sarcastic	Belligerent	Physically
Unresponsive	Surly	Inflexible	Negative	Oppositional	abusive
Downbeat	"Crabby"	Interper-	Disagreeable	Defiant	Verbally
Evasive	Sulky	sonally	Uncoopera-	Angry	abusive
Sneaky	Gruff	distant	tive	Rude	Swore
Wary	Abrupt	Suspicious	Disobedient	Rebellious	Hostile
Hesitant	Grumpy	Self-protec-	Rebellious	Disrespectful	Rageful
Restrained	Bad-tempered	tive	Mocking	Quarrelsome	Belligerent
Expression-	Short-	Resentful	Sardonic	Loud-	Intimidating
less	tempered	Noncompliant	Cynical	mouthed	Obstreperous
Unemotional	Testy	Refused to	Derisive	Confronta-	Malicious
Cagey	Irritable	participate	Nasty	tional	Violent
Hard to pin	Cranky	Unforth-	Obstinate	Spoiling for a	Destructive
down	"In a bad	coming	Contrary	fight	Hateful
Reserved	mood"	Inflexible	Stubborn	Cantankerous	Spiteful
Reticent	Cross	Obstinate	Manipulative	Irate	Malevolent
Recalcitrant	Petulant	Uncompro-	Demanding	Cross	Mean
Resistive	Resentful	mising	Imposing	Livid	Nasty
Reluctant	Sullen	Rigid	Insistent	Enraged	Cruel
Inaccessible	Broody	Intransigent	Indignant	Bad-	Sadistic
Distant	"Out of	Detached	Confronta-	mannered	Vicious
Remote	sorts"	Subtle	tional	Foul-mouthed	Disparaging
Withdrawn	"In a funk"	Hostile	Presumptu-	Vulgar	
Withholding	Snippy	Uncoopera-	ous	language	
Avoidant	Balky	tive	Frustrated		
	Pouty	"Sick and	Complaining		
	Peevish	tired"	Domineering		
	Snappish	Noncompliant	Rude		
	Grouchy		Nagging		

Response to Examiner's Behaviors

Normal/positive:

Child responded quickly to cuing from the examiner.

When psychologist provided structure to play, child became more oriented and responsive.

Child clearly benefited from redirection, praise, and positive reinforcement for his/her responses.

Was able to calm down and refocus with praise from the examiner.

Responded to firm limit setting.

Child responded well to positive reinforcement.

Child responded nicely to structure and redirection.

Demonstrated improved attention and concentration when motivational techniques (e.g., sticker chart, token reinforcement, etc.) were employed.

Overly affectionate:

> Client formed an immediate superficial attachment to evaluator/therapist.
> Upon meeting therapist, child immediately hugged him/her.
> Child initiated hug from therapist at end of each session.

Concerned/controlling:

> Child tried to negotiate with examiner how much she/he had to complete each time a new item was introduced.
> At times child became defiant and argumentative in response to praise, often denying he/she was really doing a good job.
> Child was vigilant about evaluator's behavior, frequently asking what she/he was writing on her/his clipboard.
> Child seemed to need to have some control over how examiner understood his/her answers.

Summary Statements about Rapport

> Child could engage with the examiner rather well/easily established rapport with the examiner.
> Child appeared to be at ease and happily engaged in the interview process.
> Rapport was quickly and easily/intermittently/never established and maintained.
> From the beginning, the child appeared to be comfortable with the examiner(s) and quickly engaged in conversation.
> She/he was fully cooperative during the evaluation and seemed to establish rapport fairly well.
> Rapport developed over the first few sessions.
> The child appeared relaxed and comfortable with the interview process/shared thoughts without hesitation/gave responses that appeared genuine and thoughtful.
> He/she seemed to enjoy the attention received.
> Response to authority was cooperative/respectful/appropriate/productive/indifferent/hostile/challenging/undermining/unproductive/noncompliant/contemptuous.

> Child preferred to socialize with the examiner rather than focus on the tasks at hand.
> Child displayed ambivalence toward therapist/examiner.
> Child was quiet and did not try to engage with the examiner.
> In relating to the examiner, she/he made sporadic eye contact and seemed unaware of physical boundaries.

14.3. Attention/Concentration

See also Section 16.1 "Attention-Deficit/Hyperactivity Disorder (ADHD)."
(↔ by degree across columns only)

Passive	Inattentive	Normal	Hyperactive
Quiet	Distractible	Attentive	Very active
Subdued	Intermittent	Hard-working	Wiggly
Lethargic	attention	Observant	Impulsive
Inactive	Lost concentration	Curious	Fidgeting
Unreceptive	Could not stick with	Self-directed	Problems remaining
Sluggish	task	Thoughtful	seated

Passive	Inattentive	Normal	Hyperactive
Restrained	Daydreaming	Concentrated	Constant activity
Unresponsive	Distracted	Adequate	Constantly
Slow-moving	Careless	Motivated	interrupted
Listless	Unmindful	Engaging	Squirming
Apathetic	Forgetful	Inquisitive	Restless
Dull	Absent-minded	Interested	Easily overstimulated
Uninvolved	Scatterbrained	"All ears"	"Hyper"
Uninvested	Unfocused	Focused	"Wired"
Sluggish	Dreamy	Listening carefully	Agitated
Worked slowly	Inconsistent	Alert	Restless
"In slow motion"	Varied with tasks	Paying attention	Overly energetic
Slow reactions	Low attending skills	"On the ball"	Overexcited
Slowed	Had great difficulty	Cooperative	Twitchy
Nonpersistent	following directions	Spontaneous	
		Responsive	
		Adequate	
		Good effort	

Summary Statements about Attention

(↔ *by degree*) These groups of statements are presented in order from highest to lowest quality of attention.

Excellent:

Child was focused and engaged.

Child exhibited appropriate effort, focus, and attention throughout the testing/interview.

Child never appeared clearly inattentive or distracted.

Child seemed to have a good attention span, as seen in his/her ability to sit for long periods of time without a break.

There were no behavior management issues evident.

She/he was able to stay in his/her seat and work as directed.

Good:

Child's attention to task was good, but not excellent.

Pattern of performance on tests did not indicate a consistent problem of attending to tasks.

Child was able to focus on task when reminded to do so.

Child's listening skills and ability to follow directions were inconsistent.

Child's attention was better when the task was challenging.

Some difficulties:

Child's ability to attend on tasks was variable.

At times he/she was noted to become distracted by things in his/her environment (e.g., noises, pencils).

Child often closed her/his eyes during verbal tasks as if to listen better or concentrate on the task.

Child had poorer attention when tasks were verbal/more challenging/paper-and-pencil/auditory in nature/nonverbal in nature.

Levels of attention and concentration were below age expectations in this one-to-one assessment situation.

Poor:

> Child could attend for no more than 5–15 minutes.
> Child was continually/easily distracted by objects on the table/environmental noises/his/her own thoughts.
> Child readily became distracted by internal and external stimuli.
> When asked to concentrate, she/he became oppositional.

14.4. Attitude toward Performance

Positive attitude:

> Handled failure well, demonstrated good insight about his/her performance (particularly on items he/she found difficult), made use of corrective feedback when it was provided, was willing to make guesses when material was difficult, has a good sense of the limits of her/his knowledge, will not attempt tasks judged to be beyond his/her solid knowledge.

Indifference/lack of awareness:

> Took no pride in her/his work, gave up easily when confronted with a challenging task, was not bothered by incorrect answers, often seemed unaware when he/she gave an incorrect answer or response.

Anxiety:

> Demonstrated anxiety on particular tests (e.g., timed tests, unstructured tests, projective tests), constantly asked whether answers were "right" or "okay," tried hard to determine whether answers were correct from subtle verbal and body language cues exhibited by the examiner, frequently tried to look at the score sheet, frequently made disclaimers about performance/predictions of poor performance before beginning tests for which she/he lacked confidence or ability, seemed unsure of him-/herself and seemed not to want to give a response unless he/she was absolutely sure of it.

Perfectionism/high self-criticism:

> Seemed to hold her-/himself to high standards, had difficulty making decisions/answering questions because he/she was afraid of getting something wrong, would often report an answer and then declare "oh no, that's not right" and rework the problem, sometimes arriving at the same answer later; appeared troubled/frustrated/embarrassed when she/he did not know the correct answer to a question, frequently asked whether tests were timed and how they were scored, meticulously checked and rechecked his/her answers, took significantly longer to finish a problem than the average examinee, tended to be rather perfectionistic about responses, spent more time than needed on many questions.

14.5. Coping Skills

(↔ *by degree*) These groups of descriptors are presented in order from strongest to weakest coping skills.

Good:

> Did not appear frustrated by inability to solve a problem or by repeated tasks and exercises, required only minimal encouragement when frustrated or distracted, when presented with difficult problems, child coped well.

Adequate:

> Often became discouraged by difficult items but persevered.
> Showed some frustration to difficult tasks, but was able to cope given sufficient time.

Poor:

> Exhibited low frustration tolerance, gave up easily, would begin to express self-denigrating remarks/exhibit inappropriate laughter when faced with challenging tasks, had trouble bearing the frustration of not succeeding, was aware of areas of weakness and became somewhat avoidant on these tasks, often asked to stop or end soon, was on the verge of tears when asked to complete certain test items (specify).

14.6. Effort

Summary Statements

> Child appeared to put forth his/her best effort on all the tests administered.
> Generally she/he showed strong effort, although at times needed encouragement from the examiner to continue working.
> Child craves attention and will work very hard for adult attention and reinforcement.
> Child's effort varied considerably depending on the nature of the task.
> Although _____ wanted to do well and put forth full effort, he/she was easily over-whelmed when presented with detail and complexity.
> Child did not want to put forth effort that could prove unproductive, and thus she/he gave up when an item was perceived as beyond her/his mastery level.
> Child exhibited little effort and did not care whether his/her answers were correct.
> Task persistence was diminished.
> There was low tolerance for frustration.

14.7. Motivation and Persistence

(↔ *by degree*) The following groupings of statements are presented in order from highest to lowest motivation or persistence.

High motivation or persistence:

> _____ was persistent in the face of difficulty.
> Child persevered on difficult tasks and would try his/her best until the time limit.
> Child demonstrated good attention to tasks overall, impressive perseverance, and consistently high motivation.
> During testing she/he was persistent and highly motivated to give her/his best effort and do well.
> Child was highly motivated and cooperative for the evaluation.
> Child particularly enjoyed tasks that were challenging for him/her, often requesting to complete additional items just to see whether he/she could "get it right."
> _____ was hard-working and task-oriented, proceeding like a soldier through the tests presented.
> Child maintained a high level of effort, even on tasks she/he reportedly found difficult or boring.
> Child was offered breaks several times during the testing, but refused them/was eager to continue.
> _____ concentrated on one task for a long time/finished every task.

Child was distracted only by extreme circumstances.
Child exhibited sustained/diligent/systematic/conscientious effort.

Average motivation or persistence:

Child attempted all tasks presented to him/her.
At no time did child become frustrated or ask when she/he would be done.
Child complained a little about the length of the evaluation but still persevered.
Child was candid about tests he/she did not like, but performed all tasks attentively and often enthusiastically.
Task persistence was variable, but overall well maintained.
Although she/he was cooperative, it was obvious that she/he did not enjoy certain aspects of the exam (specify).
Child was only rarely discouraged or inattentive.
On the whole, child was work-oriented/cooperative and put forth satisfactory effort on each evaluation task administered.
Child participated fully in the evaluation process, became involved in tasks, and changed tasks appropriately.

Low motivation or persistence:

Child was easily frustrated.
_____ constantly wanted to leave the testing situation/examination/therapy session.
When child was unsure of an answer, he/she asked to turn the page or go on to another item/changed the subject/became silly/spoke more softly/spoke less clearly/attempted to control the area of conversation.
Child worked without enthusiasm.
_____ tended to be persistent when challenged by tasks, but was quick to give up trying if she/he could not solve the task quickly.
Child did just the minimum to get by.
Child displayed a strong "I don't care" attitude.
Whenever a new test was introduced, child would question whether he/she had to complete it.
Child had difficulty making decisions.
Child had a tendency to give up easily.
Child needed constant prompting and persuading to keep working.
Often when challenged, she/he would develop a defeatist attitude.
Sustained effort only for _____ (specify time period).
Child preferred only easy tasks/showed no motivation to succeed with difficult tasks or perform well for examiner.
_____ offered only perfunctory cooperation.

Refusal:

Child refused some test items that were perceived as too difficult.
Even with words of encouragement, he/she preferred not to guess at a possible answer.
Child was quick to respond "I don't know" when asked verbal questions.
Child often became unsure of her-/himself and then shut down/withdrew.
Child showed irritation/became angry/complained.

15

Affective Symptoms and Mood/Anxiety Disorders

This chapter describes terms for symptomatology involving mood or affect, as well as for various mood and anxiety disorders. For more information regarding the assessment of mood and anxiety disorders and symptoms, see Chapters 2 and 3.

15.1. General Aspects of Mood and Affect

"Mood" refers to a person's overall emotional tone or quality over some period of time. "Affect" refers to the appropriateness and range of a person's moment-to-moment emotional responses.

In reports, comment on the following:

- Child's general mood.
- Fluctuation of mood/affect during interview, evaluation, or treatment.
- Appropriateness of affect for the speech and content of child's communication.
- Child's self-report of mood and affective state(s).
- Congruence of child's self-report and examiner's observations of child's mood/affect.
- Congruence of child's self-report and parent's (or other adult's) reporting and observation of child's mood/affect.

Quality/Range of Affect (↔ by degree across columns only)

Flat	Blunted	Constricted	Normal	Expansive
Bland	Detached	Tired	Appropriate range	Broad
Unresponsive	Distant	Restricted	Responsive	Highly reactive
Remote	Unspontaneous	Inhibited	Fine	Labile
Unvarying	Unattached	Shallow	Adequate levels of emotional energy	Disinhibited
Impassive	Apathetic	Low-key	Integrated	Euthymic
Aloof	Uninterested	Contained		Deep
Withdrawn	Listless	Limited range		Intense
Passive-appearing	Lacking energy	Repressed		Pervasive
Affectless	Stoic	Subdued		Generalized
Vacant stare	Inexpressive	Controlled		
Absent	Dispassionate	Low-intensity		
Expressionless	Uninvolved	Muted		
		Uninflected		

General Statements Regarding Affect

Affect and comportment were normal.

Affect was sweet and agreeable.

Affect and mood were appropriate at all times.

Child displayed an appropriate range of affect, though she/he tended toward a depressive/anxious/etc. presentation.

Child displayed the full gamut of emotions during the sessions/demonstrated full range of appropriate affect.

Testing reflects an affective style that matches/does not match the child's clinical presentation.

Child presented a very restricted range of affect.

Child's affect was inappropriate for content/task.

Quality/Range of Moods (↔ *by degree across columns only*)

The table below presents very general descriptions of mood states—that is, the prevailing emotional tone—ranging from depressed to angry. See later sections of this chapter for more information regarding moods as they relate to specific disorders.

Depressed	Anxious	Normal	Expansive	Angry
Agitated	Nervous	Bright	Animated	Defiant
Sad	Irritable	Happy	Overly dramatic	Aggressive
Tearful	Hypervigilant	"Fine"	Wide-ranging	Suspicious
Indifferent	Skittish	"Okay"	Overly cheerful	Annoyed
Miserable	Tense	Cheery	Exuberant	Irate
Unhappy	Perplexed	Cheerful	Extroverted	Mad
"Down in the	Restless	Lively	Elevated	Fuming
dumps"	Fretful	Optimistic	"High-spirited	Irritated
Dejected	Fearful	Positive	to a fault"	Livid
Low	Frightened	Upbeat		Cross
Sad	Worried	Jolly		Furious
"Down"	Concerned	Buoyant		Incensed
Despondent	Uneasy	Hopeful		Enraged
Weepy	Wary	Confident		Outraged
Melancholy	Jumpy			Infuriated
Mournful	Edgy			"Hopping mad"
Sorrowful	Stressed			
Upset	"Uptight"			
	On edge			
	Apprehensive			

General Statements Regarding Mood

Mood was generally pleasant.

Mood was even throughout testing/evaluation session(s).

Child had difficulty modulating her/his responses to incoming stimuli.

Shifts in mood were noted when _____ (e.g., child faced any type of frustration, was presented with affectively charged information, etc.).

Child prefers to avoid emotional stimulation.
_____ seems to restrict his/her expression and utilization of emotion, especially when making decisions or solving problems.

Appropriateness/Congruence of Affect or Mood and Behavior

(↔ *by degree*) The following groupings are sequenced by degree of increasing appropriateness/congruence.

High incongruence:

Indifferent to problems, discounted/flatly denied any difficulties/problems/limitations.

Incongruence:

Affect variable but inconsistent with the topic of conversation, modulations/shifts inconsistent and unrelated to content or affective significance of statements.

Congruence:

A range of emotions/feelings, appropriate emotions for the content and circumstances, emotions seemed appropriate for the situation/context.

High congruence:

Emotions highly appropriate to/congruent with situation and thought content/subject of discussion, facial expressions clearly reflected emotions reported.

15.2. Anger

Anger in children is sometimes a sign of underlying depression, conduct problems, or a juvenile-onset bipolar disorder. (*See Sections 15.5, 16.3, and 15.4, respectively, for more information regarding these disorders.*)

General Aspects

In reporting anger in children, note the following:

Aggression as a result of angry affect:

Verbal abuse (screaming, lying, swearing, etc.), physical (hitting, fighting, property destruction), etc.

Resolution of anger:

The child can/cannot self-soothe, can/cannot resolve angry feelings with/without adult assistance.

Targets of angry behaviors:

Parents, teacher, siblings, peers, etc.

Any factors that appear to have precipitated or triggered the anger and aggression.

Tantrums

Angry feelings never/sometimes/often/always result in/accompany tantrums.

Aggressive Behaviors in Children

Look for and/or comment on the following:

Location/place:

Home, school, other (specify).

Timing:

Frequently throughout the day.
During particular times of the day (specify).
When other children "crowd" his/her space.
When child is not getting any attention.
During structured activities.
During unstructured activities (e.g., playground, free choice, etc.).
During transition times.
During unsupervised times.
On the weekends.
At custodial/noncustodial parent's house.
Other (specify).

Precipitating factors:

Child has had limits placed on her/him.
Child is in close proximity to other children.
Child is pushed or threatened physically.
Child is provoked by another child or adult.
Child is frustrated with inability to complete/begin/etc. a task.
Child does not want to do what he/she has been asked to do.
There is no apparent trigger to the aggressive actions.

Targets:

Parents/family members/a particular family member.
Peers at school/a particular peer.
Anyone who places limits on child.
Only timid/shy/younger/smaller children.
Only assertive/older/bigger children.
Other (specify).

Aggressive actions:

Hitting, kicking, scratching, biting, slapping, punching, pinching, pulling hair, pushes/
  pokes/knocks down others, jumps on others, wrestles.
Verbal abuse, name calling, swearing/cursing, insulting, threatening, shouting.
Illegal behaviors (stealing, drug use, etc.).

Descriptors of Angry Behaviors/Moods (↔ *by degree across columns only*)

Annoyed	Unpredictable	Irate	Hostile
Irritated	Temperamental	Explosive	Provocative
Aggravated	High-strung	Infuriated	Antagonistic
Upset	Moody	Maddened	Aggressive
Bothered	Volatile	Riled	Intimidating
"Snippy"	Excitable	Incensed	Argumentative
Complaining	Erratic	Very angry	Seething

Annoyed	Unpredictable	Irate	Hostile
Cranky	Ill-tempered	Mad	Threatening
Resentful	"Whiny"	Livid	Belligerent
Grouchy	Short-tempered	Outraged	Bullying
Grumpy		Enraged	Menacing
Disagreeable		"Beside him-/herself"	Harassing
Ill-humored		Piqued	
"Prickly"		"Burned up"	
Grudging		Chronically angry	
Bristled			
Restive			
"Bothered"			
Sarcastic			
Disgruntled			
Miffed			
Displeased			

15.3. Anxiety   *See also Section 15.7, "Obsessive–Compulsive Disorder."*

Relevant DSM-IV-TR Codes

300.23	Social Phobia
300.29	Specific Phobia
300.02	Generalized Anxiety Disorder
300.3	Obsessive–Compulsive Disorder
309.81	Posttraumatic Stress Disorder
308.3	Acute Stress Disorder
293.84	Anxiety Disorder Due to a General Medical Condition (GMC)
300.00	Anxiety Disorder Not Otherwise Specified (NOS)
309.24	Adjustment Disorder With Anxiety
300.01	Panic Disorder Without Agoraphobia
300.21	Panic Disorder With Agoraphobia
300.22	Agoraphobia With History of Panic Disorder
309.21	Separation Anxiety Disorder

General Aspects

Common childhood phobias or fears include fear of spiders; thunderstorms/lightning; loud noises; animals (e.g., dogs, cats, horses, zoo animals); being alone; blood/injection/shots; clowns/people in costumes; crowds; darkness; ghosts/monsters; insects (e.g., bees, wasps); water; snakes; height; closed spaces; airplane travel; and dentists.

Agoraphobia symptoms in children can include fear of public places, shopping, crowds, travel, bridges, elevators, or the like. Agoraphobia is often associated with school refusal or school avoidance.

Social phobia symptoms in children can include fear of speaking (e.g., answering questions in class, reading out loud); performance anxiety (e.g., playing at piano recitals, participating in sports, writing on the chalkboard, appearing in a play); fear of eating in public or using public restrooms; fear of asking someone on a date; or fear of negative evaluation.

For panic disorder in children, include information about length of attacks (seconds, minutes, etc.); whether attacks are linked to specific activities or symptoms (e.g., driving in a car, school situations); and frequency of attacks (e.g., four attacks in 2 weeks).

General Statements about Anxiety

The child reports high levels of anxiety.

The child experiences fatigue as a result of high perceived stress.

Because of high levels of anxiety and tension, she/he may not be able to meet even minimal role expectations without feeling overwhelmed.

The child's/adolescent's anxiety is so significant that his/her ability to concentrate and attend are significantly compromised.

Relatively mild stressors will not feel mild to the child because of his/her high levels of general anxiety.

Subjective Symptoms of Anxiety

Discomfort	Fear	Dread	Panic
Uneasy	Trepidation	Scared	Horrified
"Uptight"	Distressed	Frightened	Petrified
Embarrassed	Stressed	Distraught	Paralyzed
Nervous	"Keyed up"	"Unnerved"	"Out of control"
Worried	Foreboding	Alarmed	"Go to pieces"
Irritable	Tense	Frazzled	Terrified
Restless	Apprehensive	Flustered	Hysterical
Disquieted	Agitated	Harried	Frenzied
Jittery	"The creeps"		Panic-stricken
Flighty	On edge/edgy		Frantic
			"Everything goes black"
			"The world is not real"

Physiological Symptoms

Sweating/excessive perspiration, chills/sweaty face/forehead, flushing, cold/clammy/sweaty hands/palms, "goose bumps," hot and cold flashes, pallor/"as white as a ghost."

Dry mouth, lump in the throat, decreased salivation.

Chest pain/discomfort, tight chest.

Headaches/temples pounding.

Nausea/sickness/queasiness, unsettled/upset/churning stomach, frequent stomachaches/abdominal discomfort, stomach "butterflies," diarrhea, "dry heaves," frequent urination, loss of bladder/anal sphincter control.

Dizziness/giddiness/faintness/lightheadedness/"wooziness,"/vertigo, shaking unsteadiness/trembling/"wobbly"/tremulous/quivering/"fluttery," ears ringing, room spinning, faintness/syncope, overall weakness.

Sleep disturbances, trouble falling or staying asleep, insomnia.

Tense muscles (especially neck and shoulder), diffuse limb/muscle aches, eyelid or other twitching, numbness/tingling in hands or feet, no control over limbs/legs felt leaden, incapable of moving.

Pupils dilated.

Rapid/racing heartbeat/pulse rate, pounding heart, palpitations, tachycardia.

Respiratory difficulties, shortness of breath/fast and shallow respiration, difficulty breathing/could not catch breath, choking/smothering sensations, "air hunger," hyperventilation.

"Everything looks funny/blurry/shimmering/far away."

Behavioral Symptoms

Avoidance behaviors, school refusal.

Breathing disturbances, took deep breaths between sentences, had trouble catching his/her breath, periodically exhaled audibly, sighing.

Swallowing frequently between words, frequently gulping before speaking, repeated requests for water.

Crying, clinging, bedwetting/enuresis, encopresis, regressive behaviors (e.g., thumb sucking, baby talk, immature speech).

Fainted, passed out, fell unconscious, collapsed, "blacked out."

Fatigue, tiredness, overall weakness.

Fidgeting, couldn't sit still; tapped pencil/foot/fingers, frequently changed position in seat, jittery, restless, paced.

Frequent trips to the school nurse.

"Freezing," unable to move or respond.

Nervousness/nervous habits, easily distracted, agitated, impatient, wide-eyed, nail biting, chewed on pencil/pen, picked at skin, wringing hands, coughing, cleared throat, played with clothes/hair, chewed on shirt/hair, repetitive movements (specify).

Voice cracked, stuttered, stammered, tremulous/shaky voice.

Cognitive Symptoms

Depersonalization/derealization/sense of unreality, preoccupation with bodily sensations.

Trouble concentrating/lessened concentration, increased confusion.

"I'm going to die/go crazy/lose control/collapse/have cancer,"etc.

"Worry wart," constant worrier, apprehensive about all possible disasters, ruminates.

Fears losing parents/dying/being attacked/being rejected by peers/illness/disability, worries about schoolwork/integrity of family (e.g., possibility of parental divorce), upset by fantasies, obsessive thoughts.

"My mind goes blank."

Feels the need to escape.

Misinterprets symptoms and events in a negative way that exacerbates feelings of anxiety.

Catastrophic misinterpretation of normal bodily changes.

Consequences of Anxiety

Problems in interpersonal relationships, few friends, reluctant to attend playdates/sleepovers/summer camp/parties.

Clingy, insecure, self-doubting/lacking confidence, timid, unsure of him-/herself.

Ill at ease, socially anxious.

Inflexibility, rigidity, upset by little things, cannot cope unless everything is "just right."

Oversensitivity/excessively sensitive.

Self-induced pressures, perfectionism.

Assessment Instruments for Anxiety

The tests listed below specifically measure anxiety in children and youth (*see Chapter 28 for more details about one of these, the RCMAS*). General behavior rating scales and projective measures are also commonly used (*see Chapters 28 and 27, respectively, for more information regarding these latter types of assessment instruments*).

Depression and Anxiety in Youth Scale (DAYS)
Revised Children's Manifest Anxiety Scale (RCMAS)
Internalizing Symptoms Scale for Children (ISSC)

Multidimensional Anxiety Scale for Children—Revised (MACS-R)
Screen for Childhood Anxiety-Related Emotional Disorders—Revised (SCARED-R)
State–Trait Anxiety Inventory for Children (STAIC)

15.4. Bipolar Disorders

Relevant DSM-IV-TR Codes

296.0x	Bipolar I Disorder, Single Manic Episode
296.40	Bipolar I Disorder, Most Recent Episode Hypomanic
296.4x	Bipolar I Disorder, Most Recent Episode Manic
296.6x	Bipolar I Disorder, Most Recent Episode Mixed
296.5x	Bipolar I Disorder, Most Recent Episode Depressed
296.7	Bipolar I Disorder, Most Recent Episode Unspecified
296.89	Bipolar II Disorder
301.13	Cyclothymic Disorder
296.80	Bipolar Disorder NOS

General Aspects of Childhood-Onset Bipolar Disorders

The next three subsections provide more specific descriptors for the manic, depressive, and sexual symptoms of childhood-onset bipolar disorders, but the following is a general summary:

- Abnormal mood states (mania and depression).
- Distractibility.
- Increase in activity.
- Grandiosity (often in the form of defiance, reckless activities).
- Decreased need for sleep.
- Increased interest in sex.
- Poor judgment (e.g., attempting to exit a moving vehicle, jumping out of a window or off a high ledge).

House (2002) notes that initial symptoms may include depression, anxiety, irritability, mood swings, problems with concentration, alcohol and/or drug abuse, legal problems, relationship difficulties, problems with impulse control, and insomnia.

Common Symptoms of Childhood-Onset Mania

Periods of extreme silliness.
Immature states where child exhibits "baby talk" or acts like a baby.
Extreme irritability, which may include being demanding or bossy.
Impatience to the point of being highly agitated.
Often interrupting others.
Disregard for authority of parents/school personnel/other adults.
Quick temper/proneness to intense emotional displays.
Aggressive behaviors (e.g., hitting/pushing/kicking people, throwing things, attempting or expressing desire to kill someone, verbal abuse/swearing).
Fits/explosive behaviors/tantrums, child is unable to calm him-/herself.
Narcissistic features (self-focusing).
(In some adolescents:) Manic symptoms accompanied by psychosis.

Common Symptoms of Depression in Children with Bipolar Disorders

See Section 15.5 for general information about depression in children.

Depression in children with bipolar disorders is often severely impairing and may have an angry quality that includes self-destructive acts. Commonly seen behaviors include the following:

Severely impairing depressive states.
Acts of self-harm while feeling depressed (e.g., biting/scratching/cutting self, suicide attempts).
Attempts to harm others, obsessive thoughts about harming others.

Sexual Behaviors

✓ Note: Whenever sexualized behaviors are displayed in young children, there is a need to rule out potential sexual abuse or trauma.

In Preschool and School-Age Children

Increased masturbation, particularly in public.
"Doctor" play that is abnormal for age.
Increased interest in sexual matters, initiating sexual conversations inappropriate for age.
Exposing self to other children.

In Adolescents

Obsessive interest in pornography.
Increased sexual activity and/or masturbation.
Frequent and unwelcome sexual overtures to others, sometimes in public places.

Differences between Adult-Onset and Childhood-Onset Bipolar Disorders

- Irritability often with prolonged and aggressive temper outbursts, is a more common mood change in children. Between outbursts, the children are often described as persistently irritable or angry.
- Very rapid cycling is more common, particularly in children under 8 years of age. Regular cycling (as would be seen in adults with bipolar disorders) is very uncommon before adolescence.
- Abnormal mood in children with mania is seldom characterized by euphoria.

Comorbidity of Bipolar Disorders and ADHD

Almost by definition, a child with a bipolar disorder will meet criteria for ADHD, and distinguishing between the two in children and adolescents is difficult. House (2002) has noted some important distinctions:

- A bipolar disorder diagnosis should include symptoms of elation or grandiosity, whereas a diagnosis of ADHD does not.
- A bipolar disorder diagnosis is more likely when a case of apparent ADHD appears to worsen and remit, independently of interventions.
- A bipolar disorder is more common in children with a family history of mood disorders.
- Poor response to treatments that have been found to be effective in ADHD (e.g., stimulant medication, behavior treatments) may be more indicative of a bipolar disorder.

Cyclothymia

Symptoms of cyclothymia are similar to those seen in the more severe bipolar disorders (DSM's Bipolar I and Bipolar II Disorders), but the symptoms are less intense and, by definition, longer-lasting. The symptoms include periods of depression/lethargy alternating with periods of energy/irritability/agitation.

Summary Statement about a Childhood-Onset Bipolar Disorder

Evaluation revealed findings consistent with a bipolar disorder, including intense mood lability, grandiosity, narcissistic features, significant irritability, etc.

15.5. Depression

Relevant DSM-IV-TR Codes

296.2x	Major Depressive Disorder, Single Episode
296.3x	Major Depressive Disorder, Recurrent
300.4	Dysthymic Disorder
311	Depressive Disorder NOS
309.0	Adjustment Disorder With Depressed Mood

General Information on Depression in Children

Depression in childhood is often mixed with a broader range of behaviors than in adulthood. Behaviors that are associated with depression in children include aggression, school failure, problems with peer relationships oppositional/antisocial behaviors, poor peer relationships, substance use, lack of motivation, decreased physical well-being, encopresis, enuresis, extreme fear of school or refusal to go to school, and talk of suicide.

According to DSM-IV-TR, somatic complaints, irritability, and social withdrawal are more common symptoms in children than in adults, while psychomotor retardation, hypersomnia, and delusions are less common in prepubescent children than in adolescents and adults (American Psychiatric Association, 2000).

Approximately 4–6% of children suffer from symptoms of depression, with fairly equal prevalence in boys and girls until adolescence, when twice as many girls as boys report experiencing depression (Merrell, 1999).

Although there is a general lack of consistency between self-reports and parent reports of depression in children, the reporting of a child's depressive symptomatology by parents is associated with more severe symptoms and poorer outcome (Braaten et al., 2001).

Affective Symptoms (↔ by degree across columns only)

Sad	Very sad/irritable	Despairing	Suicidal
"Down in the dumps"	Unhappy	Despondent	Anguished
Bored	Self-derogatory	Demoralized	Desperate
Brooding	Anhedonic	Dejected	Self-destructive
Glum	Temperamental	Bitter	In the depths of
despair	Changeable	Grave	"Nothing to live for"
"Blue"	Melancholic	Beaten down	Tormented
Down-hearted	Volatile	Explosive	Unbalanced
"Low"/low-spirited	Angst-ridden	Disconsolate	Giving up hope

Sad	Very sad/irritable	Despairing	Suicidal
Troubled	Distressed	Profoundly unhappy	"No light at the end of the tunnel"
Somber	Gloomy	"On the edge"	Hopeless
"Down"	"Fed-up"	Inconsolable	In grave pain
Tearful	Desolate	Miserable	Funereal
Cheerless	Distraught	Sorrowful	Morbid
Dour	Unstable	Suffering	
Dispirited	Forlorn	Morose	
Dismayed	Bitter	Woeful	
Downcast	Unpredictable		
	Highly strung		
	"Wiped out"		
	"Up and down"		

Physiological Symptoms

Appetite absent/poor, cannot stop eating/is hungry all the time, appetite/hunger increase/decrease, fasting, binges.

Bowel/bladder/stomach symptoms, encopresis/enuresis, diarrhea/constipation/stomachaches, increased frequency of urination, overconcern with elimination, chronic use or abuse of laxatives, sensations of abdominal distention or incomplete evacuation of bowels.

Lethargy/physical weakness.

Low/depleted energy, lacks energy to get things done, loses stamina easily, listless, needs to be constantly pushed to do schoolwork/chores, tired, deenergized, weary.

(In adolescents:) Loss of libido, no interest in sex/opposite sex.

Poor general health, often complains about not feeling well.

Psychomotor retardation, absence of/lessened spontaneous verbal/motor/emotional expressiveness, long reaction time to questions (indicate number of seconds), slowed pace of thinking/acting/speaking.

Vegetative symptoms: fatigue, anergia, sleep disorders/terrors, appetite changes, weeping, abdominal pains, alopecia areata, tics, eczema, allergies.

Behavioral Symptoms

Agitation, hypersensitivity, temper tantrums.

Appearance indicative of poor self-care, looks "worn."

Cannot get out of bed, has to force him-/herself to get out of bed.

Crying spells, never smiles/smiles infrequently, teary/tearful, cries openly and often inappropriately.

Concentration problems/difficulties, unable to concentrate.

Downward gaze, dejected look.

Grooming problems, difficulty grooming self, lacks good grooming habits.

Helplessness.

Lack of interest in playing/favorite activities/sports, boredom.

School problems, learning difficulties, school refusal/"phobia," fails to perform up to her/his normal academic standards, school failure.

Substance use/abuse (particularly in adolescents).

Shuffling gait, wrings hands, rubs forehead.

Uncommunicative, flat/expressionless/monotonous voice.

Unmotivated.

Other: Irrational fears (e.g., parent's dying, terrorist attacks, etc.), clingy, aggression.

Social Effects of Depression

Alienation from friends.
Belief that there is little or no social support system.
Gradual or sudden decline in interaction with friends.
Isolation from others/social isolation, withdrawal from social relationships.
Loneliness.
Plays alone, does not join in games.
Spends free time alone.

Depressive Cognitions

Arbitrary inference: Drawing a negative conclusion not supported by the evidence (e.g., thinks other children often make fun of him/her).
Automatic thoughts that reflect a sense of inefficacy and hopelessness.
Catastrophizing: Automatically assuming that the worst-case scenario will occur.
Discouraged about the future.
Dissatisfied with life.
Emotional reasoning (e.g., "Because I feel afraid, there must be danger").
Exaggerated concerns with bodily functions.
Guilt, blames self for setbacks.
Indecisiveness.
Lack of optimism about future, sees any prospects for future successes as dependent on actions of others, has considerable uncertainty and indecision about her/his plans and goals for the future.
Low self-esteem, loss of self-esteem, negative attitudes that result in low self-esteem, poor self-concept.
Mind reading: Assuming one knows another's thoughts (usually negative).
Negative self-worth when compared to others (often associated with imagined rather than real experiences), tends to judge him-/herself unfavorably.
Overgeneralizing: Basing a general conclusion on too few data or one incident, jumping to conclusions.
Personalization: Relating negative events to self without an empirical or rational basis.
Pervasive pessimism, self-pity.
Preoccupation with death (more often seen in older than in younger children), concern with separation.
Ruminations.
Selective abstractions: Attending to only the negative aspects of a situation and ignoring the other (positive) ones, mental filter, selective attention, disqualifying the positive.
Self-critical, dwells on past failures and lost opportunities, engages in self-inspection to a fault, ruminates on personal features that she/he perceives to be undesirable.
Sensitivity to criticism, thinks others do not like him/her.
Sense of helplessness/hopelessness.
Sense of worthlessness.

Common Triggers of Depression in Children

Chaotic and/or punitive home environment.
Death of a loved one.
Rejection by peers.
School failure.
Separation from parents.

Developmental Factors

In infants and toddlers, common symptoms of depression include withdrawal; slow growth or weight loss; general health problems such as frequent infections; dazed, immobile facial expressions and/or flat affect; problems with social interactions; decline in previously mastered developmental tasks; self-stimulation; and decreased play.

Preschool-age children with depression are often more tearful, clingy, and physically slowed down; are less talkative; and exhibit weight loss. Because most children in this age group cannot verbalize feelings of depression, it is important to examine physical and external symptoms (e.g., flat voice, sad facial expressions, low energy level/tiredness, unwillingness to engage in play, slow speech, and irritability).

✓ Although relatively rare, suicidal ideation does occur in the preschool-age population.

In school-age children with depression, somatic complaints (e.g., headaches, stomachaches), failure to make appropriate weight gains, low activity level, excessive sleeping, complaints of feeling bored or stupid, and decreases in school or sports performance are often common.

✓ Children this age are more able to verbalize depressive symptoms and cognitions.

Adolescents have even better capacity to describe their symptoms, which often include guilt, hopelessness, problems with schoolwork and friendships, conduct problems (e.g., promiscuity/sexual acting out, drug use, criminal activities), rageful behaviors, and decreased self-esteem. Sleep problems (either oversleeping or insomnia) are more common in this age group.

Summary Statements about Depressive Symptoms

Child's/adolescent's responses indicated that she/he is not suffering from a clinical depression at this time and that she/he has no thoughts of suicide.

Although he/she did not report experiencing significant depression, he/she does appear to have some depressive symptomatology, including _____ (specify).

The child/adolescent appears to be severely depressed, discouraged, and withdrawn.

The child's/adolescent's symptoms meet criteria for a major depressive episode.

The adolescent's/child's thinking tends to be pessimistic, and she/he approaches life with a sense of doubt and discouragement.

The child's/adolescent's responses suggest that he/she is experiencing a chronic and serious depression.

Child has a negative sense of her/his own self-worth compared to others.

Child has a sense of dissatisfaction with him-/herself and views him-/herself with a marked sense of damage or inadequacy.

Child does not perceive her-/himself as being frequently happy.

Child tends to approach life with a sense of pessimism, doubt, and discouragement and is likely to anticipate gloomy outcomes.

His/her self-concept involves much negative self-evaluation and harsh self-criticism.

She/he is plagued by thoughts of worthlessness, hopelessness, and personal failure.

_____ admits openly to feelings of sadness, a loss of interest in normal activities, and a loss of sense of pleasure in things that were previously enjoyed.

He/she is showing significant difficulties with sleep patterns and a general decrease in his/her level of energy.

Results indicate that the child/adolescent has been experiencing a chronically depressed mood for a long period of time.

Assessment Instruments for Depression

The tests listed below specifically measure depression in children and youth (see Chapter 28 for more details about one of these, the CDI). General behavior rating scales and projective measures are also commonly used (*see Chapters 28 and 27, respectively, for more information regarding these latter types of instruments*).

Children's Depression Inventory (CDI)
Children's Depression Rating Scale–Revised (CDRS-R)
Hopelessness Scale for Children (HSC)
Internalizing Symptoms Scale for Children (ISSC)
Reynolds Child Depression Scale
Reynolds Adolescent Depression Scale

15.6. Grief in Children

Descriptors include the following:

Distress, anguish, sorrow, despair, heartache, pain, woe, suffering, affliction, troubles.
Preoccupation with loss/loved one/memories.
Easily becomes tearful, slowed thinking and responding with long latencies of response, stares into space.
Feels helpless/vulnerable/useless, has lowered self-esteem.

Jarratt (1994) describes the grief process in children as having three phases: early grief, acute grief, and subsiding grief. In early grief, common reactions include denial, dissociation, hyperactivity, irritability, regressive behaviors, increased sleep, and separation anxiety. Acute grief's components include "yearning and pining"; searching (either literally searching for the person who has left/died or being preoccupied with the person); dealing with emotions such as sadness, anxiety, guilt, shame, and anger; and disorganization (e.g., lack of focus, reduced ability to concentrate). Subsiding grief includes acceptance of the grief trauma and the ability to "move on."

15.7. Obsessive–Compulsive Disorder

Relevant DSM-IV-TR Code

300.3   Obsessive–Compulsive Disorder

✓ Compulsions are repetitive, ritualistic behaviors, whereas obsessions are recurring and persistent thoughts.

Common Obsessions in Children

Fears of being dirty/touched/contaminated, bodily excretions, trash/dirt/contaminants, animals, resulting illness of self or other.
Ideas about cartoon characters/superheroes.
Concerns about the future, worries about making decisions/future plans.
Need for orderliness.
Religious concerns.
Worries about sexuality.
Somatic concerns, fears of illness or disease, ideas about body parts.

Worries about world events (possibility of war, poverty, crime, homelessness, terrorism, environmental destruction).

Other: Ideas/concerns/worries about colors, sounds/music, names/titles, numbers, phrases, memories, unpleasant images, impulses (to hurt, blurt, harm, steal, cause disaster), saying/not saying certain things, not losing things, remembering things, etc.

Common Compulsions in Children

Checking door locks, important papers, details of a story or an event, items of potential danger (e.g., kitchen knives, iron, stove, gas taps, etc.).

Completing sequence of activities correctly, restarting from the beginning if necessary (e.g., homework project, chores, etc.).

Frequent cleaning/handwashing/showering (note number of times per hour/day).

Counting number of things seen or number of times something is completed, counting out loud, repeating a ritual behavior a certain number of times.

Hoarding (particularly food) or collecting objects (frequently objects of little or no value).

Need for symmetry/order/balance: must have clothes/books/foods/etc. in certain order, will rearrange objects in room over and over again, demonstrates compulsive straightening.

Touching certain items whenever child sees them.

Verbal compulsions (repeats expressions, phrases, etc.).

Summary Statements

Child denied experiencing any obsessive thoughts or compulsive behaviors.

Child reported experiencing recurring thoughts, such as _____ (specify), that he/she cannot control and that cause him/her marked distress.

Child feels need to wash hands/count things/silently repeat words/etc.

15.8. Suicidality

Degree of Suicidal Risk

(↔ *by degree*) The following groupings are sequenced in order of increasing suicidal risk.

No risk:

Highly unlikely, improbable, never considered suicide, implausible, inconsistent with strongly held religious beliefs, no thoughts of giving up or harming self.

Ideation:

Fleeting thoughts of suicide, thoughts/ideation/wishes to end life, expressed ambivalence about living, smoldering ideation, wonders whether she/he can "make it through this," raises questions about what happens to people after they die, suicidal "flashes."

Verbalizations:

Discusses other people's suicides, talks about plans, discusses methods/means, states intent, thoughts of self-mutilation, asks others to help kill him/her, reunion wishes/fantasies.

Behavioral gestures:

Says goodbye to others, gives away possessions, writes suicide note, nonlethal/low-lethality/nondangerous method, acts of self-mutilation, symbolic/ineffective/harmless attempts, command hallucinations with suicidal intent, assembles method(s) to be used, tells others of intent.

Attempts

Deliberateness, action planning, method/means selected/acquired, medium- or high-lethality method.

Persistent attempts:

Continuous/continual efforts, unrelenting preoccupation.

Data on Suicide in Adolescents

Suicide is the third leading cause of death in the 15–19 age group in the United States, preceded only by accidents and homicide (Anderson, 2002). Completed suicides are five times more common among adolescent boys than among girls. Suicide *attempts* are two to four times more common in girls than in boys, in part because girls use less "successful" methods (e.g., pills) than boys (Grunbaum et al., 2002).

European American youth have higher suicide rates than African American youth. Asians and Pacific Islanders have the lowest rates, and Native American youth have the highest suicide rates of all (Anderson, 2002). Suicide attempts are often preceded by a number of warning signs, such as those listed below. A family history of suicide or severe psychiatric disorder increases the risk for suicide. There is greater risk in rural areas.

Suicide is not always linked to depression in adolescents; rather, suicide is often preceded by personal stressors, conflicts, or crises. These may include the breakup of a love affair, loss of a parent or other loved one, recent suicide of a peer or family member ("social contagion"), an unwanted pregnancy, contraction of a sexually transmitted disease, recent changes in school, birth of a sibling, or remarriage of a parent.

Warning Signs of Suicide in Adolescents

The following warning signs are mentioned by Schaughnessy and Nystul (1985) and Merrell (2001): emotional apathy, social withdrawal, poor grooming habits, loss of interest in recreational activities, giving away cherished belongings, blatant suicide threats, suicide notes, preoccupation with death, heavy substance abuse, losses and severe stressors (as described above), and unusual changes in behavior.

Shaffer, Garland, Gould, Fisher, and Trautman (1988) suggest that these three elements are important:

1. A triggering stressful event, such as a disagreement over parental rules or discipline, or some rejection or humiliation, such as breaking up with a boyfriend/girlfriend or a real or perceived failure.
2. A mental state that has been altered by something such as extreme hopelessness (particularly in girls), rage (*see Section 15.4, "Bipolar Disorders," for more information*), or alcohol or drug use.
3. A readily available opportunity, such as a loaded gun, medications, or other lethal means in the home.

Continuum of Suicidal Behaviors

House (2002, p. 101) sees suicidal behaviors as a continuum from ideation to completed suicide, as follows. (Note the similarity between House's continuum and the groupings of descriptors ordered by degree of risk, above.)

1. *Ideation,* ranging from "infrequent, passive thoughts to frequent, intrusive, active planning."
2. *Precursor behaviors,* such as "saying goodbye, giving away possessions, writing note, communicating intent, assembling elements of method to be used."
3. *Attempts,* ranging from low-lethality with "delayed or little risk" (e.g., "overdoses of pills, superficial wounds") to medium-lethality with "more rapid, destructive" risk (e.g., "specific drug combinations, slashing wounds") to high-lethality with "rapid, very dangerous" risk (e.g., "hanging, firearms").
4. *Completion.*

Suicide Contract

A suicide contract is used when a child or adolescent is not in imminent danger of self-harm, but there is still concern about the possibility. The contract should include a written statement that the client will not engage in self-harm, as well as names of persons the child or adolescent can call if she/he experiences a wish or urge to engage in self-harm, and/or a plan that she/he has agreed to follow.

Confidentiality issues need to be considered. If you feel that a child or adolescent is at reasonable risk for self-harm, inform him/her that you will need to notify the parents, and then take appropriate steps to notify them.

Summary Statements about Suicidality

She/he was not feeling suicidal at the time of the evaluation.
_____ denied suicidal ideation.
Suicidal and homicidal ideation was denied.
The child denied any current wish to hurt him-/herself.
The child specifically denies any suicidal ideation, intent, or plan.

Child denied any suicidal or homicidal ideation at the time of admission/evaluation, but acknowledged significant depression and very severe mood lability.
Child had some thoughts of suicide, but agreed to a contract for safety.

The child/adolescent is at moderate/high risk for harming her-/himself.
The child/adolescent was feeling suicidal at the time of evaluation and had a well-formulated plan.

Assessment Instruments for Suicidality

Although there are few assessment instruments that specifically measure suicidality in children and adolescents, general behavior rating scales and projective measures (*see Chapters 28 and 27, respectively*) are used to assess a child's level of depression and stress, and subsequent risk for suicidal ideation and behavior.

16

Childhood Behavioral and Cognitive Disorders

This chapter provides ways to describe and report information about the DSM-IV-TR disorders that are most commonly seen in childhood and adolescence. For more information regarding affective symptoms and mood/anxiety disorders, see Chapter 15. For more information about assessing these disorders, see Chapters 2–3 and Chapters 20–28. For more information regarding recommendations for treatment, see Chapter 31.

16.1. Attention-Deficit/Hyperactivity Disorder (ADHD)

Relevant DSM-IV-TR codes

314.00	ADHD, Predominantly Inattentive Type
314.01	ADHD, Predominantly Hyperactive–Impulsive Type
314.01	ADHD, Combined Type
314.9	ADHD NOS

Diagnostic Notes

Primary symptoms of ADHD include impulsivity, inattention, and hyperactivity. Other diagnoses can be masked by ADHD, and ADHD is frequently comorbid with oppositional defiant disorder (ODD), conduct disorder (CD), anxiety, depression, learning disorders, and cognitive processing disorders (Root & Resnick, 2003). A sudden onset of ADHD (as opposed to lifelong characteristics that are present before the age of 7 years) would rule out true ADHD. Thus developmental history is crucial, and other potential causes of the symptoms (e.g., trauma, depression) need to be ruled out.

Developmental Aspects of ADHD

Infants/Toddlers/Preschoolers

Because toddlers and preschoolers are naturally active, it is important to distinguish between normal activity level and ADHD.

Frequently reported ADHD behaviors include:

Cried more than other babies, was colicky/irritable/hard to console/difficult to soothe, difficulty sleeping, "once _____ learned to walk, he/she immediately started run-

ning," was incredibly active, accident-prone/clumsy, slow to establish eating and sleeping patterns, temperamental.

School-Age Children

Problems in school are frequently the most impairing.

Problems in establishing friendships begin to occur at school age, because the children's behavior is annoying to others.

The majority of children with ADHD are identified in the first three grades of elementary school (Santrock, 1997).

Boys frequently display more hyperactive–impulsive behavior, while girls display more inattentive symptoms. This is one possible reason why girls are frequently underdiagnosed.

Frequently reported behaviors in this age group include the following:

> Overactivity, impulsivity, inattention, fidgeting, poor/inconsistent school achievement, low self-esteem, disorganization, failing to complete homework/schoolwork.

Adolescents

Hyperactive symptoms tend to remit or decrease or feel more like "restlessness."

Schoolwork continues to suffer.

Risk-taking behaviors are more common than in peers (speeding, traffic accidents); rebelliousness is also more common.

These adolescents have more problems finishing high school than teens without ADHD.

Frequently reported symptoms in adolescents include the following:

> Restlessness, poor concentration, "spaciness," disorganized, shows poor follow-through, difficulty working independently, impulsivity, alcohol/drug use/abuse, antisocial personality patterns, low self-esteem, emotional/behavioral problems.

Inattentive Symptoms

Avoids tasks requiring sustained effort, difficulty with the mobilization and maintenance of effortful attention, "can't get started on tasks."

Cognitive sluggishness/slowing.

Daydreams, stares out the window/into space.

Distractible/easily distracted/self-distracting, problems staying on task, attends to background noises (voices, footsteps, traffic noises, etc.), lessened ability to sustain attention/concentration on school tasks/work/play, poor attending skills.

"Doesn't listen," seems not to listen.

Doesn't complete chores or must be constantly reminded to complete chores, fails to finish tasks.

Easily diverted from a task at hand, unable to find and attend to the relevant components of a task, tends to focus on whatever catches his/her attention rather than on the most salient parts.

Forgetful, forgets to write down homework assignments/bring homework home/bring completed homework to school or turn it in.

Frequently says "I don't know" and "I forget" when asked a question, needs/asks for repetitions of instructions, gets confused, misses announcements.

Homework difficulties, can't finish homework unless someone is standing next to her/him, does not study/prepare/organize/protect own work/do problem's steps in sequence, does not complete assignments on time, starts work before receiving full instructions, unprepared for school assignments, does not make good use of study times.

Inability to shift or move from one event to another.

Inability to divide attention or pay attention to two or more events simultaneously.
Inefficient use of time, underestimates the amount of time it will take to complete a task or assignment.
"Loses everything" (e.g., backpack, homework, mittens, coat), loses things necessary for an activity (e.g., toys, pencils, keys, assignments, books, equipment).
Makes careless errors, inattentive to details.
Organizational difficulties, difficulty organizing him-/herself/schoolwork.
Working memory difficulties, poor short-term memory skills (two- or three-step instructions), fails to remember sequences.

Impulsive Symptoms

Acts "in the moment" without considering the consequences.
Blurts out answers.
Difficulty controlling how she/he responds to a variety of situations.
Fails to consider possible alternatives.
Interrupts others, answers questions before persons asking them have finished, tends to jump into a task before hearing all the instructions.
Low frustration tolerance.
Responds quickly but incorrectly, reacts without considering, acts before thinking, limited self-regulatory functions.
Risk taker, engages in physically dangerous activities.
Senseless/repetitive/eccentric behaviors, darts around aimlessly.
Shoots rubber bands/paper airplanes/spitballs.
Shows off own work when not called on by the teacher.
Trouble/difficulty waiting turn.

Hyperactive Symptoms

Clumsiness.
Constantly/always in motion, changes seating position or posture frequently, prefers to run rather than walk, climbs on furniture, hops/skips/jumps rather than walking.
Difficulty engaging in leisure activities quietly, does not/cannot sit through an interview or meal.
Drums/taps fingers on table, constantly taps foot, swings/shakes legs.
Feels "driven by a motor," "on the go all the time."
Frequently gets up to go to bathroom/get a drink from water fountain, can't stay in seat/slides in seat, frequently "roams the classroom," moves about constantly, climbs furniture.
Makes popping sounds with mouth, hums/clicks teeth/whistles, frequently yawns loudly, makes sounds that inadvertently disturb anyone nearby.
Makes noise by slamming books, banging objects, tapping pencil, etc.
Plays with/twists hair, fiddles with objects.
Sleeplessness, hard time falling asleep.
Squirms/fidgets/twists/turns/wiggles, physically active, a "whirlwind" of activity.
Restlessness.
Talks excessively/incessantly, repeatedly asks irrelevant questions, talks about things that are not related to the task at hand, engages in lengthy conversations when he/she is supposed to be working.

Associated Problems

Adaptive skills deficits:

Poor self-help skills, trouble assuming personal responsibility and independence.

Aggressive behaviors:

Destroys (tears/crumples/etc.) others' work, destroys classroom materials (e.g., breaks pencils/crayons, writes in books, rips books), writes on other children's papers/on the desks/classroom walls/textbooks, hits others, grabs other children's materials, uses inappropriate/abusive language, curses, threatens/teases/criticizes/bullies others.

Cognitive deficits:

Weak working memory, visual/auditory memory.

Discipline problems (besides aggression):

Noncompliant, hostile, demonstrates signs of or has comorbid CD/ODD.

Emotional problems:

Poor self-esteem, anger, emotional lability, comorbid mood disorder, low tolerance for frustration, temper outbursts.

Family difficulties:

Argumentative with parents, disrupts shopping and family visits/family vacations, babysitters complain about her/his behavior, interrupts/intrudes butts in, fights with siblings/parents.

School problems:

Poor quality of schoolwork, difficulty sitting still to take tests, grades that are lower than expected or erratic, performs below ability level, grade retention/failure to graduate/expulsion, special education placement, comorbid learning disability, refractory to usual instructional approaches, may seem unresponsive to punishment or rewards.

Social skills deficits:

Poor peer relationships because of ADHD behaviors (e.g., impulsive aggression, excessive talking, poor listening skills), failure to comply with rules that leads to poor participation in sports or clubs, difficulty with authority figures, less socially competent, tactless/bossy/obstinate, unwilling to take turns, provokes/disrupts other children's activities, betrays friends, peers avoid/reject him/her, has great difficulty keeping friends.

Summary Statements about ADHD

No evidence of attention deficit was indicated on the parent report symptom checklists/teacher reports/etc.

The child's/adolescent's mother/father/teacher completed the _____ (give name of measure). Their ratings were not consistent with a diagnosis of ADHD.

The child's/adolescent's parents and teachers also completed the _____ (specify instrument), where their responses indicate that she/he does not have ADHD, either Inattentive Type or Hyperactive–Impulsive Type.

The child's/adolescent's difficulty concentrating does not fit the profile of ADHD because _____ (specify).

The child's/adolescent's mother/father/teacher completed the _____ (specify instrument). His/her responses indicate that the child/adolescent demonstrates many of the symptoms common to ADHD, but not at a significance level that meets formal diagnostic criteria.

The child/adolescent does exhibit some subthreshold symptoms of ADHD, which do not meet diagnostic criteria at the present time but do need to be monitored.

Consistent with a diagnosis of ADHD, the child/adolescent was found to have difficulty with sustained auditory attention, visual organization, and shifting set.

The overall results of testing support the existence of a primary attentional and organizational disorder that is consistent with frontal lobe impairment. A diagnosis of ADHD is therefore appropriate.

Behavior rating scales and history indicate that the child/adolescent is exhibiting significant symptoms of inattention, impulsivity, and hyperactivity consistent with a diagnosis of ADHD.

Behavior rating scales indicate that the child/adolescent meets the criteria for ADHD, Combined Type/Inattentive Type/Hyperactive–Impulsive Type. In addition she/he demonstrates difficulties on tasks requiring sustained concentration and focus and presents with organizational difficulties and impulsive responding.

The child/adolescent exhibits symptoms consistent with a diagnosis of ADHD. His/her symptoms are quite severe and interfere with his/her functioning in all areas, including academic/social/family functioning.

The child/adolescent performed in the clinically significant range on several tasks requiring sustained attention, consistent with her/his previous diagnosis of ADHD.

Assessment of ADHD

Behavior Rating Scales   *See Chapter 28 for more details about many of these scales.*

BROAD-BAND SCALES

Behavior Assessment System for Children, Second Edition (BASC-2)
Child Behavior Checklist (CBCL), Teacher's Report Form (TRF), and Youth Self-Report (YSR)—all components of the Achenbach System of Empirically Based Assessment (ASEBA)
Personality Inventory for Children, Second Edition

NARROW-BAND SCALES

ADD-H Comprehensive Teacher Rating Scale (ACTeRS), Second Edition
ADHD Rating Scale–IV
Behavior Rating Inventory of Executive Functions (BRIEF)
Child Symptom Inventory
Conners' Rating Scales–Revised (CRS-R)
Home Situations Questionnaire
School Situations Questionnaire
SNAP-IV Teacher and Parent Rating Scale

Classroom Observation Forms

ADHD School Observation Code
Revised ADHD Behavior Coding System

Tests of Attention and Other Executive Functions

See Chapter 26 for more details about many of these scales.

Brief Test of Attention (BTA)
Conners' Continuous Performance Test II (CPT-II)
Conners' Kiddie Continuous Performance Test (K-CPT)
d2 Test of Attention
Gordon Diagnostic System (Gordon, 1983)
Stroop Color and Word Test
Test of Variables of Attention (T.O.V.A and T.O.V.A.-A)
Trails A and B
Visual Search and Attention Task (VSAT)
Wisconsin Card Sorting Test

16.2. Communication Disorders   *See also Section 13.6, "Speech and Language Skills."*

Relevant DSM-IV-TR Codes

315.31	Expressive Language Disorder
315.31	Mixed Receptive–Expressive Language Disorder
315.39	Phonological Disorder
307.0	Stuttering
307.9	Communication Disorder NOS
313.23	Selective Mutism

General Information

The American Speech–Language–Hearing Association (1982) groups speech and language problems according to the following subsystems of language:

Phonology (e.g., substitution/omission of speech sounds, unintelligible speech).
Morphology (e.g., problems understanding/producing word forms, use of inappropriate prefixes/suffixes).
Syntax (e.g., problems ordering elements of a sentence).
Semantics (e.g., trouble understanding word or sentence meaning).
Pragmatics (e.g., difficulty in social use of language).

Sattler (1992) describes the following as language problems often seen in preschool/early school years:

- Ages 3–5 years: Lack of speech, speech that is unintelligible or incoherent, and an inability to speak in sentences.
- Ages 5–6 years: Substitution errors, dropping of word endings, problems with sentence structure, and nonfluency/dysfluency.

Problems with Language Quality

Poor/limited vocabulary, confabulations, stereotyped phrases, poverty of amount/content of speech, tangential, telegraphic speech, word-finding errors/problems with word recall, shortened sentences, problems with grammatical structure of language, errors in tense, poor conversational skills.

Expressive Language Difficulties

Limited/small vocabulary, speaks in short/simple sentences, vocabulary errors, simplified grammar, unusual word order; slow rate of language development.

Receptive Language Difficulties

Problems understanding words/specific types of words, difficulty understanding sentences/statements, problems with auditory processing, fails to respond to speech, seems deaf.

Problems with Vocal Quality

Loud, soft, monotonous, high/low-pitched, harsh, hoarse, nasal/hypernasal/hyponasal.

Aphasia

Types of Aphasia

Congenital/developmental/acquired, expressive/receptive/auditory.

Subcategories of Aphasia

Agraphia, agnosia, apraxia, alexia, anomia.

Symptoms in Children

Reduced spontaneous speech (often beginning as mutism and followed by limited speech), hesitations, impoverished speech, difficulty understanding verbal commands (Satz & Bullard-Bates, 1981), problems with word order/word choice, word omissions, problems comprehending verbal commands, errors of circumlocution, semantic approximations.

Articulation Problems

Abnormal production of speech sounds, unintelligible speech, difficulty saying certain speech sounds, poor diction, lisp, dysarthria.

Word sounds omitted/substituted/distorted/added/poorly produced, substitutes certain sounds for other sounds, reverses order of sounds within words, uses incorrect sounds in the place of more difficult ones (e.g., "wabbit" for "rabbit"), omits difficult phonemes (e.g., "bu" instead of "blue").

Stuttering

Andrews et al. (1983) and the American Psychiatric Association (2000) note the following developmental aspects of stuttering:

Most stutterers are identified between ages 2 and 7 years, with peak onset at 5 years, and nearly all are identified by age 10 years.

Disturbance usually begins gradually, with a waxing and waning course.

Characteristics of stuttering are as follows:

Vocal behaviors:

Abnormal hesitations in speech, prolongations/prolonged sounds, repetitions, disordered/impaired rate/rhythm/fluency, interrupted speech flow, repeats/repetitions, blocking.

Physical symptoms:

> Grimaces/clenches fists, gestures, bodily movements indicating struggle to speak/struggle behavior, blinking/eye blinks, tics.

Associated problems:

> Fear of speaking, avoiding certain situations (public speaking, talking on phone, speaking up in class), anxiety, frustration.

Other Speech Difficulties

Dysprosody, neologisms, echolalia, "word salad," disorganized, pedantic, formal/stilted, overly familiar, slow reaction times, circumstantiality, illogicality, paraphasia, perseverations, misnamings, pressured.

Summary Statements about Language

The general array of the child's language testing indicates that she/he has an average/below-average/above-average ability to use and understand language.

The child's linguistic difficulties seem more related to construction and mechanics than to comprehension and understanding.

Overall, language is an area of strength/weakness for this child.

Performance on oral language measures was within the average/below-average/above-average range.

Articulation was generally normal, with fluent speech.

The nonverbal attributes of communication were age-appropriate, including intonation, prosody, volume, and the expression of affect in tone of voice.

The child's speech is appropriate in terms of articulation, volume, modulation, and prosody (range of intonation).

Literal paraphasic errors (mispronunciations) were heard/not observed during fluent speech.

Verbal paraphasic errors (word substitutions) were heard/not observed during fluent speech.

No significant word-finding difficulties or symptoms of dysnomia were heard during fluent speech.

Verbal and situational pragmatics (the use of language as a tool of communication) were generally appropriate/inappropriate.

Spontaneous speech was virtually absent throughout the examination.

Expressive/receptive language skills were found to be within normal limits/moderately delayed/severely delayed.

Both expressive and receptive language skills are quite underdeveloped relative to potential.

The child's performance was indicative of significant problems with word retrieval.

Assessment of Language Functioning

The following are commonly used measures of language functioning in children. (*For more information about many of these tests, see Chapter 23.*)

Comprehensive Receptive and Expressive Vocabulary Test—Second Edition
Expressive One-Word Picture Vocabulary Test (EOWPVT), 2000 Edition
Expressive Vocabulary Test (EVT)
Multilingual Aphasia Examination
Oral and Written Language Scales (OWLS)
Peabody Picture Vocabulary Test—Third Edition (PPVT-III)
Receptive One-Word Picture Vocabulary Test (ROWPVT), 2000 Edition
Test of Early Language Development, Third Edition (TELD-3)

Test of Language Development–Primary: Third Edition (TOLD-P:3)
Test of Language Development–Intermediate, Third Edition (TOLD-I:3)
Test of Word Finding–Second Edition (TWF-2)

16.3. Disruptive Behavior Disorders

See also Section 16.1, "Attention-Deficit/Hyperactivity Disorder (ADHD)."

Relevant DSM-IV-TR codes

312.81	Conduct Disorder, Childhood-Onset Type
312.82	Conduct Disorder, Adolescent-Onset Type
312.89	Conduct Disorder, Unspecified Onset
313.81	Oppositional Defiant Disorder
312.9	Disruptive Behavior Disorder NOS

ODD Symptoms

Argumentative, annoys others, touchy, overreacts to appropriate rule setting, swears at parents/teacher, "hell on wheels," defiant, rude, talks back/"sasses," insubordinate, challenges/disputes.

Blames others for mistakes or problems, denies all responsibility, persistently resists others' ways of doing things.

Temper outbursts/loses temper, is spiteful/vindictive/disobedient, volatile, stubborn/noncompliant, irritability, resentfulness, negativism, provokes others.

Refuses to cooperate/follow rules during group activities, frequently cheats during games or makes up own rules to games, refuses to do what others tell him/her to do.

(Associated symptoms:) Low self-esteem, low frustration tolerance, drug/alcohol/tobacco use, mood lability, school suspensions.

CD Symptoms

Aggression:

Physically aggressive to peers/parents/teachers/animals, bullies others, uses weapons, rape, gets into frequent fights with others on the playground/on the bus/in the neighborhood/anywhere, fist fighting, gang fighting, is mean to other children, "foul mouth," uses derogatory/insulting language, violent/dangerous, assaults, threatens/intimidates/bullies, physical cruelty to animals or people.

Destruction of property:

Sets fires, writes graffiti (particularly hate graffiti), blows up mailboxes with firecrackers, vandalism, deliberate destruction of property known to belong to others.

Deceitfulness

"Often lies to get out of trouble," places blame on others, a "pathological liar"/"born liar," will cheat/lie in order to win/be seen as the winner, makes an effort on a task or toward others only if it serves his/her interests, selfishly accepts favors without any desire to return them.

Theft

Shoplifts, forges checks, breaks into people's homes/cars/stores, auto theft/joyriding, mugging, extortion/blackmail, armed robbery, stealing, burglary, purse snatching.

Violations of rules:

> "Always in trouble," truant from school, has run away from home ____ times, violates curfew, stays out all night, disobeys school rules, driving a car without a license, trades sex for money/goods/drugs, coerced others into sexual activities, substance use before age 13 and recurrent use after 13 years of age.

Associated emotional symptoms:

> Low self-esteem, poor frustration tolerance, "short fuse," temper outbursts, irritability, superficial bravado, belief that people "pick on" her/him.

Associated academic symptoms:

> Poor school achievement/drop in grades, expelled from school/school probation, special education placement, repeating a grade.

Other associated symptoms:

> Substance abuse/dependence, sexually active from an early age/multiple sex partners, gang membership, history of sexual/physical abuse, insecurity, juvenile delinquency.

Assessment of ODD and CD

> *See also the broad-band scales listed for assessment of ADHD in Section 16.1.*

Antisocial Process Screening Device (APSD)
Conduct Disorder Scale (CDS)
Jesness Behavior Checklist (JBC)
Jesness Inventory—Revised (JI-R)

16.4. Eating Disorders

Relevant DSM-IV-TR codes

307.1	Anorexia Nervosa
307.51	Bulimia Nervosa
307.50	Eating Disorder NOS

Anorexia Nervosa

Physical Presentation and Symptoms

Emaciated appearance

> Protruding ribs/hipbones, "skull-like" face, "broomstick" limbs, cachexia/cachectic, emaciation, weight loss of at least 15% without disease.

Physiological consequences

> Amenorrhea/menstrual irregularities/disruption/cessation, degeneration of muscle, cardiac stress/arrhythmia/bradycardia/heart failure, edema, electrolyte imbalance, hair loss, low blood pressure, reduced body temperature/hypothermia, growth of thick soft hair over the body.

Behavioral Symptoms

Excessive exercising/overexercising.

Laxative/diuretic misuse/abuse.

Reduces food intake to only a few vegetables/crackers/etc. a day, eating only low- and no-calorie foods, ritualizes food habits/eating (e.g., cutting food into very small pieces, chewing for long periods).

Refusal to eat/self-starvation/fasting.

Spends hours observing body in mirror.

Cognitive Symptoms

Distorted body image (believes she/he is always too fat, despite significant weight loss), loses ability to see body realistically, sees self as grossly overweight even if actually emaciated, dissatisfied with bodily appearance.

Fear of becoming obese, food phobia, fear of pubertal changes.

"Good child," well-behaved, conscientious, quiet, intense drive to be perfect or please others.

Morbid fear of gaining weight/becoming fat, distorted and implacable attitudes toward food, avoidance of "fattening" foods, overvalued ideas of/dread of fatness.

Obsession with thinness, preoccupied with food, excessive interest in food preparation/trying new recipes/cooking elaborate meals for others.

Perfectionistic, overly self-disciplined/controlled, pride in weight management, overly critical of self and/or others.

Sees family in overly positive light, denies any family conflict, idealized view of family, enmeshment with a parent, family does not reveal feelings/emotions.

Emotional/Social Aspects

Dependent/compliant.

Depression, anxiety, difficulty sleeping.

Difficulty expressing feelings (particularly negative ones).

Low self-esteem.

Socially inactive.

Bulimia Nervosa

Physical Presentation and Symptoms

Appearance:

Normal body size, near-normal weight (sometimes obese), great body fluctuations.

Physiological consequences:

Frequent sore throats, swollen glands, dental problems due to destruction of tooth enamel, intestinal problems/constipation, nutritional deficiencies, intense hunger, dehydration, lowered body temperature, disturbances of body chemistry/electrolyte imbalances, loss of hair, insomnia, amenorrhea.

Behavioral Symptoms

Alternates between binge eating and periods of fasting/normal eating behavior, eats food in secret, purchases large quantities of food that suddenly "disappear," other people's food "disappears."

Engages in gross overeating followed by purging (self-induced vomiting or overdoses of laxatives), consumes enormous amounts of high-calorie food, frequently eats high-calorie foods without gaining weight.

Excessive exercising.
Frequent weighing, attendance at weight control clinics.
Impulsivity, hyperactivity.
Junk food consumption.
Makes attempts to lose weight, is a lifelong dieter.
Perfectionism.
Self-induced vomiting, uses laxatives/diuretics/appetite suppressants/thyroid preparations.

Cognitive Symptoms

Abnormal concern with body size, weight central to self-evaluation, feels powerless about controlling weight.
Difficulty thinking clearly, rationalizes eating/symptoms, dichotomous thinking, overpersonalization, rationalization of eating/symptoms.
Fear of obesity/morbid fear of becoming fat.
Negative/distorted/irrational body image, overconcern with body appearance/shape/weight, dissatisfied/disgusted with bodily appearance.
Perfectionism.
Preoccupation with food.
Shame about abnormal behavior.

Emotional Aspects

Depression, anxiety, mood swings, masked anger.
Feelings of disgust/helplessness/panic/guilt over inability to control binges/purging.
Impulsivity.
Low self-esteem, oversensitive to criticism from others.
Suicidality.

Social Aspects

Difficulty with interpersonal relationships, refuses to date because of self-consciousness about looks.
Eats alone due to embarrassment over amount eaten/eating rituals, frequent trips to bathroom (for purging).
Family problems.
High achievement, academic success.
Restriction of social activities.
Work impairment.

Assessment of Eating Disorders

The Eating Disorder Inventory-2 (EDI-2) can be used for specifically assessing eating disorders. (*See Chapters 27 and 28 for projective measures and general behavior rating scales, respectively.*)

16.5. Elimination and Intake Disorders

For eating disorders, see Section 16.4, "Eating Disorders."

Relevant DSM-IV-TR codes

787.6   Encopresis With Constipation and Overflow Incontinence
307.7   Encopresis Without Constipation and Overflow Incontinence
307.6   Enuresis

307.52   Pica
307.53   Rumination Disorder
307.59   Feeding Disorder of Infancy or Early Childhood

Enuresis

Enuresis is wetting after the age of 5 years. "Primary" enuresis occurs when symptoms have been present throughout childhood (i.e., toilet training was never successfully accomplished). "Secondary" enuresis occurs after at least 6 months of successful toilet training.

Associated medical conditions:

Juvenile-onset diabetes, sickle cell disease, urinary tract infection, kidney infection, minor neurological impairments, structural anomalies.

Associated emotional and behavioral symptoms:

Social stigma related to bedwetting at friends' houses, reluctance to have sleepovers or go to sleep-away camp, trauma or separation from parents (often associated with secondary enuresis).

Encopresis

Encopresis is soiling after age 4 years.

Associated medical conditions:

Constipation, anal fissures, refusal to eat, weight loss, dehydration, leakage of unformed stool around impaction, Hirschsprung disease/aganglionic megacolon.

Associated emotional and behavioral symptoms:

Hiding/smearing stool or feces, high family stress/psychopathology, disorganized household, physical/sexual abuse, increased anxiety, toilet phobia, stressful events (e.g., birth of sibling, separation from parents, starting school).

General Intake/Feeding Difficulties

Snow (1998) states that problems related to infant nutrition and feeding practices can include the following:

- Iron deficiency anemia.
- Adverse/allergic reactions to food.
- Dental caries (e.g., "bottle-mouth syndrome," "nursing-bottle syndrome," or "baby-bottle tooth decay").
- Obesity.
- Malnutrition (including protein energy malnutrition, kwashiorkor, and marasmus).

Snow (1998) also notes these positive signs of growth in infancy:

- Normal growth rate.
- Good appetite.
- Firm muscle tone.
- Curiosity.
- Alertness.

Problematic eating behaviors:

Finicky eater, verbally expresses dislike for many foods, shows distress/cries when certain foods are on his/her plate, tries to remove food from plate/throws food, holds food in mouth for long periods of time/doesn't swallow food, plays with food, complains that something is wrong with the food.

Problems specifically associated with overeating:

Physical health problems (e.g., cardiovascular problems, diabetes), social problems, difficulty in physically keeping up with peers (e.g., may run out of breath when she/he walks, tires easily during movement/exercises, prefers sedentary activities), poor self-esteem.

Pica

Pica is the ingesting of non-nutritive substances such as dirt, chalk, plaster, soap, glue, matches, feces, clay, charcoal, baking soda, ashes, coffee grounds, laundry starch, or hair. It usually begins between the ages of 1 and 2 years; it is also seen in pregnant women (including pregnant teens). It may be associated with iron deficiency, and it can cause lead poisoning and intestinal obstruction.

Rumination Disorder

In rumination disorder (also called "merycism"), a child regurgitates and rechews food. Medical complications may include malnutrition or failure to thrive in infants (which can be fatal), and the act of ruminating may be associated with a hiatus hernia. It is more common in children with mental retardation than in those with normal intelligence.

16.6. Learning Disabilities

See Chapter 33, "Writing for the Schools," for more information regarding the determination of a learning disability according to the Individuals with Disabilities Education Act (IDEA).

Assessment of Learning Disabilities

See Chapters 21 and 22 for more information about many of the tests mentioned below.

Tests of intelligence, academic skills, relative cognitive abilities, and (often) emotional skills are usually needed to make a diagnosis of a learning disability. There is no one standard battery for any of the learning disabilities described in this section, as the selection of tests should be based on the referral question, the child's age and grade level, and the severity of the disability's impact. Listed below are general tests of intelligence and academic achievement.

Tests of Intelligence

Differential Ability Scales (DAS-II)
Kaufman Assessment Battery for Children, Second Edition (KABC-II)
Kaufman Brief Intelligence Test, Second Edition (KBIT-2)
Stanford–Binet Intelligence Scale, Fifth Edition (SB5)
Wechsler Adult Intelligence Scale–Third Edition (WAIS-III)
Wechsler Intelligence Scale for Children–Fourth Edition (WISC-IV)
Wechsler Preschool and Primary Scale of Intelligence–Third Edition (WPPSI-III)
Woodcock Johnson III (WJ III) Tests of Cognitive Abilities

Tests of Academic Achievement

DABERON Screening for School Readiness–Second Edition
Diagnostic Achievement Battery–Second Edition
Diagnostic Achievement Test for Adolescents–Second Edition

Wechsler Individual Achievement Test–Second Edition (WIAT-II)
Wide Range Achievement Test, Fourth Edition (WRAT4)
Woodcock–Johnson III (WJ III) Tests of Achievement
Young Children's Achievement Test (YCAT)

Associated Emotional and Behavioral Symptoms

Anxiety, depression, comorbid ADHD.
Low motivation, perception of lack of ability, less likely to credit successes to his/her ability.
Negative attitudes shown by teachers/students/parents toward child, child is teased by other children because she/he can't read.
Poor impulse control, juvenile delinquency, aggressive behaviors.
Poor social competence.

Summary Statements about Ability–Achievement Discrepancies

Academically, the child's overall level of educational achievement is significantly higher than his/her overall level of intellectual development, based on his/her performance on the _____ (give name of test).
The child's academic testing performance is comparable to or exceeds her/his cognitive test performance.

On each of the achievement tests, the child/adolescent scored at expected levels based on IQ (a measure of aptitude) and performed at grade level as compared to age-mates on tests of reading/spelling/mathematics.
His/her academic achievement was commensurate with expectations based on cognitive ability.

Although performance in a number of domains was not significantly discrepant from that of same-age peers, achievement in some areas (specify) was below what would be expected, given the child's overall intellectual abilities.
The child's performance on most measures of academic performance was at/slightly below/far below expectations, given his/her overall intellectual abilities.
A regression-based discrepancy analysis indicates a significant ____-point difference between reading/math/spelling/writing/etc. ability on achievement tests and the child's expected abilities. This difference occurs in only ____% of her/his same-age peers ($p <$ ____).
Various dimensions of reading/writing/math/listening/speaking/etc. were evaluated, and certain aspects (specify instrument) were discrepant from intellectual functioning as measured by the _____ (give name of test).

Mathematics Disorder (Dyscalculia)

Relevant DSM-IV-TR Code

315.1   Mathematics Disorder

Assessment of Mathematics Disorder

Comprehensive Mathematical Abilities Test
KeyMath–Revised: A Diagnostic Inventory of Essential Mathematics
Test of Early Mathematics Ability–Third Edition (TEMA-3)
Test of Mathematical Abilities–Second Edition (TOMA-2)

Symptoms

Difficulty performing mathematical operations (addition/subtraction/multiplication/division), trouble counting, problems with identifying/using money, cannot tell time, unable to consistently add/subtract single-digit numbers, unable to complete any multiple-digit items.

Difficulty comprehending mathematical terms/operations, trouble understanding story problems, cannot analyze word problems and make the correspondence between manipulative and abstract numbers.

Misreads operations signs, does not acknowledge corresponding signs.

Problems learning math facts (e.g., multiplication tables).

Transposes numbers.

Associated Emotional and Behavioral Symptoms

Academic problems, comorbid dyslexia, problems with conceptual aspects of learning.
Attention deficits.
Depression.
Difficulties with social cognition, social withdrawal.
Opposition to written work.

Summary Statements

The child's performance on the current testing is consistent with a diagnosis of math disorder, as achievement scores in math were discrepant from expected performance and showed a ____-year grade delay.

(For a younger child:) Academic achievement skills fall well below current grade level for math, where the child shows an insecure grasp of basic concepts (e.g., 1:1 correspondence, number recognition, appreciation of number magnitude) and has difficulty manipulating numbers, even for very simple problems and concepts.

Reading Disabilities (Dyslexia/Reading Disorder)

The terms "dyslexia," "reading disabilities," and "reading disorder" are often used interchangeably. However, the DSM uses "reading disorder," and much of the research literature uses "dyslexia." The term "reading disabilities" encompasses everything.

Relevant DSM-IV-TR Code

315.00   Reading Disorder

Assessment of Reading Disabilities   *See Chapter 22 for more details about several of these tests.*

Classroom Reading Inventory—Eighth Edition
Comprehensive Test of Phonological Processing (CTOPP)
Gates–MacGinitie Reading Tests, Fourth Edition (GMRT-4)
Gray Oral Reading Tests, Fourth Edition (GORT-4)
Gray Silent Reading Tests
Lindamood Auditory Conceptualization Test, Third Edition (LAC-3)
Nelson–Denny Reading Test
Rosner Auditory Analysis Test
Test of Early Reading Ability—Third Edition (TERA-3)
Test of Reading Comprehension—Third Edition (TORC-3)
Woodcock Reading Mastery Tests—Revised (WRMT-R)

Reading Skill Deficits

Auditory discrimination problems, unable to identify beginning/ending sounds in words, cannot recognize initial consonants/consonant clusters, cannot recognize vowel sounds.

Comprehension problems/difficulty comprehending what has just been read, relied on pictures for sentence comprehension.

Decoding problems, inaccurate reading, difficulty in the ability to recognize sounds and their sequences in words, difficulty with tasks of nonword/nonsense word reading, unable to accurately read the simplest of stories, unable to provide correct sounds for consonants/consonant digraphs/consonant blends/short vowels/long vowels/vowels embedded in three-letter consonant–vowel–consonant words, often added letters and rearranged letters within words when reading single words.

Fluency problems/dysfluent reading, hesitations, slow reading.

Letter-naming problems, unable to match upper- to lower-case letters.

Limited basic sight word vocabulary.

Oral reading errors, omission/insertion, mispronunciation/phonemic substitution, skipped words, lost place, reversed words, repetition, visual errors/whole-word guesses, lexicalizations, errors on function words, consistent word-decoding errors at the middle to end of words, guessed at words based on the first few letters.

Rhyming problems, unable to provide rhymes for specific words (e.g., "cat–hat").

Spelling impaired/limited, made letter reversals, struggled with basic sound–symbol association for both vowels and consonants.

Associated Difficulties

Academic problems in math.

Attentional difficulties.

Articulation problems.

Delinquency.

Language-processing difficulties.

Poor short- or long-term memory, difficulty with rote auditory memory (e.g., learning math facts, such as multiplication tables).

Self-esteem problems.

Visual–spatial difficulties.

Word-finding problems.

Summary Statements

FOR YOUNGER CHILDREN AND EARLY READERS

The child's performance indicates that she/he is at risk for developmental dyslexia.

The child demonstrated a pattern of scores typical of young children with dyslexia: Reading tests that depended on phonics were very difficult for him/her.

Academic achievement skills fall well below current grade level for reading and spelling.

The child's recognition of letters (visual skill) is more developed than her/his ability to associate sounds with letters (phonemic/auditory skill); the child has only the beginning of phonemic awareness at this time.

FOR SCHOOL-AGE CHILDREN

The child's test results indicated that he/she has a specific learning disability, dyslexia. Children with dyslexia have an early deficit in phonological processing (ability to recognize sounds and their sequences in words), which affects the ease with which letter–sound correspondences are learned and automatized. This results in slowed progress in learning to read and even more striking difficulties in learning to spell. The child's educational history and tests results clearly reflect this pattern.

In summary, the child is a _____-year-old boy/girl with a learning disability in the area of reading.

School history, early developmental history, and present test results all indicate that this is a child with a specific reading disability (dyslexia).

Results are highly consistent with a specific learning disability (dyslexia), with a significant weakness in phonological processing.

Test results and prior history indicate that she/he has a reading disorder (dyslexia). Specifically, achievement in reading and spelling is significantly below grade level and discrepant from what would be expected on the basis of her/his general intellectual ability.

The child's school history and present test results indicate that he/she has a specific reading disability (dyslexia), as phonological processing skills (a core deficit in dyslexia) are weaker than would normally be expected for a child of his/her educational experience and intellectual ability.

The child performed significantly below expectations with respect to reading and spelling skills. Analysis of her/his performance indicated significant difficulties with basic phonemic decoding (reading) and encoding (spelling) skills. Reading comprehension is also significantly below expectations.

The child's overall reading ability (composite of reading comprehension and word recognition) as well as his/her basic reading skills (word recognition), differed significantly from expectations based on his/her overall intellectual abilities.

FOR OLDER CHILDREN/ADOLESCENTS

The pattern of this adolescent's scores and the types of errors she/he made are both highly characteristic of young adults with dyslexia who have compensated well/partially compensated.

The adolescent's history and pattern of scores indicate a previously undiagnosed dyslexia.

Nonverbal Learning Disability (NLD)

NLD is not a DSM-IV-TR diagnosis, although it can be coded as 315.9, Learning Disorder NOS.

Assessment of NLD

Assessment of NLD typically involves administering tests of intellectual ability, visual–spatial ability, achievement measures, and executive functioning. Listed below are tests that specifically measure nonverbal intelligence. (*The CTONI and the TONI-3 are discussed further in Chapter 22. See other chapters in Section E, "Test Results," for more information regarding other types of measures.*)

Comprehensive Test of Nonverbal Intelligence (CTONI)
Raven's Progressive Matrices
Test of Nonverbal Intelligence, Third Edition (TONI-3)
Universal Nonverbal Intelligence Test

Symptoms

Higher Verbal IQ/Verbal Comprehension Index than Performance IQ/Perceptual Reasoning Index.
Academic difficulties in math, reading comprehension.
Coordination (fine motor, gross motor, and/or psychomotor) difficulties.
Problems with visual–spatial organization.

Social relationship difficulties, trouble reading nonverbal cues (such as gestures or facial expressions).
Tactile or sensory integration problems (or history of such problems), dislike of loud noises/touch/specific foods/certain smells.

Associated Difficulties

Anxiety, obsessional thinking/tendencies.
Difficulty organizing and conceptualizing verbal material, difficulty conceptualizing abstract mathematical and scientific concepts, trouble learning grammatical structures of foreign languages.
Emotional problems, oppositional behavior.
Executive function impairment, variable attention, impulsivity, perseverative tendencies, organizational problems.
Hyperlexic.
Trouble adjusting to new situations/shifting set (e.g., changes in classroom, teachers).

Summary Statements

Results of the current testing do not indicate the presence of NLD, as the difference between the child's verbal and nonverbal abilities was not at a level consistent with this diagnosis.
Although this child demonstrates better-developed verbal than nonverbal skills, test data do not indicate that she/he meets full diagnostic criteria for NLD.

In light of the _____-point discrepancy between the child's Verbal IQ and Performance IQ scores, the possibility of NLD was explored via further testing. Indeed, he/she was found to meet most of the primary criteria for NLD, including relatively weaker performance in calculation skills, visual–motor integration delays, motor planning and graphomotor output difficulty, problems reading social cues, etc.
Test results indicate a pattern typical of individuals with NLD. People with this type of learning disability have difficulty with the perception, analysis, integration, and storage of nonverbal information.
The child's current performance and past history indicate that she/he meets the primary criteria for NLD, including a significantly lower Performance IQ than Verbal IQ score; academic weaknesses in reading comprehension (due to problems making inferences) and calculation skills; visual–motor integration delays; motor planning and graphomotor output difficulties; and problems in reading nonverbal/social cues, which affect social reasoning.

Disorder of Written Expression (Dysgraphia)

Relevant DSM-IV-TR code

315.2   Disorder of Written Expression

Assessment of Written Expression

Test of Early Written Language—Second Edition
Test of Handwriting Skills
Test of Written Language—Third Edition (TOWL-3)

Symptoms

Letter reversals, substitution of upper- for lower-case letters (and vice versa) in words.
Misspellings of common/uncommon words.

Organization of writing was poor/confusing.

Pencil grip was poor/variable, inconsistent/soft/hard pencil pressure.

Poor handwriting, difficulty copying, difficulty in the mechanics of writing, poorly formed letters, retraced letters, too much/too little space between words, does not separate words, prints letters with significant difficulty, has idiosyncratic manner of producing letters.

Poor motor speed/sequencing.

Poor spelling/punctuation/capitalization, run-on sentences, omitted apostrophes in contractions, used upper-case letters incorrectly.

Problems composing text, poor paragraph construction, grammatical errors, added and missing words in sentences, inability to formulate phrases/complete sentences from a picture, sentences are not grammatically formulated, had difficult time coming up with connected ideas that were according to a given topic.

Utilized overly short/concrete/simple sentences, no sentence coherence or story development in his/her writing, vocabulary was basic, sentences lacked variation in structure and word use, more impoverished writing content than would be expected from child's intellectual abilities and educational level.

(Difficulties seen in middle and high school:) Problems with note taking, difficulty taking essay exams (including problems organizing and expressing thoughts effectively and in a limited time period), persistent problems with handwriting, slow writing speed, failure to complete work on time.

Summary Statements

Assessment of academic achievement revealed a significant weakness in written language abilities, as the child's performance on tests assessing writing/spelling/capitalization/punctuation/word usage fell below grade and age expectations.

Within the academic domain, a significant discrepancy was seen between the child's general intellectual ability and his/her performance on academic measures of written language.

16.7. Mental Retardation

Relevant DSM-IV-TR Codes

317	Mild Mental Retardation
318.0	Moderate Mental Retardation
318.1	Severe Mental Retardation
318.2	Profound Mental Retardation
319	Mental Retardation, Severity Unspecified

Characteristics of Mental Retardation by Diagnostic Category

Mild Mental Retardation

IQ of 50–55 to 70.

Speech is typically similar in structure to that of individuals without mental retardation, but is often concrete in content.

Individuals can expect to achieve up to sixth-grade level in academic skills.

They can work and live independently, usually with some support from family or community.

About 85% of those diagnosed with mental retardation have the mild form.

Moderate Mental Retardation

IQ of 35–40 to 50–55.

Individuals are typically able to communicate needs to others through speech, but slow to develop language skills.

They can work if significant oversight is provided, but typically cannot live independently.

About 10% of individuals diagnosed with mental retardation have the moderate form.

Severe Mental Retardation

IQ of 20–25 to 35–40.

Language typically consists of vocalizations, single words, or two- to three-word phrases.

Individuals can often perform simple jobs with appropriate supervision, although they cannot live independently.

About 5% of individuals diagnosed with mental retardation have the severe form.

Profound Mental Retardation

IQ below 20–25.

Individuals lack verbal language, but may be able to indicate needs through vocalizations/behaviors.

About 1–2% of individuals diagnosed with mental retardation have the profound form.

Categories of Adaptive Functioning

Life skills:

Can/cannot manage money/use the telephone/tell time.

Safety:

Can/cannot be left alone at home or in backyard.

Self-care:

Can/slow to learn/cannot tie shoes/brush teeth/get dressed/use a knife and fork, no problems/problems with feeding/dressing/toileting/personal hygiene.

Social skills:

Social skills adequate/deficient (e.g., difficulties interacting with peers at an age-appropriate level).

Causes of Mental Retardation

Pregnancy and birth:

Maternal infections (e.g., cytomegalovirus [CMV], rubella, toxoplasmosis, syphilis), maternal substance abuse (e.g., fetal alcohol syndrome [FAS]), anoxia during birth process, extreme prematurity.

Environmental toxins or causes:

Severe malnutrition, severely deprived environment/understimulation, lead poisoning, meningitis, encephalitis.

Hereditary or congenital conditions:

Down syndrome, fragile X syndrome, tuberous sclerosis, Tay–Sachs disease, phenyl-ketonuria (PKU), trisomy 18, Prader–Willi syndrome, Wilson disease, anencephaly, hydroencephaly, porencephaly, microcephaly, hydrocephalus.

Trauma:

Anoxia, infections, head injury.

Common Medical and Developmental Problems

Epilepsy.
Growth difficulties as a fetus or developing child, low birth weight.
Physical handicaps, paralysis, problems with coordination, cerebral palsy, fine and gross motor delays, abnormal muscle tone.
Sensory problems, blindness, deafness.

Associated Emotional, Behavioral, and Cognitive Problems

Mood-related symptoms, depression, low self-esteem, problems with mood regulation, vulner-ability to emotional/psychiatric disorders.
Aggression, self-injurious behaviors, verbal abusiveness, tantrums, noncompliance, unpredict-able behavior.
Passivity, easily led by others.
Inappropriate behaviors (e.g., stripping, vocalization, fetishes).
Low frustration tolerance.
Poor judgment.
Poor attentional skills, hyperactivity, impulsivity.
Stereotypies/stereotypic behavior.
Stubbornness.

Summary Statements

In summary, this child/adolescent is a ____-year-old male/female with Down syndrome/etc. (specify) and mild/moderate/severe/profound mental retardation.
The results of today's evaluation place the child's overall level of intellectual functioning with-in the mild/moderate/severe/profound range of Mental Retardation, with performance on tests of intelligence, language, visual–motor, and adaptive skills all converging on this level of functioning.
The child is a ____-year-old girl/boy who is currently functioning in the mildly/moderately/ severely/profoundly mentally retarded range of intelligence, with widespread cognitive and adaptive difficulties consistent with this picture.

Assessment of Mental Retardation

Assessment of mental retardation typically involves the administration of a standard intelligence test. (*See Chapter 21 for more information about IQ tests.*) Since a diagnosis of mental retardation also must include problems in everyday functioning, the first list below covers tests of adaptive function-ing (*see Chapter 28 for more details about most of these*). The second list covers assessment measures for children with severe mental impairment.

Tests of Adaptive Functioning

AAMR Adaptive Behavior Scales–Residential and Community: Second Edition (ABS-RC:2)
AAMR Adaptive Behavior Scales–School: Second Edition (ABS-S:2)
Adaptive Areas Assessment (AAA)
Vineland Adaptive Behavior Scales, Second Edition (Vineland-II)

Assessments for Children with Severe Disabilities

A Developmental Assessment for Students with Severe Disabilities–Second Edition (DASH-2)
Assessment for Persons Profoundly or Severely Impaired (APPSI)

16.8. Movement and Tic Disorders

Relevant DSM-IV-TR Codes

307.23	Tourette's Disorder
307.22	Chronic Motor or Vocal Tic Disorder
307.21	Transient Tic Disorder
315.4	Developmental Coordination Disorder
307.3	Stereotypic Movement Disorder

Developmental Coordination Disorder

Clumsy; has difficulty tying shoes/buttoning shirt/zipping pants or jacket/trouble assembling puzzles, playing games or sports, difficulty with writing, abilities well below others of his/her age in daily activities requiring motor coordination, has not achieved motor milestones on time.

Tourette's Disorder and Other Tic Disorders

Motor tics

Stereotypic movements (see below), eye blinking, grimaces, taps hands/feet, touching, twirling when walking, retracing steps, knee bending, picking.

Verbal tics:

Makes strange noises (barks/growls/clicks/snorts/sniffs), uses inappropriate words or phrases/obscene language (coprolalia), coughs/clears throat, repeats words/phrases/sounds.

Merrell (2001) describes depressed mood, social discomfort, shame, self-consciousness, and obsessive–compulsive behaviors as associated characteristics of Tourette's disorder.

Stereotypic Movement Disorder

"Endless" body/head rocking, repetitive twirling/spinning, mouthing, wall patting, ritualistic hand movements, grimacing, "blindisms," hand waving, playing with hands/fingers.
Self-injurious behaviors (e.g., head banging, biting, pinching, hitting, face slapping, poking/rubbing the eyes, skin picking).

16.9. Pervasive Developmental Disorders

Pervasive developmental disorders have essentially the same core features: delays in development (particularly language and communication skills), impaired social skills, and difficulty with symbolic play and imagination. Differential diagnoses can be difficult with these disorders, but some generalities are as follows. Children with Asperger's disorder are typically recognized later than those with autism (in whom symptoms are seen before age 3 years), those with Rett's disorder (in whom there is normal development for 5–12 months), or those with childhood disintegrative disorder (CDD) (in whom development is normal for up to 2 years). Normal or above-average IQ is typical in children with Asperger's disorder, while children with autism frequently have low to below-average IQ, and children with Rett's and CDD exhibit a loss of previously acquired skills. Communication is typically not significantly delayed in children with Asperger's disorder, while children with autism and Rett's have impaired communication, and children with CDD have a loss of previously acquired skills. Stereotypies are common to all of these disorders. The NOS diagnosis (see below) is used when a child does not meet criteria for a more specific pervasive developmental disorder, but when there are some symptoms present.

Relevant DSM-IV-TR Codes

299.00	Autistic Disorder
299.80	Rett's Disorder
299.10	Childhood Disintegrative Disorder
299.80	Asperger's Disorder
299.80	Pervasive Developmental Disorder NOS

Developmental Deficits in Infancy and Toddlerhood

Does not enjoy close physical contact/cuddling, does not respond to voices of others.

Has failed to develop appropriate smiling.

Has failed to develop appropriate attachment to parents, develops "mechanical" or "inflexible" attachment to single adult.

Lack of eye contact, unresponsive infant.

Lacking in normal fear of strangers.

Social Interaction Deficits

Cries in unfamiliar settings or among unfamiliar people, no affection or interest when held, goes limp/stiff when held.

Does not need caregiver, unaware of caregiver's absence.

Fails to develop attachment, emotionally distant.

Lack of spontaneous sharing of interests/pleasures/achievements with others, "happiest when left alone," does not seek comforting from others or seeks it in strange ways when distressed/upset/frightened, ignores people.

Little or no social reciprocity, prefers solitary activities, impaired awareness of others, has no concept of others' needs, absence of sharing behaviors, lacks social give and take.

Peer relationship difficulties, little interest in other children, problems understanding the conventions of social relationships.

Poor eye contact, gaze avoidance, looks "through" people, lack of appropriate facial expressions, little use of appropriate gestures, no social smile.

Inability to infer mental states in self and others/theory-of-mind deficits, unawareness of the existence of feelings in others.

Communication Deficits

Delayed/undeveloped language skills, lack of verbal spontaneity/sparse expressive speech, does not imitate speech or does it strangely/mechanically.

Difficulty with nonverbal communication.

Echolalia, affirmation by repetition.

Either extreme literalness or "metaphorical language."

Intonation/pitch/rhythm problems, monotonous voice, "woodenness" in speaking.

Language comprehension difficulties, unable to understand humor/jokes/questions/satire, problems with higher-order language functions/inferencing/abstractions.

Neologisms.

Play skills delayed/impaired/nonexistent, lack of spontaneous play, unable to engage in imaginative play, struggles with initiating and sustaining play with peers.

Pragmatic difficulties: fails to use appropriate greetings when meeting other people, asks inappropriate questions, interrupts others, difficulty with appropriate turn taking.

Pronoun reversals, never uses first-person pronouns, refers to self as "you," refers to others as "I" or "me."

Repeats requests excessively (to the point of being socially inappropriate).

Tends to talk excessively on the same topic without taking peers'/other people's point of view into account.

Unable to sustain a conversation.

Uses stereotyped/idiosyncratic language, repeats TV shows/commercials/movies verbatim.

Baker (1983) mentions the following typical language deficits in autism:

- Receptive language skills may be better developed than expressive skills.
- Echolalia or repetition of rote phrases often does not constitute meaningful language (e.g., a child who often repeats the phrase "Come here" may not actually want someone to come near her/him).
- Language skills often do not generalize from one setting to another.
- Language skills may not follow a normal developmental trajectory.

Stereotyped Behaviors

Fascination with parts of objects, more interested in objects than in people, obsessively fascinated with unusual things for age (e.g., bus schedules, numbers).

Has restricted pattern of interests that is abnormal for age.

Inflexibility, has apparent need to perform specific rituals/patterns of behavior, becomes extremely distressed over minor changes in environment, becomes defiant when others try to redirect his/her play or social behavior, preservation of sameness.

Play is rigid/lacking in imitation/imagination.

Repetitive motor mannerisms, repetitive play habits.

Stereotyped body movements (e.g., spinning, clapping, hand gestures/flapping, rocking, swaying, twirling, head banging, tiptoe walking), staring at spinning things (e.g., fans, spinning tops).

Associated Behavioral and Cognitive Symptoms

Aggressiveness toward others, self-injurious behaviors.

Demonstrates splinter skills (e.g., mathematical ability, musicality, rote memory), savantism.

Gross and fine motor difficulties, trouble moving body in space, will often inadvertently bump into people/things or fall off chairs.

Hyperactivity, impulsivity.

Inattention, short attention span.

Masturbation.

Mood dysregulation, absence of emotional reactions, inappropriate emotional reactions, depression.

Sensory integration difficulties, insensitivity/oversensitivity to pain/sounds/touch/foods/smells, perceptual deficits, does not show normal startle response, hates bright lights/loud noises/certain types of clothing.

Sleeping difficulties.
Temper tantrums.

Summary Statements

The tests of cognitive, behavioral, and neuropsychological functioning did not indicate a pattern consistent with a pervasive developmental disorder, such as autism or Asperger's disorder.

Although the child has some symptoms that are consistent with Asperger's disorder she/he does not appear to meet full diagnostic criteria.

Current testing is consistent with a diagnosis of Asperger's disorder, as the child has generally demonstrated relative weaknesses in visual–motor integration, executive functions, higher-order language, pragmatics, and social reasoning. His/her behavioral concerns (e.g., rigidity/oppositionality, anxiety, moodiness) are also associated with Asperger's disorder.

Results from this testing, and previous history, indicate that the child meets criteria for an autism spectrum disorder such as Asperger's disorder. In review, her/his social skill weaknesses (including problems in social awareness, social comprehension, and emotional insight; inflexible adherence to routines; and obsessional tendencies) are all consistent with this diagnosis. In addition, her/his poor gross motor coordination and sensory integration problems are also frequently observed in people with Asperger's disorder.

Given the test data, historical information, and behavioral observations, a diagnosis of autistic disorder appears to be warranted. The key features of autistic disorder include a marked and sustained impairment in communication; markedly abnormal or impaired development in social interactions; and restricted, repetitive, and stereotyped patterns of behavior, interests and activities.

The child exhibits behavior consistent with a diagnosis of a pervasive developmental disorder, in that he/she shows severe and pervasive impairment in reciprocal social interaction skills, a restricted pattern of interests and activities, and a failure to develop peer relationships appropriate to developmental level. The child's abnormal functioning in the areas of social interaction and communication is long-standing.

Results of the evaluation indicate that the child meets criteria for autism, including impaired use of language, a lack of social interest and responsiveness, and stereotypies; she/he also exhibits an uneven cognitive profile, odd responses to sensory stimuli, and atypical body use.

Assessment of Pervasive Developmental Disorders

Asperger Syndrome Diagnostic Scale (ASDS)
Autism Behavior Checklist
Autism Diagnostic Interview—Revised (ADI-R)
Autism Screening Instrument for Educational Planning—Second Edition (ASIEP-2)
Behavioral Observation Scale (BOS) for Autism
Childhood Autism Rating Scale (CARS)
Gilliam Asperger's Disorder Scale (GADS)
Gilliam Autism Rating Scale (GARS)

16.10. Schizophrenia and Other Psychotic Disorders

Relevant DSM-IV-TR Codes

295.30	Schizophrenia, Paranoid Type
295.10	Schizophrenia, Disorganized Type

295.20	Schizophrenia, Catatonic Type
295.90	Schizophrenia, Undifferentiated Type
295.60	Schizophrenia, Residual Type
295.40	Schizophreniform Disorder
295.70	Schizoaffective Disorder
297.1	Delusional Disorder
298.8	Brief Psychotic Disorder
297.3	Shared Psychotic Disorder
293.xx	Psychotic Disorder Due to a GMC
298.9	Psychotic Disorder NOS

General Information

According to Barker (1990), psychotic disorders of childhood or adolescence fall into four groups:

- Schizophrenia.
- Disintegrative psychosis, usually as a result of an organic disease of the brain (this can be progressive or nonprogressive).
- Reactive psychosis.
- Psychosis caused by an infection, a metabolic disorder, or intoxication with drugs (marijuana, LSD/acid, cocaine, opiates).

Very-early-onset schizophrenia begins before age 13 years. Early-onset schizophrenia begins in either late childhood or adolescence. Schizophrenia most often manifests itself during late adolescence or early adulthood.

Symptoms

Affective symptoms:

Extreme mood changes, inappropriate affect, flat affect, behavioral passivity, indifference, euphoria, irritability, agitation, catatonia, depressed mood.

Negative symptoms:

Unmotivated, alogia, avolitional/lack of volition, flat affect, blocking.

Behavioral symptoms:

Disorganized/bizarre/incoherent speech, loose associations, tangentiality, circumstantiality, derailment, either poverty of content or flood of ideas, mumbles considerably, inappropriate responses to questions, stops talking in the middle of a sentence and does not continue, excitability, either hyperkinesis or immobility, rigidity, muteness, sudden shifts from immobility to excitability, social or occupational dysfunction.

Cognitive symptoms:

Confusion, spatial/temporal, disorientation, disordered thinking, bizarre ideation, illogical thinking, thought disorder, loss of contact with reality/real world.

Delusions:

Paranoid delusions, feelings of being persecuted, ideas of reference/grandiosity/control, other distortions of thought content (specify).

Hallucinations:

Auditory/visual/olfactory/tactile disturbances, specific perceptual distortions (specify).

16.11. Sleep Disorders

Relevant DSM-IV-TR Codes

307.47	Nightmare Disorder
307.46	Sleep Terror Disorder
307.46	Sleepwalking Disorder
780.59	Breathing-Related Sleep Disorder
780.5x	Sleep Disorder Due to a GMC

Nightmare Disorder

Child has long/vivid/frightening dreams, awakens repeatedly during sleep, is able to recall many details of dreams.

Sleep Terrors

During sleep child suddenly begins to have episodes including screaming/heart palpitations/ sweating, child is inconsolable/does not respond to others' attempts to comfort him/her, child cannot recall dreams or episode.

Sleepwalking

Child gets up and walks about during sleep (usually during first third of sleep), child is not awake during episode and can only be awakened with difficulty.

D. The Child or Adolescent in the Environment

17

Home and Family

See Chapter 11, "Developmental and Family History," for more information regarding family functioning and relationships.

17.1. Living Situation

Indicate whichever of the following factors are relevant to a child's assessment/treatment: family structure (include parents, stepparents, and siblings who do not live in the home); length of time the child has spent in the current living situation; and primary caregivers (indicate the relationship of each to the child, the number of hours per day the child is in a child care setting, and the number of different people who care for the child). If the parents are separated or divorced, indicate who has custody of the child and how often the child sees the other parent.

Types of Family Structure

Intact, mother–stepfather, father–stepmother, single mother/father (never married/widowed/divorced).

Lives with parents, mother, father, siblings, relatives, guardian, mother/father and her/his spouse/live-in partner, etc.

Types of Housing

Single-family home, apartment, trailer, duplex, "double/triple-decker," condo, townhouse, row house, mobile home.

Home is owned/rented, family is living with relatives/living in shelter/homeless.

Family lives in unsafe neighborhood, inadequate housing, adults are concerned they may lose their home/rental support/housing support.

If relevant, note number of bedrooms; whether child shares a room or bed, and if so, with whom; and presence or absence of books, televisions, computers, and age-appropriate toys.

Routines

Mealtimes

Family/caregiver maintains routine times for breakfast/lunch/dinner.

Family eats no/some/most meals together.

Atmosphere at mealtimes is happy/angry/quiet/noisy/filled with frequent fighting/animated conversations/arguments.

Chores

Setting table, washing dishes, taking out trash, help with grocery shopping, laundry, ironing, putting clothes away, emptying garbage, babysitting younger children, care of pets (walking the dog).

✓ Also comment on appropriateness of chores for age/developmental level, frequency of chores, punishment/reward for chores not done/done.

Sleep

Does/does not take morning/afternoon naps, naps usually last _____ hours/minutes.
Has/does not have a regular night bedtime, has a bedtime but it is inconsistently/infrequently/rarely enforced.

Family Activities

Church/synagogue/mosque/temple attendance, meals, movies, sports/games, vacations, volunteer work, watching television together, etc.

17.2. Parents

Identify which parent (or both) takes primary responsibility for the child regarding school, health problems, doctor visits, discipline, housework.

Employment/Financial Status

✓ Note the parents' employment status as it affects family/child care (e.g., dual-career family, stay-at-home mother/father); also note the effect on the child when a stay-at-home mother/father returns to work.

Flexible/inflexible hours/schedule/working situation.
Happy/unhappy with present employment.
Work stress negatively affects quality of family life.
Father/mother is laid off/unemployed.
Family finances/financial resources are adequate/inadequate.
Family receives public assistance.

Relationship between Parents

Positive, loving/warm, peaceful, affectionate, close, functional.
Critical/accusatory, frequent yelling, controlling, unstable, parents always "dwell on the negative," lack of affection between parents, parents frequently belittle each other, stormy, distant, mismatched.
Abusive (physically/verbally), frequent screaming, slamming doors, physical threats (to divorce/cause harm to someone/leave/leave and take the kids), throwing things, brutal.

17.3. Parenting

Styles

Maccoby and Martin (1983) describe four kinds of parenting styles; these styles, with appropriate descriptors, are as follows:

Authoritarian:

> Rely on coercive techniques (e.g., punishment, threats) for controlling child's behavior, value utmost respect for authority, impose rules and expect obedience, often say things such as "Why? Because I said so."

Permissive:

> Set few limits, make few demands on child, permits child to make his/her own decisions about many routine activities (e.g., amount of TV and video time, mealtimes, bedtimes).

Authoritative:

> Expect child to behave in mature manner, use rewards more than punishment, communicate expectations clearly to child, encourage communication to and from child, explain reasons for rules, allow exceptions when making rules.

Uninvolved:

> Neglectful, uninterested in events or people in child's life (e.g., school, friends), expect little and invest little, are psychologically unavailable to child.

Behaviors/Emotional Tone toward Child

Accepting, friendly/gregarious, helpful, affectionate, courteous/respectful, warm, parent frequently expresses affection toward child, shows enthusiasm toward child's activities, puts child's needs first, responds to child with empathy, is responsive to child's needs, initiates play.

Rejecting, little empathy toward child, affection rarely expressed toward child, child's needs are rarely responded to, punitive response to crying, muted/no demonstration of affection.

Dysfunctional, neglectful, angry, negative, violent/abusive.

Discipline

✓ Note who is primarily responsible for disciplining the child, as well as the level of agreement between parents on discipline techniques. For use of a curfew, note its type, its reasonability for age, and the child/teen's reaction to the curfew.

Limits:

> Overprotection/excessive restriction, overpermissiveness/indulgence, unrealistic demands.

Strictness/leniency:

> Rules/no rules on mobility, feeding/eating, interruption by child(ren), table manners, neatness/cleanliness, bedtime, noise, radio/TV, chores, obedience/compliance/aggression, nudity/modesty, masturbation/sex play.

Aggression:

> Inhibit/redirect aggression, encourage child to fight back/defend self, different responses to aggression toward parents/siblings/peers.

Parental differences:

> High/low ratio of maternal to paternal discipline, mother/father views other parent as overly strict, parental conflicts over discipline.

Praise:

Use praise for table manners/obedience/nice play, use praise frequently/often/occasionally/rarely, make no use of praise.

Problematic discipline:

Lack of discipline, inconsistent discipline, harsh/overly severe discipline, fear/hatred of parent, decreased initiative/spontaneity, unstable/erratic values.

Consistency of discipline:

Clear and consistent enforcement of rules, inconsistent in administering punishment, unclear and inconsistent rules, lack of rules/limits.

Methods of discipline:

Ignore problem behavior, redirect child's attention, assign extra chores, time out/send child to room/make child sit on chair, scold, spank, take away toy/activity/special food/television/play dates/allowance/money/access to car, set curfew.

Problematic methods of discipline:

Verbally/physically threaten child, punitive/erratic discipline, unrealistic expectations, isolation, child is hit/kicked/bitten/beaten with/without an object (belt, shoe, paddle, etc.), child is threatened/assaulted with a weapon (knife, gun, etc.), neglect.

17.4. Social Support

Family receives wanted/unwanted support from extended family/friends.

Family has adequate/some/little/no access to practical/logistical/emotional assistance from family/friends, family lacks adequate social support, family has difficulty with acculturation/discrimination.

17.5. Sibling Relationships

Relationship with brother(s)/sister(s) is normal.

Typical sibling rivalry is noted.

Child is picked on/picks on other siblings, often teases/is teased by siblings, siblings are verbally abusive/physically violent toward one another.

Parental expression of favoritism/dislike toward certain child/children in family results in tense/anxious/stressed/strained/negative/confrontational/violent sibling relationships.

18

School

18.1. Physical Environment

School Building

Building is well/poorly maintained, clean/unkempt, is/is not wheelchair-accessible, is located in high-crime/unsafe/safe area, playground is well/adequately/poorly maintained, (no) outside play areas.
School is small/medium/large in size, with a total student population of _____.

Classroom

Note any problematic aspects of the physical classroom environment, such as temperature, lighting, noise level, or condition/cleanliness; also describe the classroom's physical arrangement.

18.2. Classroom Climate

Class Size

Note number of students, teachers, aides, and/or other adults.

Schedule

Note length of classroom day, number of days per week (for preschool/kindergarten), subjects taught (length of sessions), and amount of free time/playground time.

Classroom Resources

Adequate/inadequate number of chairs/desks/tables/chalkboards/bulletin boards.
Room arranged in rows of desks with teacher in front, desks arranged in circle, no desks/only tables in classroom, open classroom.
Classroom resources are/are not adequate/appropriate for children's academic needs.
Classroom resources include computers, TVs, radios, audiocassette and/or videocassette players/CD players (specify number of each), adequate/inadequate number of textbooks/library books/worksheets/instructional materials.

18.3. Classroom Group Dynamics

General Group Climate

Nature of relationships between children:

Children tend to get along with one another well/poorly, very cohesive/noncohesive class of children.

Child's position in group climate:

Leader/follower, bossy, has difficulty/no difficulty entering group situations, is frequently angry/annoying/agitated/irritating/bothersome/passive/calm/relaxed/quiet in group activities.

Reaction of group toward teacher:

Positive/negative/etc. (specify).

Transitions(i.e., routines for finishing/beginning work, putting away or getting out materials, and lining up for recess/lunch):

Smooth/easy, well-structured/well-ordered, uneventful/without incident, chaotic/disordered/disorganized, confusing to some/most/all students, hectic/frenzied, topsy-turvy, resulted in unruly behavior from a few/some/all students.

Child's reaction to transition times:

Has no/some/much difficulty transitioning from one activity to another, reacts to transitions by crying/refusing to participate/shutting down/having tantrums.

18.4. Child's/Parents' Attitudes

Child's Attitudes toward School

Child comes to school ready to learn, curious/interested/energetic/eager, distracted/anxious, uninterested/bored, angry/hostile, wanting/not wanting to learn new things, fearful of failure.

✓ As appropriate, note not only the child's general attitude toward school, but her/his favorite/least favorite subjects and easiest/hardest subjects. Are the subjects offered at the school appropriate/inappropriate for this child's needs?

Child's Attitudes toward Academic Achievement

Child feels that the quality of his/her schoolwork matches his/her abilities/efforts/is satisfactory, views self as underachieving/overachieving, perceives schoolwork as challenging/overwhelming.
Child's school achievement is consistent with/higher than/lower than ability level would indicate.

Child's Attitude toward Teacher

Child likes/does not like/feels neutral about teacher, child feels liked/favored/punished/"picked on"/disliked/treated unfairly by teacher.

Parental Involvement in School

Parents do/do not regularly attend parent–teacher conferences/open houses/other school events, mother/father/both parents active/inactive in school activities, never/rarely/sometimes/often volunteer for classroom/school roles/projects.
Parents uninvolved in school/have never been in contact with teacher, teacher has never tried to contact parents.
Teacher has tried but been unable to contact/meet with parents.

Dropping Out of School

Note whether child/teen dropped out of school before completing high school, along with factors contributing to dropping out of school:

Suspension, poor grades, lack of motivation, dislike of school, pregnancy, marriage, other (specify).

Also note last grade completed, as well as date/month/year of last date of school attendance.

18.5. Teacher

Expectations

Teacher has overly high/high/low/appropriate/inappropriate expectations for students, teacher teaches "down" to students/"over their heads."

Quality of Teaching

Excellent/good/poor, mismatch between child and teacher's style/academic level.

Teaching Style

Authoritative, permissive, authoritarian, interactive/involving, academically challenging, reinforcing, teacher frequently/sometimes/rarely/never praises students, expresses warmth toward students/is personable with students, is distant/cool with students.

Discipline

Teacher spends much/little time in discipline, teacher has good/poor control of classroom and thus little/much time is spent on disciplining students, teacher imposes appropriate/inappropriate/excessive discipline.

Homework/Assignments

As relevant, note the frequency, regularity, quality, and quantity of homework assigned.

Homework is regularly/irregularly/often/sometimes/rarely assigned.
Assignments generally require an excessive/large/average/moderate/small/negligible amount of study time in school/out of school.
Assignments are usually/often/sometimes/rarely/almost never relevant to classwork, assignments tend to be busywork.

Special Education Services   *See Section 12.16, "Special Education," services.*

19

Social and Work Relationships, Recreational Activities

19.1. General Social and Developmental Considerations

The initial descriptions at each bullet below are normal developmental patterns in children's social relationships and are drawn from Bee (1997) and Bukato and Daehler (1998).

Infancy

- Infants show signs of being interested in other infants beginning at age 6 months.

    Looks at other infants with interest/curiosity/attention/awareness/inquisitiveness/alertness/responsiveness, does not look at other infants, shows no interest in other infants, responds to other infants with indifference/unresponsiveness/apathy/lack of interest.

Preschool

- Activities with friends usually consist of pretend play, game playing, object sharing.

    Engages in pretend play/game playing/etc. with friends, shares objects with friends, is unable to engage in pretend play with friends, prefers to play alone, does not share with other children.

- By age 3 or 4 years, children prefer to play with peers rather than alone.

Elementary School

- Playing or being with friends occupies much of children's nonschool time.

    Frequently/infrequently plays with friends out of school, plays with friends outside of school for approximately _____ hours/afternoons/days per week, rarely/never has play dates after school.

- Most play is segregated by sexes.

Middle School

- Friendships are motivated by desire for peer acceptance and avoidance of peer rejection.
- Cross-sex friendships are rare, but begin to appear as children enter adolescence.

Adolescence

- Intimacy is important in friendships.
- Adolescents value the ability to self-disclose and share feelings with friends.
- Prefer same-sex friends, although cross-sex friendships are more common than in middle school.

19.2. Play

Parten (1932) has classified children's play as follows:

Unoccupied play—child is unengaged, may stand in corner, looks around room.
Solitary play—child plays alone, engrossed in activity but independent of other children (common at ages 2–3 years).
Onlooker play—child avidly watches other children's play without entering into their experience.
Parallel play—child plays separately from other children, but with similar materials to other children (e.g., two children independently playing on the floor with trucks).
Associative play—play that involves social interaction with very little organizational quality.
Cooperative play—play with social interaction that includes a sense of group identity and organization.

Types of Play

The following grouping includes several of Parten's types (see above), as well as several others.

Solitary play, parallel play, cooperative play, social pretend play or sociodramatic play, rough-and-tumble play, sensory–motor play, practice play, pretend/symbolic play, social play, constructive play, game playing.

Common Difficulties

Often ends up playing alone but would prefer to play with other children.
Becomes anxious in social gatherings with peers (e.g., birthday parties, playground).
Can play fairly well with another child on a one-to-one basis.
Engages frequently in rough play.
Fights frequently with playmates.
Is controlling when playing with friends.
Is easily overstimulated in play.

19.3. Friendships

Child initiates/accepts/enjoys play dates with peers, is able to compromise well with friends, is a child who can both follow and lead, is well liked and accepted by a wide range of children/most children in the class, has extremely good social skills, makes friends easily, has no difficulty making friends, is seen as a leader by her/his peers, is frequently invited for play dates, social interactions with peers are satisfactory, _____ is said to have many friends.

The child does not make the best choices regarding his/her friendships, is a follower to inappropriate friends, becomes obsessed with certain friends.

Fights frequently with playmates, prefers to play with younger children, has a few adequate friendships/has only one friend, has a history of problems playing with other children.

Child has "no" friends, has difficulty making/keeping friends due to extreme angry outbursts/inability to share/problems reading nonverbal cues/difficulty modulating affect/other (specify).

Has a pervasive pattern of detachment from social relationships.

19.4. Peer Groups/Dating

Types of Peer Social Groups

Popular children, neglected/rejected children, cliques, athletes/"jocks," "druggies," "geeks," "Goths," "dweebs," "brains"/"nerds," "preppies," "loners," "losers," "partyers."

Positive Peer Group Experiences

Stands up for the "underdog" in peer settings, is well liked/popular/accepted/admired by peers.

Problems with Peer Relationships/Groups

Is often the last to be chosen as a partner in school.

Is teased/"picked on" by several of her/his peers, is bullied, has trouble fitting in with classmates.

Shows relational aggression (e.g., "You can't come to my birthday party").

Substance Use in Peer Groups

Report frequency of drug use, smoking, and underage drinking, as well as the effects of these on functioning. Asking initially about friends'/peer group's substance use is less threatening. Note quantity of each substance consumed per episode.

Dating

Note the age at which dating began; the frequency or pattern of dating behavior and whether the pattern is appropriate/inappropriate for age/developmental level; and whether the adolescent has an exclusive boyfriend/girlfriend relationship (i.e., is "going steady").

Dating intensity:

Never, seldom/rarely, only for special times (e.g., prom, special dances), "gets together with," interested in more dates but _____ (specify), frequently, compulsively/promiscuously, many dating partners, has many/only brief relationships, has had a long-term monogamous relationship since age ____, "going steady."

Other qualities:

Experiences physical/verbal/emotional abuse, is exploited by boyfriend/girlfriend (describe), is in relationship that is inappropriate/too serious/too sexual in nature for age, unsatisfying, symbiotic, stable, functional, adequate, satisfying, rewarding, close/tight, intimate, enhancing, loving/fulfilling.

19.5. Work/Employment

Note the employer's name; numbers of hours worked outside of school; type of job; appropriateness of work/job for developmental age; effects of work on school performance (i.e., whether grades are same/lower/higher); and relationship with supervisors/coworkers.

Attitude toward Work

Conscientious/average/negligent, is responsive/resistant toward supervision or constructive feedback, dislikes working, prefers working to attending school.

Work Skills

Performance is/skills are poor/average/good/exceptional, exhibits quite mature/immature work skills/habits for age.

Motivation to Work

Refuses, apathetic/indifferent, is only minimally motivated/compliant/positive/eager, willing to work at tasks seen as monotonous or unpleasant.

Work Attendance

Unreliable/inadequate/minimal/spotty/deficient, has unusual/large number of unexcused absences/calls in sick, seldom/generally punctual for arrival/breaks/lunch hours, performs without excessive tardiness/rest periods/time off/absences/interruptions from psychological symptoms, dependable/responsible.

Relationship to Peers/Coworkers

Avoidant/distant/shy/self-conscious, nervous, conflictual, domineering, submissive, competitive, suspicious, attention-seeking, clowning/immature/provocative, inappropriate, dependent, troublemaker, ridiculing/teasing, friendly.

19.6. Recreational Activities

General Statements

Favorite activities include _____ (specify).
Least favorite activities are _____ (specify).
Recent changes in activity level from _____ to _____ (specify).
Child has no hobbies/no recreational activities, does nothing for relaxation/fun, very few pleasurable activities.
Child takes typical interest in recreation, has active and satisfying recreational life.
Recreation is integrated into school and social life.

Types of Activities

Collections:

Baseball/Yu-Gi-Oh/etc. cards, dolls, books, shells, rocks, etc.

Friends:

"Hanging out" with, playing with, going to the movies/the mall/etc. with, playing sports/ etc. with.

Games:

Chess, Yu-Gi-Oh, computer games, video games, Game Boy/Nintendo/PlayStation, board games. puzzles, other (specify).

Hobbies:

Art/drawing/painting, building things/models, crafts, watching TV, sewing, photography, writing, cooking/baking, other (specify).

Music:

Likes listening to music, enjoys playing the piano/guitar/etc., takes piano/guitar/etc. lessons.

Pets:

Plays with pet dog/cat/bird/fish/rabbit/etc., cares for pet.

Playing:

Dolls/dollhouse, playing on scooter/trampoline/other (specify), outdoor play, make-believe play, playing at the park, playing dress-up.

Reading:

Enjoys reading/likes being read to, favorite book is _____ (specify), favorite types of reading materials are books/magazines/comics/anime/picture books/mysteries/horror/adventure/science fiction/nonfiction/other (specify).

✓ Note amount of time child reads in a week, as well as number of books read in last month.

Sports:

Watches on TV, attends/spectates, reads about, discusses.
Participates in ballet, baseball, basketball, biking, bowling, cheerleading, dancing, fishing, golf, gymnastics, hockey, in-line skating, jogs, karate, lacrosse, runs, skateboarding, skiing, snowboarding, soccer, softball, swimming, Tai kwon do, t-ball, tennis, walks, weightlifting.

Quality of sports participation:

Is talented in sports; was noted to be a very good athlete; is star player on the _____ team.
Loves sports and is very coordinated.
Has trouble with good sportsmanship/losing/playing fair/playing within the rules because of problems with emotional arousal/lack of competitive drive/difficulty with social skills/other (specify).
Has difficulty participating in sports because of poor gross motor skills and lack of coordination.

Toys:

Legos, K'NEX, dolls, stuffed animals, blocks, cars/trucks, other (specify).

Volunteering:

Volunteers in church-related activities, with charity-based organizations, other (specify).

Organizations

Boy/Girl Scouts, Boys and Girls Clubs, Camp Fire, Cub Scouts/Brownies, 4-H, Future Farmers of America (FFA), Junior Achievement, school newspaper, Young Democrats/Republicans, Little League, school clubs (specify).

E. Test Results

20

General Guidelines
for Presenting Test Results
in a Report

This chapter covers general aspects of presenting test results in a report, including the reporting of scores. It provides the reader with general descriptors common to many tests/evaluations, while Chapters 21–28 address more specific areas of testing/evaluation.

20.1. Validity Statements

The following validity statements apply specifically to test results. (*For general statements about validity, see Section 7.6.*)

Adequate Validity

Throughout the evaluation process, the child appeared to put forth the necessary effort to consider this an adequate interpretation of his/her functioning level and abilities.

During the testing sessions the child exhibited good effort and motivation, and these findings are therefore considered a valid estimate of her/his current cognitive/neuropsychological/psychological status.

_____ (give name of test) appears to be a valid measure of intellectual/language/visual–spatial/emotional/other (specify) functioning, as the child was an attentive and cooperative participant.

Concentration and attention to the test items were noted to be consistent and appropriate, and thus test results are felt to be an accurate assessment of his/her current level of functioning.

Inadequate Validity

The severity of this child's inattentiveness/hyperactivity/impulsivity/etc. had a negative impact on her/his test performance; consequently, these data are likely to represent an underestimate of her/his current capacity.

The child did not appear motivated on the testing, and the examiner therefore questions whether the scores are true indications of his/her ability.

When confronted with more difficult tasks, the child refused to continue or did not appear to try her/his best, and consequently the results should be viewed with caution.

20.2. Test Scores: Description

Test results are computed in various ways: as grade equivalents, as percentile ranks, and as scaled and standard scores. When you are reporting test scores, always include an explanation of which type(s) of scores you are using (standard, scaled, etc.), including the mean and standard deviation.

There are no hard and fast rules for how to describe test results. Much depends upon the results; sometimes it may be to the child's advantage to present the scores within a range, but at other times a specific score may be indicated. This is similar for the question of grade equivalents and standard scores: Some tests give results using standard scores, while others give grade equivalents, and still others provide both. There are no specific times when either is appropriate or not appropriate. The decision really depends on personal preference and the type of scores provided by the test itself.

Grade Equivalents

A grade equivalent indicates that a child's performance resembles the average performance at a particular grade level. Grade equivalents are typically presented in decimal form; for example, 4.2 means that the child is functioning at a level typical for a student in the second month of fourth grade.

Percentile Ranks

A percentile rank score compares the child's performance to that of other children his/her age. It represents the percentage of the population who did less well than the child being tested—that is, the percentage of same-age or same-grade peers in a norm group who were found to score below the score obtained by the tested child. For example, a percentile rank of 70 indicates that an individual performed better than 70% of peers taking the test.

Scaled Scores

Scaled scores on subtests are based on comparison with the scores of same-age peers in a norm group and can range from 1 to 19, with an average of 10 and a standard deviation of 3. Scaled scores between 8 and 12 fall within the average range.

Standard Scores

Standard scores for IQs on the Wechsler scales (the WAIS-III, WISC-IV, and WPPSI-III), and also on the most recent revision of the Stanford–Binet (SB5) have a mean of 100 and standard deviation of 15. Roughly two-thirds of all individuals will obtain a score between 85 and 115. Standard scores between 85–90 and 110–115 are often considered "average," although these may be significantly below or above expectations for a particular individual. (*Section 20.5 presents more detailed classification ratings for IQs on the Wechsler scales and the SB5.*)

Confidence Intervals

A confidence interval (CI) encompasses a standard score plus and minus 1 standard error of measurement (SEM). This range is a ____% confidence band. In other words, one can be confident that ____% of the time the subject's "true score" will fall within this range.

20.3. Sample Statements of Test Results

On the _____ (give name of the test), the child achieved a Full Scale IQ of ____. The likelihood that his/her true score falls between ____ and ____ is about ____%. This score places him/her in the _____ range of psychometric intelligence. His/her Verbal Comprehension Index was ____ (____ percentile), in the _____ range; his/her Nonverbal/Perceptual Reasoning Index was ____ (____ percentile) in the _____ range. The difference between the two IQ/Index scores was/was not statistically significant.

The child's scores are as follows and are reported as standard scores and percentile ranks for each of the tests. Standard scores have a mean of 100 and a standard deviation of ±15. Her/his scores range from the ____ to the ____ percentile.

20.4. Describing Verbal–Nonverbal Discrepancies

There is a ____-point discrepancy between the child's Verbal IQ/Verbal Comprehension Index and Nonverbal/Performance IQ/Perceptual Reasoning Index, which is statistically significant.

Verbal and NonverbalPerformance IQ scores were significantly different (difference = ____; frequency = ____), with Verbal IQ falling in the _____ range and Nonverbal Performance IQ falling in the _____ range.

A significant discrepancy exists between the two scales, denoting better development of one set of skills (verbal reasoning skills/nonverbal problem-solving abilities) than of the other.

The child demonstrated a significantly higher Verbal IQ than Performance/Nonverbal IQ. These scores indicate that his/her performance was much better on tasks requiring verbal abstractive skills and information gained from the environment than on tasks requiring spatial reasoning and immediate problem-solving skills

20.5. IQ Classification Ratings

Wechsler (2003) provides the following classification ratings for IQs on the Wechsler Scales, which are reproduced here with permission. (These now also apply to the SB5.)

130+	Very superior
120–129	Superior
110–119	High average
90–109	Average
80–89	Low average
70–79	Borderline
69 and below	Intellectually deficient or extremely low

Lezak (1995) gives this classification of ability levels, which is also reproduced here with permission:

Classification	z-score*	Percent included	Lower limit of percentile range
Very superior	+2.0 and above	2.2	98
Superior	+1.3 to 2.0	6.7	91
High average	+0.6 to 1.3	16.1	75
Average	±0.6	50.0	25
Low average	−0.6 to −1.3	16.1	9
Borderline	−1.3 to −2.0	6.7	2
Retarded	−2.0 and below	2.2	—

*z-score represents how many standard deviations the score deviates from the mean.

21

Tests of Intellectual Functioning

This chapter lists and briefly describes the most commonly used tests of intellectual functioning for children. These descriptions can be used in report writing.

21.1. General Facts about Intelligence Test Scores

Intelligence test scores reflect the following:

- Factual knowledge.
- Learned abilities.
- Problem solving.
- Memory.
- Attention.
- Future learning and academic success.

Intelligence test scores do *not* measure these qualities:

- True innate ability or absolute learning potential.
- Motivation, curiosity, creativity, drive, or determination.
- Study skills.
- Achievement in academic subjects.

✓ Note that schools in California cannot use results from IQ tests to assign African American children to any special education program, with the exception of gifted and talented programs (*Larry P. v. Riles*, 1984).

21.2. Bayley Scales of Infant and Toddler Development, Third Edition (Bayley-III)

✓ Note that although it is listed here in the chapter on intellectual functioning, the Bayley-III is not a measure of specific intellectual ability.

General Description

The Bailey-III is a standardized measure of infant development that determines whether a child is progressing normally or in need of intervention.

Scales

The Cognitive Scale provides a measure of how a child explores the world around her/him and a measure of problem solving skills.

The Language Scale measures expressive and receptive communication through observing the child's communication skills and asking him/her to identify pictures and objects, follow directions, and answer questions.

The Motor Scale measures a child's fine and gross motor skills through having her/him complete fine motor tasks such as stacking blocks or reaching and manipulating objects or by assessing gross motor skills such as head control, crawling, walking, and balance.

The Social Emotional Scale measures a child's social–emotional milestones via caregiver report.

The Adaptive Behavior Scale measures (through caregiver report) a child's daily living skills such as communication skills, functional pre-academic skills, and self-direction.

21.3. Detroit Tests of Learning Aptitude—Fourth Edition (DTLA-4)
(Hammill, 1998)

General Descriptions

The DTLA-4 is a measure of general intellectual ability that includes a General Mental Ability Composite, a Linguistic Domain Composite, an Attentional Domain Composite, and a Motoric Domain Composite.

Subtests

Word Opposites measures knowledge of antonyms).
Sentence Imitation measures short-term auditory memory for sentences.
Story Construction assesses short-term auditory memory for stories.
Basic Information covers general factual information.
Word Sequences assesses attention and short-term memory.
Design Sequences measures visual discrimination ability and short-term visual memory.
Reversed Letters assesses attention, memory, and fine motor skills.
Design Reproduction covers attention, short-term memory, visual motor skills)
Symbolic Relations measures abstract reasoning and problem-solving skills.
Story Sequences assesses sequential processing.

21.4. Comprehensive Test of Nonverbal Intelligence (CTONI)
(Hammil, Pearson, & Wiederholt, 1997)

General Description

The CTONI is a test of nonverbal reasoning abilities that is particularly useful with children for whom other intelligence tests are either inappropriate or biased.

Subtests

Pictorial Analogies.
Pictorial Categories.
Pictorial Sequences.

Geometric Analogies.
Geometric Categories.
Geometric Sequences.

Composite Scores

Scores are generally reported as one or more of three composites or Quotients as follows:
The Nonverbal Intelligence Quotient measures analogical reasoning, category classification, and sequential reasoning.
The Pictorial Nonverbal Intelligence Quotient measures problem-solving and reasoning skills, using pictures of familiar objects.
The Geometric Nonverbal Intelligence Quotient is a measure of problem-solving and reasoning skills, using unfamiliar designs.

21.5. Differential Ability Scales, Second Edition (DAS-II)   *(Elliott, 2006)*

General Description

The DAS-II is a measure of overall cognitive functioning.

Sample Statements

The child was administered the DAS-II to assess his/her overall intellectual functioning. The Cognitive Battery of the DAS-II is composed of subtests that yield a General Conceptual Ability (GCA) score, as well as Verbal, Nonverbal Reasoning, and Spatial Cluster scores. These scores have a mean of 100 and a standard deviation of 15. In addition, the DAS-II includes a set of diagnostic subtests, which test memory and information-processing abilities, and a set of achievement tests. Subtest scores are reported as T-scores, which have a mean of 50 and a standard deviation of 10.
On the DAS-II the child achieved a GCA score of ____, which places her/him at the ____ percentile relative to age-mates. This index is a composite score of three factors on which she/he scored as follows: Verbal Cluster of ____, ____ percentile; Nonverbal Reasoning Cluster of ____, ____ percentile; and Spatial Cluster of ____, ____ percentile.

Factors

The Verbal Cluster is a measure of verbal concepts, vocabulary development, expressive language ability, and general knowledge base.
The Nonverbal Reasoning Cluster is a measure of fluid intelligence and nonverbal ability.
The Spatial Cluster is a measure of spatial perception, visual–spatial imagery, and visual–motor coordination.

Core Subtests

Early Number Concepts is a measure of early mathematical ability (e.g., counting, identifying numbers).
Matching Letter-Like Forms is a test of the ability to match items that are similar to letters.
Matrices is a test of nonverbal inductive reasoning and the perception of visual detail and spatial orientation in drawings.
Naming Vocabulary is a test of the ability to name pictorial stimuli.
Pattern Construction is a test of nonverbal reasoning and spatial visualization skills, where the child is asked to construct block designs in response to a stimulus picture.
Phonological Processing measures knowledge of sounds and ability to manipulate sounds.

Picture Similarities is a test of inductive reasoning ability, where the child is asked to match pictures based on their conceptual similarities.

Rapid Naming assesses ability to quickly integrate visual symbols with phonological naming skills.

Recall of Designs assesses short-term visual–spatial memory, perception of spatial orientation, and retention and retrieval of whole visual images.

Sequential and Quantitative Reasoning is a test designed to assess a child's ability to understand sequences of numbers and abstract symbols.

Verbal Comprehension is a measure of the ability to perform simple one- and two-step directives (e.g., "Put a house on each side of the car" or "Give me all the things that have hair").

Verbal Similarities is a test of verbal inductive reasoning.

Word Definitions is a test of a child's knowledge of word meanings as demonstrated through spoken language.

Diagnostic Subtests

Recall of Digits is a test of short-term auditory memory.

Speed of Information Processing is a subtest requiring rapid and efficient visual search.

Recall of Objects (Immediate and Delayed) is a task that requires the child to learn a visually presented list of items over a course of three trials.

Achievement Tests

See Section 22.3, "Differential Ability Scales, Second Edition (DAS-II) Achievement Tests."

21.6. Kaufman Adolescent and Adult Intelligence Test (KAIT)
(Kaufman & Kaufman, 1993)

The KAIT is a test of intelligence for individuals ages 11–85+ years. It assesses crystallized and fluid abilities, as well as mental status and memory.

Core Battery Scales

The Crystallized Scale assesses word knowledge, verbal concept formation, acquired knowledge, and verbal comprehension.

The Fluid Scale measures the ability to learn and apply new information and logical reasoning.

Additional Measures

Four Extended Battery subtests measures immediate versus delayed memory.

A Supplementary Mental Status measure permits an estimate of mental functioning for severely impaired individuals.

21.7. Kaufman Assessment Battery for Children, Second Edition (KABC-II) *(Kaufman & Kaufman, 2004)*

General Descriptions

The KABC-II is a test of intelligence and achievement.

Scales

The Sequential Processing and Short-Term Memory Scale measures a child's ability to solve problems by remembering sequentially presented information.

The Simultaneous/Visual Processing Scale measures a child's ability to solve problems that require the processing of many stimuli at once.
The Learning Ability/Long-Term Storage and Retrieval Scale measures a child's ability to store and retrieve newly learned information.
The Planning/Fluid Reasoning Scale measures a child's nonverbal reasoning skills such as inferential thinking and inductive/deductive reasoning skills.
The Knowledge/Crystallized Ability Scale measures a child's ability to store general knowledge and information, such as vocabulary.

21.8. Stanford–Binet Intelligence Scales, Fifth Edition (SB5) *(Roid, 2003)*

General Description

The SB5 is an assessment instrument that provides a Full Scale IQ, a Verbal IQ, a Nonverbal IQ, and five Composite Scores. Scores are provided as standard scores with a mean of 100 and a standard deviation of 15.

Content Areas

Fluid Reasoning: Measures verbal and nonverbal reasoning skills.
Knowledge: Measures acquired knowledge, such as vocabulary, as well as procedural knowledge.
Quantitative Reasoning: Measures numerical reasoning ability.
Visual–Spatial Processing: Measures visuospatial and nonverbal concept formation.
Working Memory: Measures verbal and visual auditory attention and memory skills.

21.9. Test of Nonverbal Intelligence—Third Edition (TONI-3)
(Brown, Sherbenou, & Johnsen, 1997)

General Description

The TONI-3 is a test that measures nonverbal intelligence, such as nonverbal problem-solving and abstract reasoning abilities

21.10. Wechsler Abbreviated Scale of Intelligence (WASI)
(Psychological Corporation, 1999)

General Description

The WASI provides an estimate of IQ and includes those subtests from the WISC-III and WAIS-III that have the highest loadings on g (general intelligence). It is a brief test of intelligence designed for individuals ages 6–89 years.

Subtests   *See Sections 21.11 and 21.12 for more information on these subtests.*

Vocabulary.
Similarities.
Block Design.
Matrix Reasoning.

21.11. Wechsler Adult Intelligence Scale—Third Edition (WAIS-III)
(Wechsler, 1997a)

General Description

The WAIS-III is a test of intellectual ability for individuals ages 16–89 years.

Sample Statement

This adolescent's WAIS-III profile indicates a Full Scale IQ of ____. His/her Full Scale IQ falls in the _____ range, higher than ____% of peers in his/her age group. The Full Scale IQ can be further broken down into Verbal IQ, Performance IQ, and four Index scores (Verbal Comprehension, Perceptual Reasoning, Working Memory, and Processing Speed).

Index Scores   *See Section 21.12 for information about the Index scores.*

Subtests

Arithmetic is a test of mental arithmetic and numerical reasoning ability.
Block Design is a test of visual–spatial ability and nonverbal concept formation.
Comprehension is a measure of social judgment.
Digit Span is a test of immediate auditory attention and memory.
Digit Symbol/Coding is a test of visual–motor coordination, attention, visual scanning and tracking, and cognitive flexibility.
Information is a test of a person's fund of general information and long-term memory for information.
Letter–Number Sequencing is a test of short-term auditory memory, attention, and information processing.
Matrices is a test of nonverbal reasoning.
Matrix Reasoning is a test of perceptual reasoning ability.
Object Assembly is a test of visual organization ability.
Picture Arrangement is a test in which the individual is asked to use pictures in order to tell a story; it provides a measure of nonverbal reasoning.
Picture Completion is a measure of visual attention to detail, as well as the ability to discriminate between essential and nonessential details.
Similarities is a test of conceptual reasoning, as defined by the capacity to ascribe commonalities between two objects or concepts.
Symbol Search is a test of perceptual discrimination, attention and concentration, and cognitive flexibility.
Vocabulary is a test of word knowledge, fund of information, verbal concept formation, and language development.

21.12. Wechsler Intelligence Scale for Children—Fourth Edition (WISC-IV)   *(Wechsler, 2003)*

General Description

The WISC-IV is a test of intellectual ability for children and adolescents ages 6 years, 0 months to 16 years, 11 months.

Sample Statements

In order to assess overall level of intellectual functioning, the child was administered the WISC-IV. This instrument comprises a set of subtests that yield a Full Scale IQ score, as well as Verbal Comprehension, Perceptual Reasoning, Working Memory, and Processing Speed Index scores. IQ and Index scores share the same scale (i.e., mean of 100 and standard deviation of 15).

The results of the current examination indicate that she/he is performing within the _____ range of overall intellectual functioning (WISC-IV Full Scale IQ = ____, ____ percentile).

The WISC-IV is a battery of 10–15 subtests that provide a profile of intellectual strengths and weaknesses as well as overall intellectual functioning. It is divided into five to eight subtests that require a spoken response, and five to seven subtests that require the child to do something with her/his hands.

Index Scores

The Verbal Comprehension Index measures the ability to make sense of complex verbal information and use verbal abilities to solve novel problems

The Perceptual Reasoning Index measures the ability to analyze visual materials and to solve problems nonverbally, using concrete visual materials.

The Working Memory is a measure of attention, concentration, working memory, and mental alertness.

The Processing Speed Index measures the ability to process simple or routine information rapidly without making errors; it calls for cognitive flexibility, psychomotor speed, and visual selective attention.

Subtests

Arithmetic is a measure of numerical accuracy, reasoning, and mental arithmetic.

Block Design measures visual organization and analysis of part–whole spatial relationships.

Cancellation is a measure of visual alertness and visual scanning ability.

Coding assesses visual–motor coordination, speed, and concentration.

Comprehension provides a general measure of verbal reasoning, comprehension of social situations, and social judgment, as well as knowledge of conventional standards of social behavior.

Digit Span is a measure of immediate auditory memory and sequencing.

Information measures the ability to recall factual information.

Letter–Number Sequencing is a measure of a child's short-term memory, as well as concentration and attention skills.

Matrix Reasoning is a measure of nonverbal problem-solving ability, inductive reasoning, and visual processing.

Picture Completion measures the ability to detect essential details in a visual picture and to differentiate essential from nonessential details.

Picture Concepts is a measure of fluid reasoning and perceptual organization.

Similarities measures the ability to abstract meaningful concepts and relationships from verbally presented material.

Symbol Search is a measure of visual discrimination, scanning speed, and sequential tracking of simple visual information without a primary motor component.

Vocabulary assesses word knowledge, verbal comprehension, ability to verbalize meaningful concepts, and long-term memory.

Word Reasoning provides information about a child's verbal comprehension and general reasoning abilities, as well as the ability to integrate different types of information.

21.13. Wechsler Preschool and Primary Scale of Intelligence—Third Edition (WPPSI-III)   *(Wechsler, 2002)*

General Description

The WPPSI-III is a test of intellectual ability for children ages 2 years, 6 months to 7 years, 3 months.

Sample Statement

The child is currently functioning in the _____ range of intelligence, with a Full Scale IQ of ____ on the WPPSI-III. This places him/her at the ____ percentile relative to others in his/her age group. He/she achieved a Verbal IQ of ____ (____ percentile) and a Performance IQ of ____ (____ percentile), indicating somewhat/significantly better/similar performance on verbal comprehension tasks than on nonverbal tasks such as perceptual organization/immediate problem-solving ability.

Scales

The Verbal Scale assesses a child's ability to reason with words and process verbal information.
The Performance Scale measures a child's understanding of perceptual organization and non-verbal reasoning. On subtests within this scale, the child is asked to manipulate visually abstract and concrete materials.

Subtests

The following are the WPPSI-III subtests for children ages 2 years, 6 months to 3 years, 11 months. The subtests for children ages 4 years, 0 months to 7 years, 3 months include the ones described below plus Vocabulary, Word Reasoning, Matrix Reasoning, Picture Concepts, Coding, Symbol Search, Similarities, Comprehension, and Picture Completion (*see Section 21.12 for descriptions of these*).

Block Design is an abstract visual–motor task, where the child is asked to assemble a design with the help of a visual model.
Information requires the child to answer a broad range of questions dealing with factual information; performance on this test may be influenced by cultural opportunities, outside interests, reading, and school learning.
Object Assembly requires a child to assemble puzzles; it measures a child's skill at synthesis (i.e., the ability to put things together to form familiar objects), as well as visual–motor coordination.
Picture Naming is a test of expressive language ability.
Receptive Vocabulary is a test of word knowledge.

21.14. Wide Range Intelligence Test (WRIT)   *(Glutting, Adams, & Sheslow, 2000)*

General Description

The WRIT is a brief measure of cognitive ability.

Subtests

Vocabulary is a measure of verbal knowledge, where the child is asked to define words.
Verbal Analogies is a measure of conceptual ability, where the child is asked to complete a series of analogies.

Matrices is a measure of nonverbal reasoning ability, where the child is asked to complete a maze by picking one from a group of choices.

Diamonds is a test of visual–spatial ability, where the child is asked to use diamond-shaped pieces to construct designs.

21.15. Woodcock–Johnson III (WJ III) Tests of Cognitive Abilities

(Woodcock, McGrew, & Mather, 2001)

General Description

The WJ III Tests of Cognitive Abilities constitute a battery for measuring general intellectual ability and specific cognitive skills in persons ages 2–90+ years.

Sample Statements

On the standard battery of the WJ III Tests of Cognitive Abilities, the child received a General Intellectual Ability score of _____ (_____ percentile), which placed her/him in the _____ range for children her/his age.

The WJ III Tests of Cognitive Abilities was administered to provide a general overview of the child's cognitive abilities and of strengths and weaknesses in his/her learning style.

The WJ III Tests of Cognitive Abilities were given in order to further assess the child's ability to process information through different learning channels.

Clusters

The Auditory Processing Cluster measures the ability to comprehend auditory patterns and synthesize them into words.

The Comprehension–Knowledge Cluster measures the depth and breadth of knowledge and reasoning, based upon previous learning experiences.

The Fluid Reasoning Cluster measures the application of inductive and deductive reasoning and problem skills in novel tasks.

The Long-Term Retrieval Cluster measures the ability to store and retrieve information from long-term memory.

The Processing Speed Cluster measures the ability to perform automatic cognitive tasks quickly, under pressure to maintain focused attention.

The Short-Term Memory Cluster measures the ability to remember and use auditory information within a short time period.

The Visual Processing Cluster measures the ability to perceive items visually and process visual information, as well as short-term visual recall.

Subtests

Analysis–Synthesis asks a child to apply information from a key available to solve problems.

Concept Formation evaluates a child's ability to find commonalities and rules in a series of items, and the ability to draw conclusions or make inferences.

Cross Out asks a child to match geometric forms.

Delayed Recall—Memory for Names assesses the ability to recall the information presented on the Memory for Names subtest after a delay of several days.

Listening Comprehension measures a child's breadth and depth of knowledge and its effective application.

Memory for Sentences asks a child to listen and repeat a series of sentences that increase in length and complexity; it provides a measure of short-term auditory memory.

Memory for Words asks a child to listen and then repeat a series of unrelated words; it provides another measure of short-term auditory memory.

Numbers Reversed asks a child to repeat a series of digits backward.

Oral Vocabulary asks a child to provide synonyms and antonyms for words presented orally by the examiner; it tests the breadth and depth of previously learned information.

Picture Recognition is a test of short-term visual recall, where the child is asked to scan a series of pictures and then identify previously observed items.

Picture Vocabulary asks a child to identify pictures.

Sound Blending asks a child to blend isolated sounds to form words.

Spatial Relations presents a child with two or three shapes that represent parts of a whole figure, which then need to be identified as parts of the figure.

Verbal Analogies is a measure of comprehension, knowledge, and fluid reasoning skills through the completion of verbal analogies.

Visual Auditory Learning asks a child to associate a name with an illustration.

Visual Closure asks a child to identify illustrations with missing parts.

Verbal Comprehension is a test of word knowledge.

Visual Matching evaluates a child's ability to recognize two similar numbers in a row of six numbers composed of one, two, or three digits; it measures scanning speed or accuracy.

22

Achievement Measures

This chapter lists and briefly describes the most commonly used tests of intellectual functioning for children. These descriptions can be used in report writing. The chapter also includes descriptors for achievement–ability discrepancies.

22.1. Academic Performance Descriptions

Overall Performance

_____ performed well within/significantly above/significantly below intellectual, age, and grade expectations across measures of single-word reading, reading comprehension, spelling, and math calculation.

Reading

Good Performance

The child's reading skills are quite well developed, as indicated by his/her strong performance on the _____ (give name of test).

Poor Performance

On tests of reading comprehension, she/he was noted to rely on pictures for sentence comprehension and to guess on many of the items.

The child's performance indicates that he/she is struggling with attaining the basic skills and concepts necessary to the acquisition of reading.

Her/his performance on tests of reading indicates that she/he does not have the reading skills typically acquired by the beginning/middle/end of ____ grade.

Writing

Good Performance

Writing skills were grade-appropriate/advanced for age, were within/above the average range.

Poor Performance

Writing skills were notable for letter reversals (e.g., b for d) and substitutions of upper- for lower-case letters in words and in his/her name.

Qualitative assessment of spelling performance indicated errors of letter reversal and omission, as well as vowel substitution.

22.2. Achievement–Ability Discrepancies

No Discrepancy

_____'s overall performance on the achievement tests indicates achievement commensurate with expectations in all areas and is not indicative of a formal learning disability.

Discrepancy

_____'s overall level of educational achievement is significantly higher/lower than his/her overall level of intellectual development, based on his/her performance on the _____ (name of test).

22.3. Differential Ability Scales, Second Edition (DAS-II) Achievement Tests   *(Elliott, 2006)*

See Section 21.5 for further information about the DAS-II.

General Description

The Achievement Tests of the DAS-II are administered to determine a child's current level of achievement in three areas: reading, spelling, and arithmetic.

Subtests

Basic Number Skills measures arithmetical reasoning and calculation skills.
Spelling is a measure of spelling ability.
Word Reading measures the ability to read single words.

22.4. Gates–MacGinitie Reading Tests, Fourth Edition (GMRT-4)
(MacGinitie, MacGinitie, Maria, & Dreyer, 2002)

General Description

The GMRT-4 includes measures of Prereading and Beginning reading abilities, as well as timed tests of reading that correspond to a child's grade level (e.g., Level 1 corresponds with the first-grade level). Level 1 uses multiple-choice pictures as answers, while Levels 2 through High School use multiple-choice words, phrases, or sentences as answers.

Subtests

The Vocabulary subtest presents a child with a series of written target words; for each one, he/she needs to determine which of five other words or phrases are closest in meaning to the target word.

The Comprehension subtest asks a child to read a series of written passages; following each passage, the child answers written multiple-choice questions pertaining to the passages' meanings.

Sample Statements

On the GMRT-4 (Level ____), the child was required to read several stories and answer detailed questions about the material. He/she performed above/at/below grade expectations, at a grade equivalent of ____, which placed him/her at the ____ percentile compared to same-age peers.

(For Level 1:) Ability to comprehend what she/he reads was assessed by administering the GMRT-4. On the Vocabulary subtest, the child was asked to find which of several words corresponded to the picture (in a series of items). On the Comprehension subtest, she/he was asked to read a series of short stories, and for each one, to answer questions about its meaning by selecting from three pictorial choices.

(For the Beginning Reading Skills Level:) His/her performance on this test indicated that for all areas assessed—including ability to recognize initial consonants and consonant clusters in words, ability to recognize vowel sounds, ability to utilize sentence context to read, and ability to identify final consonants and consonant clusters—he/she performed at the ____ percentile.

22.5. Gray Oral Reading Tests (GORT-4)   *(Wiederholt & Bryant, 2001)*

General Description

The Gort-4 is a timed test of oral reading rate, accuracy, fluency, and comprehension, in which the child is asked to read passages of increasing difficulty aloud.

Sample Statements

The GORT-4 was administered to evaluate the child's reading rate, accuracy, fluency, and comprehension. She/he was asked to read several passages out loud. An overall reading ability computed for each passage by combining the fluency score (rate plus accuracy) with the comprehension score.

Performance on the passage scores of the GORT-4 is far above/below grade expectations.

Performance on this test reveals that the rate and accuracy of his/her contextual reading are at the ____ percentile for children his/her age, and that his/her reading level is at/above/below what would be expected for a child at the end of ____ grade.

Poor Performance

Oral reading was labored and slow, even on simple passages.

Reading was not always fluent, because the child was impulsive/did not attend to what she/he was reading/had difficulty decoding words.

The child's performance indicated that this task was much too difficult for him/her, as he/she was unable to read any of the passages.

The child skipped words or phrases/repeated words or phrases/had trouble sounding out unfamiliar words/substituted or omitted words.

22.6. Lindamood Auditory Conceptualization Test, Third Edition (LAC-3) *(Lindamood & Lindamood, 2004)*

General Description

The LAC-3 is a test of phonological processing that requires the child to represent sounds with colored blocks and then manipulate those blocks as the order of the sounds is changed; it assesses underlying auditory analysis skills, which are important to phonetic reading skills and success.

Sample Statements

The child's phonological skills were assessed through administration of the LAC-3, where he/she was presented with phonemes in isolated patterns or syllable patterns and was asked to use blocks to indicate the number, sequence, and similarity/difference of sounds.

Poor Performance

She/he had difficulty perceiving distinct consonant, vowel, and combination sounds and then sequencing these sounds by associating them with different-colored blocks.

His/her performance was equivalent to the suggested minimum for children at the beginning/middle/end of kindergarten and far below grade expectations. Children scoring below minimum recommended scores have been found to have difficulty meeting grade-level reading expectations.

22.7. Nelson–Denny Reading Test *(Brown, Fishco, & Hanna, 1993)*

General Description

The Nelson–Denny Reading Test is a measure of vocabulary, comprehension, and reading rate for adolescents (grade 9 and up) and adults.

Subtests

The Comprehension subtest asks the individual to read a series of written passages. After each passage, the person responds to multiple-choice pictures pertaining to the passage's meaning. The first minute of the Comprehension subtest is used to determine reading rate.

The Vocabulary subtest asks the individual to read target words and determine which of five other words are closest in meaning to the target words.

22.8. Slosson Test of Reading Readiness *(Perry & Vitali, 1991)*

General Description

The Slosson is a screen of reading readiness abilities that includes the ability to name upper- and lower-case letters, match upper- and lower-case letters, match word forms, provide rhymes for words, identify beginning sounds in words, sequence a story, and provide opposites.

22.9. Test of Early Mathematics Ability (TEMA-3)   *(Ginsburg & Baroody, 2003)*

General Description

The TEMA-3 is a measure of math and premath abilities such as numbering skills, numeral literacy, understanding of number facts, calculation skills, and understanding of number concepts.

Sample Statements

The child performed in the average/above-average/below-average range on the TEMA-3, a measure of early mathematical abilities (e.g., counting, identifying numbers, simple addition).

On the TEMA-3, _____ performed at the ____ percentile, with a Math Quotient of ____.

22.10. Test of Written Language (TOWL-3)—Third Edition
(Hammill & Larsen, 1996)

General Description and Subtests

The TOWL-3 is a measure of writing competence that includes the following subtests: Vocabulary, Spelling, Style, Logical Sentences, Sentence Combining, Contextual Conventions, Contextual Language, and Story Construction.

For the Spontaneous Formats portion of the TOWL-3, a child is asked to write a story describing a scene. This story provides the scores for the Contextual Language, Contextual Conventions, and Story Construction subtests. This test is a good indicator of the child's ability to write stories/essays and take notes in class.

Good Performance

On the TOWL-3 Story Construction subtest, the child was able to formulate a reasonably coherent story.

The child's overall performance on the TOWL-3 indicated good written vocabulary and writing skills.

Poor Performance

On the TOWL-3, the child's written output was markedly below expectations based on age and grade level. His/her simple story was unreadable due to numerous spelling errors.

Qualitatively, her/his handwriting was quite poor, and her/his written narrative contained numerous spelling errors.

22.11. Wechsler Individual Achievement Test—Second Edition (WIAT-II)   *(Wechsler, 2001)*

General Description

The WIAT-II is a comprehensive individually administered battery for assessing achievement in a wide variety of curriculum areas.

Subtests

Listening Comprehension assesses receptive language skills; a child listens to a word or sentence and points to a picture that describes the word or sentence, or looks at a picture and responds with the correct word.

Math Reasoning is a test of a child's ability to solve oral or written mathematical problems regarding time, money, measurement, graph reading, and geometry.

Numerical Operations is a test of a child's ability to complete written math problems correctly, including addition, subtraction, multiplication, and division.

Oral Expression is a measure of such skills as the ability to describe a picture or to give directions; a child is asked to repeat sentences, tell a story based on a series of pictures, and list words that match a particular topic.

Pseudoword Decoding is a measure of phonetic decoding skills.

Reading Comprehension is a measure of the ability to comprehend what has been read; a child is asked to read sentences and short paragraphs and answer questions about these passages, such as the main idea, specific details, or the order of events.

Spelling is a measure of the ability to spell orally presented words correctly.

Word Reading asks a child (depending on his/her age) to read words, identify letters of the alphabet, identify letter sounds, or find rhymes for words.

Written Expression asks a child to write words, sentences, and a short essay in response to a topic; writing is evaluated on organization, vocabulary, theme development, and mechanics (e.g., spelling and punctuation).

22.12. Wide Range Achievement Test—Fourth Edition (WRAT4)
(Wilkinson & Robertson, 2006)

General Description

The WRAT4 is a measure of achievement in the areas of reading, spelling, and arithmetic.

Subtests

Word Reading measures a child's ability to read printed words or identify letters.

Sentence Comprehension measures a child's ability to comprehend written sentences through the use of a modified cloze technique.

Spelling measures a child's ability to spell dictated letters or words.

Math Computation measures a child's basic math skills such as counting, solving simple oral problems, or completing written math problems.

22.13. Woodcock–Johnson III (WJ III) Tests of Achievement
(Woodcock, McGrew, & Mather, 2001)
See Section 21.15 for information about the WJ III Tests of Cognitive Abilities.

General Description

The WJ III Tests of Achievement are individually administered tests that measure educational achievement.

Subtests

Academic Knowledge is a measure of a child's knowledge in several academic subjects.

Applied Problems is a test of quantitative ability that requires a child to analyze and solve practical problems in mathematics. The information is presented to the child both orally and in written text.

Calculation is a paper-and-pencil test of quantitative abilities, such as the ability to comprehend mathematical concepts and perform numerical operations such as subtraction, addition, multiplication, and division.

Dictation measures an individual's skill in providing written knowledge of letter forms, spelling, punctuation, and capitalization.

Editing requires a child to identify and correct errors in written passages (e.g., punctuation, word use, capitalization); it focuses on language development and English usage.

Letter–Word Identification is a measure of reading skills that asks a child to identify isolated letters and words.

Math Fluency is a timed measure of math ability.

Oral Comprehension is a test of receptive language development.

Passage Comprehension measures a child's ability to read a short passage and identify a missing key word; it assesses comprehension and vocabulary skills.

Picture Vocabulary is a measure of word knowledge.

Punctuation and Capitalization is a measure of the ability to apply punctuation and capitalization rules.

Quantitative Concepts is a measure of quantitative reasoning and mathematical concepts.

Reading Fluency is a measure of reading speed.

Reading Vocabulary measures comprehension at the single-word level; it requires a child to read isolated words and supply antonyms or synonyms in response to the words presented.

Spelling measures a child's ability to write letters and words that are presented orally to her/him.

Sound Awareness is a test of phonological ability.

Spelling of Sounds is a measure of phonological and orthographic coding ability.

Story Recall is a measure of receptive and expressive language.

Understanding Directions is a test of language development and listening ability.

Word Attack is a test that requires a child to sound out nonsense words; it measures phonics skills.

Writing Fluency is a timed (7-minute) test that requires a child to formulate as many short sentences as she/he can from words and pictures grouped to stimulate sentence production; it is a good indication of a child's ability to write stories, essays, and take notes in class.

Writing Samples measures a child's skill in writing responses to a variety of demands; the child is not judged on the mechanics of writing, but rather on the quality of his/her written expression.

22.14. Woodcock Reading Mastery Tests—Revised (WRMT-R)
(Woodcock, 1998)

General Description

The WRMT-R is a test battery of reading skills.

Subtests

Passage Comprehension is a structured test of reading comprehension; it consists of short passages (one or two sentences) with a word missing that the examinee is requested to supply.

Visual–Auditory Learning is a measure of the ability to form relationships between oral responses and visually presented stimuli.

Letter Identification is a test of the ability to identify upper- and lower-case letters.

Word Attack measures the ability to apply phonetics to written language when presented with nonsense words.

Word Identification is a test of the ability to read isolated words.

Word Comprehension measures a child's knowledge of synonyms, antonyms, and analogies.

23

Tests of Language Functioning

This chapter lists and briefly describes the most commonly used tests of language functioning for children. Suggested phrasings for reporting results are also given. See also the following sections of in Chapters 21 and 22 for descriptions of subtests and composites that measure language ability: 21.5 (DAS-II Word Definitions, Similarities); 21.11 and 21.12 (WAIS-III and WISC-IV Similarities, Vocabulary, Comprehension, Information); 21.12 WISC-IV Word Reasoning and Verbal Comprehension Index); and 22.11 (WIAT-II Listening Comprehension).

23.1. Boston Naming Test (BNT) *(Kaplan, Goodglass, & Weintraub, 1983)*

General Description

The BNT is a test of confrontation naming.

Sample Statements

Word retrieval skills on the BNT were average/high average/below average/etc. (____/60; mean = ____; standard deviation = ____).

Vocabulary knowledge was assessed by administering a test of basic expressive language skills, the BNT.

Expressive vocabulary was assessed on the BNT, a test in which the child is presented with a series of line drawings of objects (e.g., wheelchair, camel, cactus) and is asked to provide a name for each one.

On the BNT, which evaluates naming and word retrieval, the child scored within the _____ range for his/her age.

Confrontation naming on the BNT was in the _____ range.

23.2. Bracken Basic Concept Scale—Revised (BBCS-R) *(Bracken, 1998)*

General Description

The BBCS-R is a measure of children's receptive language skills and language concept acquisition.

Subtests

Colors assesses the ability to name colors.

Comparisons assesses the ability to match objects depending on their most important characteristics.

Directions and position assesses knowledge of terms related to directions.

Letters assesses upper- and lower-case letter identification skills.

Numbers and Counting is a test of the ability to recognize numbers and assign number values to groups of objects.

Quantity measures concepts regarding amounts and dimensions.

Self/Social Awareness assesses knowledge of personal–social categories and emotional values.

Shapes assesses the ability to identify shape concepts.

Sizes assesses understanding of size concepts.

Texture/Materials measures the ability to apply concepts regarding attributes of objects.

Time/Sequence assesses abilities relating to temporal or sequential events.

23.3. Clinical Evaluation of Language Fundamentals— Fourth Edition (CELF-4)

General Description

The CELF-4 assesses a child's knowledge of word meanings, knowledge of word and sentence structure (morphology and syntax), and the recall and retrieval of spoken language (memory).

Sample Statements

Language form and content were evaluated on the CELF-4.

Word meanings (semantics), word and sentence structure (morphology and syntax), and recall of spoken language (auditory memory) were evaluated on the CELF-4.

23.4. Controlled Oral Word Association Test (COWAT)   *(Benton, 1968)*

General Description

COWAT assesses verbal fluency by measuring responses to both phonemic cues (FAS) and semantic cues (Animals).

Sample Statements

The child was administered the COWAT, consisting of two tests of verbal fluency that require the individual to initiate and sustain attention. On a test of letter fluency, he/she was asked to rapidly generate a list of words beginning with each of three letters. On a category fluency task, he/she was asked to rapidly generate a list of animals within a time limit.

The child performed in the _____ range on a task that required her/him to generate words to a phonemic cue (FAS = ____ words; ____ percentile) and semantic cue (Animals = ____ words; ____ percentile).

On the FAS subtest, word fluency was low-average/average/high-average/etc. (____ words in 3 minutes).

On the Animals subtest, semantic fluency was within/below/above normal limits (____ animals in 1 minute).

23.5. Expressive One-Word Picture Vocabulary Test (EOWPVT), 2000 Edition   *(Brownell, 2000a)*

General Description

The EOWPVT measures the ability to fluently name pictures of familiar objects.

Sample Statements

On a test of expressive vocabulary (the EOWPVT), the child achieved a score of ____, indicating vocabulary skills above/at/below age level.

23.6. Expressive Vocabulary Test (EVT)   *(Williams, 1997)*

General Description

The EVT is a measure of expressive vocabulary and word retrieval skills.

Sample Statements

The EVT was given to assess the child's single-word expressive vocabulary knowledge and related word retrieval abilities. On the test, he/she was presented with a series of pictures and given this carrier phrase for each one: "Tell me another word for _____."

On the EVT, the child is shown a series of pictures, one at a time. For each picture, a word is provided to describe the picture, and the child is asked to give another word that means the same thing.

23.7. Illinois Test of Psycholinguistic Abilities— Third Edition (ITPA-3)   *(Hammill, Mather, & Roberts, 2001)*

General Description

The ITPA-4 is a measure of children's spoken and written language, including oral language, writing, reading, and spelling.

23.8. Oral and Written Language Scales (OWLS)   *(Carrow-Woolfolk, 1995)*

General Description

The OWLS is a test of receptive and expressive language.

Subtests

Listening Comprehension provides a measure of vocabulary, grammar skills, and verbal thinking skills.

Oral Expression measures the accuracy of the structure of language and the capacity to articulate and elaborate ideas.

Written Expression assesses the ability to use correct writing conventions.

23.9. Peabody Picture Vocabulary Test—Third Edition (PPVT-III)
(Dunn & Dunn, 1997)

General Description

The PPVT-III is a test of single-word receptive vocabulary.

Sample Statements

The PPVT-III tests receptive vocabulary by asking the child to select the picture that illustrates each word read by the examiner.

The PPVT-III was administered to assess the child's single-word receptive vocabulary skill knowledge. He/she was asked to point to each stimulus item named, from a field of four pictures.

The PPVT-III assesses knowledge of general word meaning by asking the child to identify words through pointing to the corresponding picture. The test is also a good indicator of verbal intelligence.

23.10. Receptive One-Word Picture Vocabulary Test (ROWPVT), 2000 Edition   *(Brownell, 2000b)*

General Description

The ROWPVT is a measure of receptive vocabulary skills.

Sample Statements

The ROWPVT was given to assess the child's single-word receptive vocabulary skills. On this test, the child was asked to choose a picture that best matched a target word given by the examiner.

23.11. Test of Adolescent and Adult Language— Third Edition (TOAL-3)   *(Hammill, Brown, Larsen, & Wiederholt, 1994)*

The TOAL-3 is a measure of language functioning that includes tests of listening, speaking, reading, writing, spoken language, written language, vocabulary, grammar, receptive language, and expressive language.

23.12. Test for Auditory Comprehension of Language— Third Edition (TACL-3)   *(Carrow-Woolfolk, 1999)*

General Description

The TACL-3 is a measure of auditory comprehension of receptive language, which assesses knowledge such as syntax, sentence structure, oral vocabulary, and morphemes.

Sample Statements

The TACL-3 was administered to further assess the child's understanding of specific word and sentence structures.

23.13. Test of Early Language Development—Third Edition (TELD-3)
(Hresko, Reid, & Hammill, 1999)

General Description

The TELD-3 is a measure of oral language for very young children.

Subtests

Expressive Language assesses a child's ability to produce oral language (e.g., semantics, syntax).

Receptive Language assesses a child's understanding of spoken language.

23.14. Test of Language Development—Intermediate: Third Edition (TOLD-I:3)   *(Newcomer & Hammill, 1997a)*

General Description

The TOLD-I:3 is a measure of overall language abilities for older children (ages 8 years, 0 months to 12 years, 11 months).

Subtests

General measures the ability to identify the relationship among three words.

Grammatic Comprehension assesses the ability to recognize ungrammatical spoken language.

Malapropisms measures the ability to recognize when a word has been incorrectly used in place of a word that sounds similar to it.

Picture Vocabulary is an assessment of the ability to understand the meaning of two-word spoken phrases.

Sentence Combining measures the ability to combine two to four short, simple sentences into one complex or compound sentence without changing the meaning.

Word Ordering assesses the ability to construct a meaningful sentence from a set of words presented orally in a random sequence.

23.15. Test of Language Development—Primary (TOLD-P:3)
(Newcomer & Hammill, 1997b)

General Description

The TOLD-P:3 is a measure of verbal comprehension and expression abilities at the single-word and sentence levels for young children (ages 4 years, 0 months to 8 years, 11 months).

Subtests

Grammatic Completion is a test of the ability to use common English morphology.

Grammatic Understanding is a test of the ability to understand sentence meaning.

Oral Vocabulary is a test that asks the child to provide definitions for words.

Phonemic Analysis measures the ability to segment words into phonemic units.

Picture Vocabulary is a test of word knowledge.

Relational Vocabulary is a test of the ability to understand the relationship between two words.

Sentence Imitation is a measure of short-term memory that asks a child to repeat sentences.

Word Articulation assesses the ability to articulate speech sounds.

Word Discrimination assesses the ability to discriminate speech sounds.

24

Memory Tests

This chapter lists and briefly describes the most commonly used tests of memory functioning for children. These descriptions can be used in report writing. For memory subtests of broader cognitive/intelligence batteries, see Chapter 21.

24.1. Benton Visual Retention Test (BVRT), Fifth Edition   *(Sivan, 1992)*

General Description

The BVRT assesses difficulties in memory, motor behavior, and spatial orientation.

24.2. Children's Memory Scale (CMS)   *(Cohen, 1997)*

General Description

The CMS is a comprehensive battery of memory tests; it includes assessment of memory in visual and verbal modalities, and in immediate and recall conditions.

Subtests

General Memory is a measure of a child's ability to recall general information.

Numbers requires the recall of numbers both forward and backward.

Sequencing includes a variety of tasks involving sequencing (e.g., listing months backward or counting backward from 20 to 1).

Stories assesses a child's immediate recall of details presented in a story that has been read to him/her. The child is then asked to recall them again following a delay.

Stories—Delayed Recognition Format presents facts in the story in a yes–no format.

Verbal Memory includes a measure of story memory, as well as a measure of ability to remember verbal paired associates.

Word Pairs presents a child with word pairs (related as well as unrelated) over three repeated trials. Memory is tested after each of the trials by cuing with the first word in each pair, as well as in a free-recall paradigm in immediate- and delayed-recall conditions.

24.3. List-Learning Tests

The California Verbal Learning Test–Children's Version (CVLT-C; Delis, Kramer, Kaplan, & Ober, 1994) is used for ages 6–17.

The California Verbal Learning Test–Second Edition (CVLT-II; Delis, Kramer, Kaplan, & Ober, 2000) is used for ages 16 and above.

The Children's Auditory Verbal Learning Test–2 (CAVLT-2; Talley, 1993) is used for ages 6–17 as an alternative to, or instead of, the CVLT-C.

General Description

The CVLT-C/CVLT-II/CAVLT-2 is a test of verbal learning and memory where the child is asked to listen to a list of words and then recall as many of the words as possible over five trials and in short and long delayed-recall conditions.

Sample Statements

The child's performance on the CVLT-C/CVLT-II/CAVLT-2, a test of learning and memory, fell above/at/below the mean for ability to recall information after short/long delays under conditions of free/cued/recognition recall.

On the CVLT-C/CVLT-II/CAVLT-2, the individual is asked to recall a list of 16 items presented repeatedly over five learning trials. Memory for the list is tested after each presentation, after presentation of an interference list (i.e., short delay), and again after a long delay, in free-recall, cued-recall, and recognition memory conditions. Normal performance on this measure is characterized by a positive learning curve—that is, with additional items recalled after successive learning trials. Also, performance is generally better on cued- than free-recall trials, and recognition is typically better than recall.

Common Errors

Passive learning strategy (e.g., reliance on serial order of list as opposed to semantic categorization), difficulty with sustained attention (e.g., shown by fewer items recalled over time), perseverations, poor retention over time, vulnerability to interference.

24.4. Rey Auditory Verbal Learning Test (RAVLT)   *(Forrester & Geffen, 1991)*

General Description

The RAVLT is a test of verbal learning where the child is asked to learn a 15-word list over five learning trials, followed by one recall and one recognition trial after an interference condition.

Rey–Osterrieth Complex Figure Test (ROCF)   *See Section 25.9.*

24.5. Wechsler Memory Scale—Third Edition (WMS-III)   *(Wechsler, 1997b)*

General Description

The WMS-III is a comprehensive test battery that assesses visual and auditory memory.

24.6. Wide Range Assessment of Memory and Learning, Second Edition (WRAML2)   *(Adams & Sheslow, 2003)*

General Description

The WRAML2 is a test battery that measures a child's ability to actively learn and memorize a variety of auditory and visual information.

Subtests

Design Memory is a test of spatial memory, where a child is asked to study sequences of geometric designs for 5 seconds and then wait 10 seconds before drawing them.

Finger Windows is a test of immediate recall for nonverbal, visual–spatial sequences.

Number–Letter asks a child to repeat strings of letters and numbers of increasing length.

Picture Memory measures visual attention and memory, as well as the ability to keep visual information in working memory; a child is asked to look at four scenes for 10 seconds each, and then immediately after presentation to identify elements that have been added or changed.

Sentence Memory is a measure of verbal memory skills for simple material.

Sound–Symbol is a test of visual and auditory memory, where a child is asked to recall the sound that is paired with a symbol.

Story Memory is a test where a child has to listen to and repeat short paragraphs.

Symbolic Working Memory is a test of visual working memory skills.

Verbal Learning is a test of auditory working memory, where information is presented in a list that the child hears four times; it includes Delay Recall and Delay Recognition conditions.

Verbal Working Memory is a test of auditory working memory, where the child hears a string of words and is asked to recall them in a certain categorical order.

25

Tests of Visual–Spatial and Motor Skills

This chapter lists the most commonly used tests of visual–spatial and motor functioning for children. Brief descriptions of many of these tests are offered and can be used in report writing.

25.1. Beery–Buktenica Developmental Test of Visual–Motor Integration, Fifth Edition (Beery VMI-V) *(Beery, Buktenica, & Beery, 2004)*

General Description

The Beery VMI asks a child to copy simple geometric forms (e.g., circle, square) that are developmentally normed. It assesses visual–motor integration, which is the degree to which visual perception and finger–hand movements (e.g., fine motor movements) are well coordinated.

Sample Statements

The Beery VMI requires the child to copy progressively complex designs. His/her performance fell in the _____ range (_____ percentile; _____-year, _____-month age equivalent).

This test consists of 24 geometrical forms that are copied in a developmental sequence, from simple to more complex. The child copied these forms with pencil and paper from examples.

On the Beery VMI, the child copied geometric figures of ascending difficulty in a structured format. His/her performance on the VMI indicated no/little/some/much difficulty on this task.

Common Problems

Spatial confusion, lack of precision in copying designs, poor attention to detail, problems reproducing angled shapes/three-dimensional designs/designs where lines change directions, difficulty paying attention to visual detail/integrating parts into whole/making diagonals.

25.2. Bender Visual–Motor Gestalt Test (Bender Gestalt)   *(Bender, 1938)*

General Description

The Bender Gestalt is a screening measure of visual–motor integration ability that requires a child to make copies on a blank sheet of paper of nine geometric and line drawings presented individually. It can be scored on two levels: perceptual processing, and social and emotional markers.

Sample Statements

The child completed the Bender Gestalt, a visual–motor skill screening that required him/her to copy several geometric figures and patterns.

The Bender Visual–Motor Gestalt Test required the child to copy a series of geometric figures on paper with a pencil. She/he made _____ error(s), according to the criteria of the Koppitz System. Such errors(s) would/would not be expected of an individual her/his age.

The Bender Gestalt test showed some/many/no signs of visual–motor difficulties, as the child copied each of the figures with minimal/several/numerous distortions.

Common Problems

Difficulties with regulating size/forming angles/spatial planning, problems with organization of figures on page, figures drawn on one small portion of page, wavy lines.

25.3. Bruininks–Oseretsky Test of Motor Proficiency, Second Edition (BOT-2)   *(Bruininks & Bruininks, 2006)*

General Description

The BOT-2 assesses a child's skill levels in the areas of gross motor performance, fine motor performance, bilateral integration, and coordination. Both quality of skill and completion within a time frame are considered; the test is normed for individuals ages 4–21.

Sample Statements

The child's motor performance was evaluated with the BOT-2, a measure of speed, agility, balance, strength, bilateral coordination, and upper-limb coordination.

Subtests

Balance requires a child to balance on one foot with eyes open and with eyes closed, to perform other balancing tasks, and to walk on the floor as well as on a balance beam.

Bilateral Coordination assesses the ability to perform reciprocal and symmetrical arm and leg motions.

Fine Motor Integration assesses the ability to copy shapes.

Fine-Motor Precision assesses the ability to coordinate precise hand and visual movements, such as cutting out a circle.

Manual Dexterity measures the ability to perform fine motor tasks quickly.

Running Speed and Agility measures speed and dexterity during a shuttle run.

Strength assesses arm, shoulder, abdominal, and leg strength through tasks such as a broad jump, push-ups, and sit-ups.

Upper-Limb Coordination includes bouncing and catching a tennis ball, as well as arm and finger coordination items.

25.4. Finger Tapping or Finger Oscillation Test   *(Reitan & Wolfson, 1993)*

General Description

The Finger Tapping/Finger Oscillation Test is designed to measure motor control and requires kinesthetic ability, motor speed, and visual–motor coordination.

Sample Statements

On the Finger Tapping Test, the child performed similarly/slightly faster/slightly slower with his/her left/right hand, at the ____ percentile, indicating below-average/normal/above-average simple fine motor speed.

The Finger Oscillation Test required _____ to repeatedly tap a device with the index finger of each hand over several repeated trials, and over these trials his/her rate of tapping was calculated.

25.5. Grip Strength or Hand Dynamometer   *(Reitan & Wolfson, 1993)*

General Description

The Grip Strength or Hand Dynamometer task requires a child to squeeze a dynamometer with each hand and is used to detect differences in hand strength.

25.6. Grooved Pegboard   *(Matthews & Kløve, 1964)*

General Description

The Grooved Pegboard task is a manipulative dexterity test consisting of 25 holes with randomly positioned slots. Pegs with a key along one side must be rotated to match the hole before they can be inserted.

Sample Statements

The child's performance was normal/abnormal on a test of fine motor dexterity and motor planning (Grooved Pegboard).

Common Problems

Filling in the pegboard in a very disorganized fashion, a significant number of drops.

25.7. Hooper Visual Organization Test   *(Hooper, 1983)*

General Description

The Hooper Visual Organization Test is a measure of visual closure; the child is asked to identify a picture (e.g., saw, flower) that has been cut up into pieces and arranged in separate parts on the stimulus page.

25.8. Judgment of Line Orientation   *(Benton, Hannah, & Varney, 1975)*

The Judgment of Line Orientation task requires a child to judge the location and directionality of a series of lines; it is a measure of pure spatial judgment.

25.9. Rey–Osterrieth Complex Figure Test (ROCF)   *(Lezak, 1995)*

General Description

The ROCF is used to assess visual–spatial constructional ability and visual memory. The copy component of this test requires a child to reproduce a complex line drawing on a blank sheet of paper while the drawing is in full view; the delayed-recall component of the test requires him/her to draw the figure from memory 30 minutes subsequent to seeing the figure.

Sample Statements

Memory performance was assessed by asking the child to draw the Rey–Osterrieth Complex Figure from memory, both immediately and again following a 30-minute delay.

Good Performance

The child utilized a configural approach in the reproduction for the ROCF, and her/his overall performance was within the average/above-average range.

He/she demonstrated a well-organized approach to his/her copy of the design.

Overall, the child demonstrated age-appropriate visual skills (visual perception, planning, and organization, and memory).

Poor Performance

The child's copy of the figure was quite segmented, suggesting that she/he does not yet have the visual-perceptual ability to appreciate the larger organizational elements in a visual stimulus, but rather processes detail by detail.

Although the child did succeed in recalling parts of the overall organizing structure, the details were placed in a haphazard manner, suggesting a loss of information regarding the organization of the design.

His/her memory of the figure was poor and evidenced difficulty in understanding the wholeness of the figure.

The child's copy of the figure was characterized by a disorganized approach; specifically, she/he failed to appreciate the figure's overall organizing structure and instead proceeded in a piecemeal fashion, indicating poor ability to grasp and encode the figural information.

Common Problems

Figure lacks a sense of coherence/gestalt, poorly organized, fragmentation, difficulty in understanding the wholeness of the figure, misalignments/distortion errors, difficulty determining where to start and how to approach the drawing, added details that were not a part of the design, impulsive style.

Problems on the ROCF may indicate difficulty with executing multistep behaviors, problems in attending to environmental complexity, trouble seeing the "big picture," problems with work completion and time management.

ROCF Scoring Systems

Bernstein, J. H., & Waber, D. (1996). *Developmental scoring system for the Rey–Osterrieth Complex Figure.* Odessa, FL: Psychological Assessment Resources.

Meyers, J. E., & Meyers, K. R. (1995). *Rey Complex Figure Test and Recognition Trial (RCFT).* Odessa, FL: Psychological Assessment Resources.

Stern, R. A., Javorsky, D. J., Singer, E. A., Singer Harris, N. G., Somerville, J. A., Duke, L. M., et al. (2002). *The Boston Qualitative Scoring System (BQSS) for the Rey–Osterrieth Complex Figure.* Odessa, FL: Psychological Assessment Resources.

Tactual Performance Test (TPT)   *See Section 26.13.*

Other Tests of Visual–Spatial Ability

See the following sections of Chapters 21 and 24 for more information about these subtests and composites that measure visual–spatial ability:

- 21.5: DAS-II Matrices, Recall of Designs, Pattern Construction, Matching Letter-like Forms, Spatial Cluster.
- 21.11 and 21.12: WAIS-III and WISC-IV Block Design, Matrix Reasoning, Perceptual Reasoning Index.
- 21.5: DAS-II Subtests: Matrices, Recall of Designs, Pattern Construction, Matching Letter-like forms, Copying, Spatial Cluster.
- 24.6: WRAML2 Picture Memory, Design Memory.

26

Measures of Executive and Neuropsychological Functioning

This chapter lists the most commonly used tests of executive and neuropsychological functioning for children, as well as descriptions that can be used in report writing. Since the number of tests in this category is quite large, and assessment in this area requires specialized training, this chapter is not meant to provide exhaustive coverage.

26.1. Definition of Executive Functions

Executive functions include skills such as attention, impulse control, working memory, and organization.

26.2. Aphasia Screening Test *(Reitan & Wolfson, 1985)*

General Description

The Aphasia Screening Test measures expressive and receptive language functioning, letter identification, and the ability to perform lateralized hand functions and copy simple shapes, and simple arithmetic problems.

26.3. Children's Category Test *(Boll, 1993)*

The Children's Category Test is a measure of nonverbal concept formation and use of feedback information to form and test hypotheses, as well as the ability to adapt behavior in response to corrective feedback.

Common Problems

Performance problems may indicate cognitive inflexibility, difficulty in the ability to develop/ test/modify hypotheses.

26.4. Conners' Continuous Performance Test II (CPT II)
(Conners & MHS Staff, 2000)

General Description

The CPT II is a computerized measure of the ability to sustain attention over time and to inhibit impulsive responses.

Sample Statements

On the CPT II, _____'s performance was within the above-average/average/below-average range for all aspects of the testing, indicating (un)satisfactory attention. (Indicate whether the child was on or off medication at the time of testing.)
_____'s performance on the CPT II was poor/good and provides strong evidence that she/he does/does not typically struggle with attentional difficulties.

26.5. Gordon Diagnostic System   *(Gordon, 1998)*

General Description

The Gordon Diagnostic System includes several tasks that test sustained attention and the ability to inhibit responses.

Subtests

The Vigilance Test requires a child to pay attention to a repetitive stimulus.
The Distractibility Task requires a child to attend to a specific set of stimuli and screen out competing stimuli.

26.6. Halstead–Reitan Neuropsychological Test Battery for Older Children and Reitan–Indiana Neuropsychological Test Battery for Children   *(Reitan & Wolfson, 1985, 1992)*

General Description

Both the Halstead–Reitan and Reitan–Indiana consist of several subtests or scales, each intended to assess one or more neuropsychological abilities.

Subtests

Children's Category Test *(see Section 26.3)*.
Tactual Performance Test (TPT) *(see Section 26.13)*.
Finger Tapping or Finger Oscillation Test *(see Section 25.4)*.
Aphasia Screening Test *(see Section 26.2)*.
Matching Pictures Test.
Individual Performance (Matching Figures, Star, Matching V's, Concentric Squares).
Marching Test.
Progressive Figures Test.
Color Form Test.
Target Test.
Seashore Rhythm Test *(see Section 26.9)*.
Speech Sounds Perception Test *(see Section 26.10)*.

Trail Making Test (Parts A and B) (*see Section 26.16*).
Sensory–Perceptual Examination.
Tactile Finger Recognition.
Fingertip Number Writing.
Tactile Form Recognition.
Grip Strength or Hand Dynamometer (*see Section 25.5*).

26.7. Luria–Nebraska Neuropsychological Battery–II (LNNB-II) and Luria–Nebraska Neuropsychological Battery—Children's Revision (LNNB-C)   *(Golden, 1987)*

General Description

Both the LNNB-II and LNNB-C are designed to assess a broad range of neuropsychological functioning and measure a variety of sensory–motor, perceptual, and cognitive abilities. There are 11 scales: motor functions, rhythm, tactile functions, visual functions, receptive speech, expressive speech, writing, reading, arithmetic, memory, and intellectual processes.

26.8. NEPSY   *(Korkman, Kirk, & Kemp, 1998)*

General Description

The NESPY is a developmental neuropsychological test battery that evaluates five domains: Attention/Executive Functions, Language, Sensorimotor Functions, Visuospatial Processing, and Memory and Learning.

26.9. Seashore Rhythm Test   *(Reitan & Wolfson, 1993)*

In the Seashore Rhythm Test, a child is presented with pairs of tone patterns and has to identify whether the patterns in each pair are the same or different; it is a measure of sustained attention and the ability to perceive and compare rhythmical patterns.

26.10. Speech Sounds Perception Test   *(Reitan & Wolfson, 1993)*

In the Speech Sounds Perception Test, a child is presented with a series of nonsense words on an audiotape and is asked to identify each spoken nonsense word from among a written list of choices.

26.11. Stroop Color and Word Test   *(Golden, 1978)*

General Description

The Stroop is a formal test of cognitive inhibition, impulse control, and concentration; it assesses the ability to filter out irrelevant information and attend to the relevant information in a given task or situation, with scores for speed and accuracy in three conditions.

26.12. Symbol Digit Modalities Test (SDMT)   *(Smith, 1982)*

General Description

The SDMT is a symbol-coding task (similar to the Coding subtest of the WISC-IV/WAIS-III) that provides a measure of processing speed and attention.

26.13. Tactual Performance Test (TPT)   *(Reitan & Wolfson, 1993)*

General Description

The TPT is a measure of tactile form recognition, psychomotor problem solving, memory for shapes, and spatial thinking.

Sample Statement

On the TPT, the child completed a formboard blindfolded three times (using his/her dominant hand, nondominant hand, and both hands on the respective trials). The task assesses form discrimination, kinesthesis, coordination of arm movement, manual dexterity, and visualization of spatial configurations. After completing the third trial, the child was asked to draw what he/she thought the board looked like without ever having seen it.

26.14. Test of Variable Attention (TOVA)   *(Greenberg, 1990)*

General Description

The TOVA is a visual and auditory performance test that assesses attention and impulse control.

26.15. Token Test for Children (TTFC)   *(DiSimoni, 1978)*

The TTFC is a test of auditory comprehension that has a child manipulate tokens in response to instructions from the examiner (e.g., "Put the red triangle next to the yellow circle").

26.16. Trail Making Test, Parts A and B   *(Spreen & Strauss, 1991)*

General Description

The Trail Making Test is a test of efficiency in following two sequential procedures; it measures higher-order executive functions such as planning, ability to change cognitive set, sequencing, and integrative abilities, as well as visual scanning skills and accuracy under the pressure of time.

Sample Statements

To further assess attention, the child was administered the Trail Making Test; this test includes two parts (A and B), both of which are basically connect-the-dots tasks involving numbers and (in Trails B) letters as well. Aside from motor planning, these tasks require a good deal of visual attention, scanning, and an ability to "shift set."

The child was given the Trail Making Test, a measure of visual scanning speed, psychomotor speed, sequencing ability, and visual attention and concentration. Part B of this test is a more specific measure of cognitive flexibility.

The Trail Making Test is an attention task that also has a perceptual–motor component. On the more simplistic Trails A, which requires the attention to a single attribute, the child's performance was superior/excellent/good/normal/average/adequate/mixed/poor. On the more complex Trails B, which requires the attention to two attributes simultaneously, the child's performance was in the superior/excellent/good/normal/average/adequate/mixed/poor range.

Good Performance

The Trail Making Test is a paper-and-pencil task that requires the child to connect randomly distributed circles in a specific order. On Trails A the circles are connected in numerical order, while in Trails B the circles are connected in alternating numerical–alphabetical order. The child's performance on both parts of the test was average/above average, indicating no problems with the executive and visual functions tapped by the test.

Poor Performance

Poor performance on Trails B indicates difficulties in shifting set. Such difficulties typically manifest as problems in making transitions, cognitively and/or behaviorally.

Overall, his/her performance times were significantly below average, indicating sequencing and visual scanning difficulties.

Results lend support to the examiner's observations of difficulty with focused and sustained attention.

26.17. Wisconsin Card Sorting Test (WCST)   *(Heaton, 1981)*

General Description

The WCST requires abstract concept formation, flexibility in thinking, and the ability to use new information in a problem-solving task. In this test, the individual is asked to sort cards according to criteria (e.g., color, form, number) that she/he must figure out from feedback provided on each sort.

Sample Statements

The child was given the computer-administered version of the WCST, a test of abstract reasoning abilities in which the individual is asked to sort computerized images of cards. The cards vary from one another in shape, number, and color or elements printed on each one. The individual is not told the sorting criteria, nor is he/she told that a criterion shifts during the task. Rather, the only feedback given is the computer's response of "right" or "wrong."

The WCST is designed to assess abstract concept formation and the ability to shift and maintain mental set. It is considered a measure of executive functions, in that it requires the ability to develop and maintain an appropriate problem-solving strategy across changing stimulus conditions in order to achieve a future goal.

The child's performance on the WCST, which requires the utilization of feedback presented in a trial-and-error method to problem solve, fell within the superior/excellent/good/average/normal/below-normal/below-average/poor/impaired range.

Good Performance

His/her overall accuracy placed him/her at the _____ percentile as compared to age-matched norms, and there was no indication of perseverative tendencies, providing evidence for a high degree of cognitive flexibility.

The child was able to complete all six categories on this task, suggesting no deficits in the areas of pattern analysis, cognitive flexibility, and tolerance for frustration.

The child was very quick to understand the organizational structure of the game, and maintained excellent attention while executing the game strategy. Overall, her/his performance on these tasks does not suggest that she/he has attentional, organizational, or planning difficulties.

Poor Performance

The child lost set _____ times (_____ percentile), suggestive of attentional difficulties.

The child was unable to continue to apply the principle required to do the task; he/she had a tendency toward perseverative thinking/responses.

Other Measures of Executive Functioning

See Chapters 21, 23, and 24 for more information about these tests, subtests, and composites that measure executive functioning:

21.5: DAS-II Speed of Information Processing, Recall of Objects (Immediate and Delayed), Recall of Digits.

21.11 and 21.12: WAIS-III and WISC-IV Processing Speed Index, Picture Completion, Digit Span, Arithmetic, Letter–Number Sequencing.

23.4: COWAT FAS and Animals.

24.3: CVLT-C, CVLT-II, and CAVLT.

24.6: WRAML2 Sentence Memory, Story Memory.

27

Measures of Emotional and Personality Functioning

This chapter lists and briefly describes the most commonly used tests of emotional and personality functioning for children. Also included are phrases that can be used to characterize children's responses on various projective measures. Phrases used to describe various emotional symptoms in children can be found in Chapter 15.

"Projective tests" are measures that are used to evaluate a child's psychological or emotional health; they are based on the assumption that individuals project their unconscious feelings and personalities when responding to ambiguous stimuli. Clinicians will often use projective testing when there are unanswered questions regarding a child's behavior or feelings about a situation. See Section 3.10 for questions used in projective assessments.

27.1. General Statements

A projective screening was done to assess underlying attitudes, concerns, and mood, as well as personality variables that might be having an impact on school/home/social performance.
The child's responses were rather short and not very descriptive. (Such responses may reflect guardedness or concrete verbal formation.)

Unimpaired Emotional Functioning

Personality test data suggest that the child is currently in adequate contact with reality and fairly well aware of the conventional.
Projective measures indicated that the child demonstrated a capacity for empathy and emotional expression.

Impaired or Compromised Emotional Functioning

Although assessment of emotional and personality functioning reveals no evidence of formal thought disorder or psychosis, she/he is clearly experiencing emotional turmoil and great difficulties with impulse control.
On measures of personality functioning, the child shows moderate similarity to individuals who present with depression/anxiety/bipolar disorders/etc.
The personality tests showed suggestions of possible functioning along the borderline–narcissistic continuum, with some self-focusing suggestive of narcissistic features.

239

Results of testing indicated an emotionally constricted young girl/boy who attempts to deny and avoid emotional needs and drives.

The child's responses on a variety of the tests indicated a concerning level of depression/anxiety/mood dysregulation/poor self-locus of control/problems with authority figures/boredom/posttraumatic stress/fears.

With regard to projective responses, the child seems to view the world as a hostile and unpredictable place where he/she often feels powerless to change.

Results of projective testing indicate that the child is likely to have fewer psychological resources than other children her/his age and may feel flustered and overwhelmed by life's ups and downs.

Evidence from a number of sources, such as _____ (specify), raised concerns about this child's level of emotional functioning.

The projective testing suggested that the child's affective world seems marked by feelings of self-doubt, sadness, and painful rumination.

Results of the personality testing suggest that the child is an anxious boy/girl who is struggling with a complex matrix of issues, including social immaturity/depression/anxiety/discomfort with strong emotions/lowered self-regard/poor self-esteem/normal developmental conflicts/etc.

27.2. Draw-A-Person or Human Figure Drawing

General Description

On the Draw-A-Person/Human Figure Drawing test, the child is asked to draw a picture of a person. It provides an indication of how the child feels about him-/herself.

Scoring and Suggestions

Qualitative scoring is based on the number of body parts presented, the proportion of various parts to the whole, and other aspects (e.g., the presence of clothing). The Draw-A-Person also gives a developmental/cognitive level; the cognitive and emotional levels are scored according to separate systems. Directions include "Draw the *whole* person" and "Draw the best way you know how" (or something to that effect).

In reports, comment on the following:

- Elaboration of figure.
- Detail of figure relative to age and intellectual expectations.
- Gender (male, female, indeterminate).
- Who is portrayed in the drawing (the child, a relative, etc.).

27.3. Kinetic Family Drawing

On the Kinetic Family Drawing test, the child is typically asked to draw a picture of her/his family doing something. It provides insight into child's perception of her/his family unit.

Suggestions

In reports, comment on the following:

- Which family members are portrayed.
- Cohesiveness of family activity.

- Emotional content in the picture.
- Whether the child spontaneously draws the family members doing something together or apart.

27.4. Kinetic School Drawing

General Description

On the Kinetic School Drawing test, the child is asked to draw a picture that includes him-/herself, his/her teacher, and a friend or two doing something at school.

Suggestions

In reports, comment on the following:

- Who and what are portrayed in the picture.
- The cohesion (or lack of cohesion) between persons in the picture.
- Emotional content in the picture.

27.5. House–Tree–Person Drawing

General Description

The House–Tree–Person drawing is used to assess visual–motor abilities and creativity.

Suggestions

In reports, comment on the following:

- Orientation of components, proportionality, space, and detail.
- Creativity (or lack of it).

27.6. Rorschach   *(Rorschach, 1921/1942)*

General Description

The Rorschach is a perceptual–cognitive task where subjects are presented with 10 inkblots and are asked about each, "What might this be?" In responding to the inkblots, the person tells what she/he sees in each one and then reports what features in the inkblot made it look that way. The subject's problem-solving approach reflects key dimensions of his/her psychological traits and states.

Rorschach Scoring Systems

Each Rorschach response is scored and interpreted according to specific criteria. The Exner system (Exner, 2002) is the most commonly used system. Norms can be found for children as young as 5 years.

Statement for an Invalid Protocol

The child's completed Rorschach protocol only contained _____ responses. This is considered invalid and should be interpreted with caution.

Sample Interpretive Statements

The possible interpretive statements for the Rorschach are nearly limitless. The following statements are only provided as examples of how Rorschach results can be used in report writing.

> The child's approach to the task revealed an ambitent coping style, indicating that she/he has a limited capacity to form and implement coping strategies for dealing with problems in life. She/he tends to switch between exerting an independent decision-making style at times of stress and withdrawing from stressors altogether.
>
> The child has a limited ability to recognize and deal with his/her feelings comfortably, and may tend to avoid or withdraw from expression of strong feelings.
>
> The child's emotional resources are less than needed and therefore create the potential for stress overload, impulsivity, and unpredictability when she/he is confronted with new and unfamiliar situations, especially when her/his poor coping strategies are taken into account.
>
> The child's responses on the Rorschach indicate that he/she has a unique way of interpreting the world, which may lead him/her to misunderstand or distort others' motives.

27.7. Selected Apperception Tests

Roberts Apperception Test for Children (RATC) *(McArthur & Roberts, 1982)*

General Description

> The RATC is a subjective instrument in which a child is asked to tell stories about various ambiguous interpersonal situations, depicted on large picture cards.

Suggestions

In reports, comment on the following:

- Social reasoning difficulties, such as trouble picking up on the nuances of social situations and/or understanding conflicting social cues.
- Trouble making sense of a particular scene in which each character seems to be having a different feeling.
- Perseverative and concrete social reasoning (e.g., carrying over the same theme from one scene to another).
- Difficulty making inferences about why people might behave or respond in the pictures.

Thematic Apperception Test (TAT) and Children's Apperception Test (CAT)
(Murray, 1971 [TAT]; Bellak & Bellak, 1949 [CAT])

General Description

> On the TAT/CAT, the child is asked to create stories about various scenes shown to him/her.

Sample Statements

> On the TAT/CAT, the child was asked to tell a story for a series of _____ different pictures. The TAT/CAT pictures depict situations and relationships related to the social and emotional development of children, as well as more ambiguous pictures. Her/his stories were then judged for emotional content and common themes.

The TAT/CAT is a projective test that attempts to illuminate issues a child may be experiencing. The child was asked to tell stories about various pictures.

The TAT/CAT asks a child to create stories based on a series of presented drawings. The child's responses and stories can be used to characterize his/her state of mind.

UNREMARKABLE PERFORMANCE

The child's responses did not indicate any evidence of cognitive or perceptual distortions.

In general, the child's responses were appropriate to the content of the pictures depicted and did not identify any problematic areas in his/her functioning.

Her/his stories show that she/he feels at ease with/interactive with peers, and that it is important for her/him to look very capable in front of peers.

His/her stories show that he/she is able to accept limits from adults.

REMARKABLE PERFORMANCE

Overall, the child's stories suggest that she/he does not perceive her-/himself as being frequently happy. In most of her/his stories, the characters were either angry or sad.

His/her stories show that he/she has a difficult time accepting and controlling aggressive feelings toward his/her peers.

Her/his stories show that she/he lacks the ability to postpone gratification of demands/to control negative impulses.

Possible Problems

Difficulty generating stories; problems with verbal expression.

Trouble making sense of scenes that included children/adults; difficulty interpreting and integrating complex social information.

Difficulty tolerating ambiguity.

Inability to complete the task because child provided concrete descriptions of scene as opposed to stories/tended to described the picture instead of telling a story.

Inability to deduce what individuals in cards may be feeling or thinking.

Common Themes

Children who hate school/are struggling with school/do not have a positive attitude toward academic learning/are unmotivated to achieve in school.

Children who are not frequently happy; characters who are typically angry/sad.

Children who demonstrate a closeness and connectedness with mother/father/parental figures and who tend to seek him/her/them out for comfort; parents and children who experience a high amount of conflict.

Adults who are perceived as having good intentions but who cannot meet a child's needs.

Children who have difficulty accepting and controlling aggressive feelings toward peers/problems with peer acceptance; children who lack strategies for learning to become group members.

Children who are disciplined/punished and feel ashamed/sad/angry at themselves for behaving in ways that they know are wrong.

Children who tend to engage in power struggles/be oppositional/have difficulty accepting limits/push the limits with adults; children who are well aware of social norms and rules, but who are not willing or able to adhere to them; main characters who are oppositional/disobey parents/act out in school and at home.

Children with feelings of low self-esteem.

Children who are unable to delay gratification of demands/control negative impulses.

Children who are bored/are depressed/are sad/exhibit morbid thinking.
(Positive themes:) Children who feel pride/happiness; when stories involve conflict, characters who are able to resolve their difficulties.

27.8. Sentence Completion Tests

Many different sentence completion tests (both published and unpublished) exist. Well-known published tests include the following:

Rotter Incomplete Sentence Blanks (Rotter & Rafferty, 1950).
Sacks Sentence Completion Test (Sacks & Levy, 1950). *A sample sentence completion test can be found in Section 40.5.*

General Description

On a sentence completion test, a child is asked to finish a number of incomplete sentence stems (either orally or in writing). It provides types of information about attitudes and social–emotional well-being that are thought to be difficult to obtain in direct questionnaire formats.

Suggestions

In reports, comment on the following:

- Self-concept.
- Level of engagement with friends and family.
- Acknowledgment of strengths and weaknesses.

Sample Statement

The child's responses on the sentence completion test raised some concerns about self-esteem/feelings of social isolation/parental conflict/negativity/abuse by family members/ etc.

28

Behavior Rating Scales and Tests of Adaptive Functioning

The first part of this chapter lists and briefly describes the most commonly used behavior rating scales that can be used by parents and teachers (and sometimes by older children or adolescents to rate themselves). The second part of this chapter lists and briefly describes tests of adaptive functioning, typically used when there are questions about developmental abilities and disabilities.

BEHAVIOR RATING SCALES

28.1. General Statements

The child's parents and teacher(s) completed a number of questionnaires related to behavior and attention. The responses on the measures were all within the normal/abnormal/etc. range.

The child's mother/father completed the questionnaires specified above/below. Her/his ratings indicated that the child is/is not experiencing any significant behavioral difficulties.

28.2. ADD-H Comprehensive Teacher Rating Scale (ACTeRS), Second Edition *(Ullman, Sleator, & Sprague. 1991)*

General Description

The ACTeRS is a checklist for ADD-H (now ADHD) diagnostic criteria.

Sample Statements *See Section 28.3, below.*

28.3. ADHD Rating Scale–IV *(DuPaul, Power, Anastopoulos, & Reid, 1998)*

General Description

The ADHD Rating Scale–IV lists each of the diagnostic criteria for ADHD and asks a parent/teacher to rate a child on each symptom.

Sample Statements

The child's mother/father/teacher completed the ADHD Rating Scale–IV. Her/his responses indicate that the child exhibits few difficulties with hyperactivity or inattention.

Scores on the ADHD Rating Scale–IV indicated significant problems with inattention/hyperactivity/impulsivity.

The parent/teacher responses indicate that the child meets the diagnostic criteria for ADHD, Combined/Predominantly Inattentive/Predominantly Hyperactive–Impulsive Type, with _____ out of 9 inattentive symptoms endorsed and _____ out of 9 hyperactive–impulsive symptoms endorsed.

28.4. Battelle Developmental Inventory, Second Edition (BDI-2)
(Newborg, 2004)

General Description

The BDI-2 measures developmental skills in children in five domains: Personal–Social, Adaptive, Motor, Communication, and Cognitive.

28.5. Behavior Assessment System for Children, Second Edition (BASC-2) *(Reynolds & Kamphaus, 2004)*

General Description

The BASC-2 assesses a child or adolescent's behavioral and emotional functioning at school and at home. It includes three measures: the Parent Rating Scales (PRS), the Teacher Rating Scales (TRS), and the Self-Report of Personality (SRP).

Sample Statements

The child/adolescent/mother/father/teacher completed the BASC SRP/PRS/TRS. His/her/their ratings indicate clinically significant/at-risk scores on the following subscales: _____ (specify).

TRS and PRS Subscales

Activities of Daily Living measures a child's self-help and self-care skills.

Adaptability measures a child's ability to adapt to changes in his/her environment.

Aggression is a measure of aggressive behaviors (fighting, etc.).

Anxiety measures the tendency to be anxious, nervous, or fearful.

Attention Problems assesses the tendency to daydream or be easily distracted.

Atypicality measures unusual behaviors, such as those associated with psychoticism (e.g., visual or auditory hallucinations) or extreme immaturity.

Conduct Problems measures antisocial or delinquent behaviors, such as truancy, alcohol/drug use, lying, and stealing.

Depression assesses feelings of depression, such as sadness, unhappiness, and stress.

Functional Communication measures a child's "real-world" communication skills.

Hyperactivity measures hyperactivity, impulsivity, and the tendency to act before thinking.

Leadership measures a child's competencies in school and social settings, such as the ability to interact well with others.

Learning Problems assesses problems with completing or understanding schoolwork.

Social Skills measures a child's interpersonal skills.

Somatization measures the tendency to have somatic complaints.

Study Skills measures the skills that are important to academic success.

Withdrawal measures a child's tendency to withdraw from or avoid social contact with others.

Additional SRP Subscales

The SRP includes self-report versions of the Anxiety, Attention Problems, Atypicality, Depression, Hyperactivity, and Somatization subscales from the PRS and TRS, as well as several additional subscales:

Alcohol Abuse measures alcohol use and tendency toward or symptoms of alcohol abuse (on the College version only).

Attitude to School measures a child's feelings about school (e.g., satisfaction/dissatisfaction); high scores are associated with feelings of resentment toward school.

Attitude to Teachers measures a child's perception of teachers, with high scores indicating dislike of teachers.

Interpersonal Relations measures a child's perception of her/his social relationships with peers.

Locus of Control measures a child's perception of who controls his/her life, with high scores indicating an external locus of control (e.g., child feels that success or failure is determined by forces outside his/her control) and low scores indicating an internal locus of control (e.g., child feels that he/she has control over his/her own destiny).

Relations with Parents indicates whether the child has positive or negative feelings toward her/his parents.

School Maladjustment measures a child's view of his/her difficulties in school.

Self-Esteem measures a child's satisfaction with her-/himself.

Self-Reliance assesses a child's belief in his/her abilities, perseverance, and persistence (or lack thereof).

Sensation Seeking measures a child's tendency to be a risk taker or engage in potentially hazardous activities.

Sense of Inadequacy assesses a child's belief in her/his ability to succeed or achieve in academic and personal endeavors.

Social Stress measures a child's stress level, such as feelings of tension and pressure, as well as his/her coping resources.

28.6. Behavior Rating Inventory of Executive Functions (BRIEF)
(Gioia, Isquith, Guy, & Kenworthy, 2000)

General Description

The BRIEF is a parent and teacher rating of executive functions.

Subscales

Emotional Control assesses a child's ability to control or modulate emotions.

Inhibit assesses a child's ability to control impulses and appropriately stop her/his own behavior.

Initiate measures a child's ability to begin a task or activity or independently generate ideas.

Monitor measures a child's ability to check his/her work and keep track of his/her performance while doing a task.

Organization of Materials assesses behaviors such as a child's leaving her/his playroom a mess, leaving a trail of belongings wherever she/he goes, or leaving messes that others have to clean up.

Plan/Organize assesses a child's ability to anticipate future events, set goals, and determine the steps needed to complete tasks.

Shift assesses a child's ability to make transitions freely from one situation or activity to another and to use flexibility in solving problems.

Working Memory measures a child's ability to stick with an activity and remember what is needed to complete an activity.

28.7. Behavior Rating Inventory of Executive Functions—Preschool Version (BRIEF-P) *(Gioia, Espy, & Isquith, 2003)*

General Description

The BRIEF-P is a parent and teacher measure of executive functions in preschool-age children.

Subscales

Inhibit, Shift, Emotional Control, Working Memory, Plan/Organize. *(See Section 28.6 above, for descriptions.)*

28.8. Child Behavior Checklist (CBCL), Teacher's Report Form (TRF), and Youth Self-Report (YSR) *(Achenbach & Rescorla, 2001)*

General Description

The CBCL, TRF, and YSR are components of the Achenbach System of Empirically Based Assessment (ASEBA); they provide a cross-informant assessment of behavior. Although each one can be used on its own, the scales are most frequently given together. The CBCL is given to parents of a child or adolescent, the TRF is given to a teacher, and the YSR is completed by an adolescent (ages 11–18).

Sample Statements

The child's mother/father/teacher completed the CBCL/TRF, which assesses many different aspects of child behavior and emotional adjustment.

The CBCL/TRF is a behavioral rating instrument completed by parents/teachers, in which numerous descriptors are rated as "not true," "somewhat true," or "very true." Descriptor ratings are quantified and indexed onto the appropriate scale.

The adolescent completed the YSR, which assessed his/her behavior as it relates to constructs such as anxiety, self-esteem, depression, attitude to school, and relations with parents.

28.9. Childhood Autism Rating Scale (CARS)
(Schopler, Reichler, DeVellis, & Daly, 1980)

General Description

The CARS is a behavior rating scale useful in identifying children with autism; the measure also helps the clinician distinguish among mild, moderate, and severe autism.

28.10. Children's Depression Inventory (CDI) *(Kovacs, 1992)*

General Description

The CDI is a self-report measure of depressive symptoms for children ages 7–17. It provides a Total score as well as five factor scores: Negative Mood, Interpersonal Problems, Ineffectiveness, Anhedonia, and Negative Self-Esteem.

28.11. Conners' Rating Scales—Revised (CRS-R) *(Conners, 1997)*

General Description

The CRS-R is a set of questionnaires for assessing a child's or adolescent's behavioral and emotional functioning. It includes long and short forms of rating scales for parents and teachers, as well as of a self-report scale for adolescents (ages 12–17).

Subscales

Oppositional measures behaviors such as whether a child is likely to break rules, have problems with authority, or become easily annoyed.

Cognitive Problems/Inattention indicates whether a child learns more slowly, has organizational problems, has difficulty completing tasks, or has problems with concentration.

Hyperactivity measures whether a child has difficulty sitting still or remaining seated, or has problems with restlessness and impulsivity.

Anxious–Shy assesses whether a child has an atypical amount of worries and fears, is prone to be emotional and sensitive to criticism, is anxious in unfamiliar settings, or is shy and withdrawn.

Perfectionism assesses a child's tendency to set high goals for her-/himself, be fastidious about the way she/he does things, or be obsessional about her/his work.

Social Problems measures a child's tendency to perceive that he/she has few friends, to have low self-esteem and self-confidence, or to feel emotionally distant from peers.

Psychosomatic reports whether a child has an atypical number of aches and pains.

Index Scores

Conners' ADHD Index identifies children at risk for ADHD.

Conners' Global Index: Emotional Lability assesses whether a child is prone to emotional responses or behaviors (e.g., anger, crying, outbursts) than would be typical for her/his age.

Conners' Global Index: Restless–Impulsive

28.12. Devereux Scales of Mental Disorders (DSMD)
(Naglieri, LeBuffe, & Pfeiffer, 1994)

General Description

The DSMD assesses whether a child or adolescent is experiencing (or is at risk for) a behavioral or emotional disorder and includes the following scales: Conduct, Attention/Delinquency, Anxiety, Depression, Autism, and Acute Problems.

28.13. Gilliam Asperger's Disorder Scale (GADS)   *(Gilliam, 2001)*

General Description

The GADS is a scale that documents behavioral characteristics of children suspected of having Asperger's disorder.

28.14. Millon Adolescent Personality Inventory (MAPI)
(Millon, Green, & Meagher, 1982)

General Description

The MAPI is a self-report measure based on Millon's theory of personality; it includes eight Personality Style scales, eight Expressed Concerns scales, and four Behavioral Correlates scales.

Subscales

Personality Style scales: Introversive, Inhibited, Cooperative, Sociable, Confident, Forceful, Respectful, and Sensitive.

Expressed Concerns scales: Self-Confident, Personal Esteem, Body Comfort, Sexual Acceptance, Peer Security, Social Tolerance, Family Rapport, and Academic Confidence.

Behavioral Correlates scales: Impulse Control, Societal Compliance, Scholastic Achievement, and Attendance Consistency.

28.15. Minnesota Multiphasic Personality Inventory—Adolescent (MMPI-A)   *(Butcher et al., 1992)*

General Description

The MMPI-A is an adolescent version of the well-known MMPI. It includes 10 basic scales and 15 content scales.

Subscales

Basic scales: Hypochondriasis, Depression, Hysteria, Psychopathic Deviate, Masculinity–Femininity, Paranoia, Psychasthenia, Schizophrenia, Hypomania, and Social Introversion.

Content scales: Anxiety, Obsessiveness, Depression, Health Concerns, Alienation, Bizarre Mentation, Anger, Cynicism, Conduct Problems, Low Self-Esteem, Low Aspiration, Social Discomfort, Family Problems, School Problems, and Negative Treatment Indicators.

28.16. Revised Children's Manifest Anxiety Scale (RCMAS)
(Reynolds & Richmond, 1985)

General Description

The RCMAS is a self-report measure of anxiety in children; it measures symptoms such as physiological symptoms of anxiety, worry, depressive symptomatology, and somatic complaints.

TESTS OF ADAPTIVE FUNCTIONING

"Adaptive functioning" refers to a child's effectiveness in areas such as social skills, communication, and daily living skills. Tests of adaptive functioning measure how well a child meets the standards of personal independence and social responsibility expected at his/her developmental stage.

28.17. AAMR Adaptive Behavior Scales—Residential and Community: Second Edition (ABS-RC:2) *(Nihira, Lel, & Lambert, 1993)*

The ABS-RC:2 assesses social behavior and living skills in children who may have mental retardation or other learning, behavioral, or emotional issues.

28.18. AAMR Adaptive Behavior Scales—School: Second Edition (ABS-S:2) *(Nihira, Lambert, & Lel, 1993)*

General Description

The ABS-S:2 is an observational rating scale that assesses school-related behavior and social adjustment in children who may have mental retardation or other learning, emotional, or behavioral issues.

28.19. Adaptive Behavior Assessment System (ABAS)
(Harrison & Oakland, 2000)

General Description

The ABAS assesses children in the specific adaptive skills areas specified in the DSM-IV diagnostic criteria for mental retardation; it includes a Teacher Form, Parent Form, and Adult Form.

Battelle Developmental Inventory, Second Edition (BDI-2)
See Section 28.4.

28.20. Scales of Independent Behavior—Revised (SIB-R)
(Bruininks, Woodcock, Weatherman, & Hill, 1996)

General Description

The SIB-R measures skills needed to function independently in home, school, and community settings.

28.21. Vineland Adaptive Behavior Scales, Second Edition (Vineland-II) *(Sparrow, Cicchetti, & Balla, 2005)*

General Description

The Vineland-II measures personal and social skills used for everyday living in four domains: Communication, Daily Living Skills, Motor Skills, and Socialization. There is also an optional Maladaptive Behavior Index. Both interview and rating scale versions of the Vineland-II are available.

Sample Statements

The Vineland-II was given to determine whether the child meets the standards of personal independence and social responsibility expected for a child her/his age.

The child's mother/father/teacher/guardian completed the Rating Form of the Vineland-II, for the purpose of determining what a child does to take care of him-/herself. It is a measure of typical performance, not maximal performance.

The Survey Interview Form of the Vineland-II was completed, with the child's mother/father/teacher/guardian as the informant. Four adaptive behavior domains were assessed: Communication, Daily Living Skills, Socialization, and Motor Skills.

Domains

Communication measures skills such as knowing one's home address, birthday, and telephone number.

Daily Living Skills measures skills such as toileting, answering the phone, looking both ways before crossing the street, and showering/bathing independently.

Motor Skills measures fine and gross motor skills.

Socialization measures skills such as the ability to follow rules in simple games, apologizing for mistakes, and responding appropriately when being introduced to someone.

F. Ending the Report

29

Diagnostic
Statements/Impressions

Diagnoses are a kind of professional shorthand for integrating many kinds of data. In most cases, your diagnosis should follow from and sum up the data you have reported earlier. Most diagnostic statements are made in the "Summary" section of the report (see Chapter 30). A diagnosis also orients your readers to the recommendations for treatment planning that typically follow it in a report (see Chapter 31).

Generally offer only the most important one or two diagnoses, unless diagnosis was the reason for the referral, you are in training, or your setting requires a fuller listing. You should include all five axes of a DSM-IV-TR (or ICD-9-CM) diagnosis, and any "rule-outs" or other qualifications (see Section 29.3 "Qualifiers for Diagnosis"). Offer a "diagnostic impression" if you are not qualified to offer a DSM-IV-TR diagnosis or if you are quite uncertain.

29.1. DSM-IV-TR

Diagnostic classification systems are useful because they provide a way for mental health practitioners to communicate with one another, offer a framework for researching disorders, and help guide treatment decisions for particular disorders (Clark, Watson, & Reynolds, 1995).

The current version (fourth edition, text revision) of the *Diagnostic and Statistical Manual of Mental Disorders* (DSM-IV-TR), developed by the American Psychiatric Association (2000), is the most widely used classification system in the United States. DSM-IV-TR uses a multiaxial system, each of which involves a unique domain of functioning:

Axis I	Clinical Disorders
	Other Conditions That May Be a Focus of Clinical Attention (*see Section 29.6*)
Axis II	Personality Disorders
	Mental Retardation
Axis III	General Medical Conditions (abbreviated in this chapter as GMCs)
Axis IV	Psychosocial and Environmental Problems (*see Section 29.7*)
Axis V	Global Assessment of Functioning (GAF) Scale (*see Section 29.8*)

29.2. ICD-9-CM

The *International Classification of Diseases*, 10th revision (ICD-10), Chapter V: Mental and Behavioral Disorders (World Health Organization, 1992) is the most widely used classification system outside the United States and is a system that covers both medical and psychological disorders. However,

ICD-10 has not been and will not soon be adopted in the United States; the Health Insurance Porta-bility and Accountability Act (HIPAA) requires the use of the Clinical Modification of ICD-9 (ICD-9-CM; U.S. Department of Health and Human Services, 1980, with updates at www.cdc.gov/nchs/datawh/ftpserv/ftpicd9/ftpicd9.htm). The various editions of DSM have been in wide use for years, and this will continue through DSM-V and beyond. DSM contains both the diagnostic labels and criteria for making the diagnosis, prognostic and prevalence data, and other information, all of which are lacking in ICD.

The bulk of this chapter (*see Sections 29.4–29.5*) lists diagnoses that can typically be applied to chil-dren and adolescents, together with the appropriate DSM-IV-TR and ICD-9-CM code numbers. The chapter does not cover all diagnoses that are found in DSM-IV-TR, just those that are typically applied to children. First, you will find "Disorders Usually First Diagnosed in Infancy, Childhood, or Adolescence," with these disorders listed in the order given in DSM-IV-TR. This list is followed by an alphabetized listing of other disorders that can be applied to children and adolescents.

The DSM-IV-TR codes are reprinted with permission from the *Diagnostic and Statistical Manual of Mental Disorders*, fourth edition, text revision. Copyright 2000 American Psychiatric Association.

29.3. Qualifiers for Diagnosis

A diagnosis may be described or qualified with one of the following terms:

> **Initial, deferred, principal, additional/comorbid, rule out** _____ (specify), **admitting, tentative, working, final, discharge, in remission, quiescent.**

When the criteria are currently met for a diagnosis, DSM-IV-TR offers these qualifiers that specify severity and course:

> **Mild** (few symptoms), **Moderate** (impairment between mild and severe), **Severe** (symptoms in excess of those required to make diagnosis or symptoms that are severely impairing), **In Partial Remission, In Full Remission, Prior History.**

29.4. Disorders Usually First Diagnosed in Infancy, Childhood, or Adolescence

Mental Retardation

All of these are coded on Axis II of DSM-IV-TR. The middle column gives the IQ equivalents of these categories.

DSM-IV-TR		IQ equivalents	ICD-9-CM	
317	Mild Mental Retardation	50–55 to about 70	317	Mild mental retardation
318.0	Moderate Mental Retardation	35–40 to 50–55	318.0	Moderate mental retardation
318.1	Severe Mental Retardation	20–25 to 35–40	318.1	Severe mental retardation
318.2	Profound Mental Retardation	Less than 20–25	318.2	Profound mental retardation
319	Mental Retardation, Severity Unspecified	Not testable	319	Mental retardation, unspecified

Learning Disorders

DSM-IV-TR		ICD-9-CM	
315.00	Reading Disorder	315.0	Specific reading disorder
		315.0	Reading disorder, unspecified
		315.01	Alexia
		315.02	Developmental dyslexia
		315.09	Other Specific spelling difficulty
315.1	Mathematics Disorder	315.1	Mathematics disorder
315.2	Disorder of Written Expression	315.2	Other specific learning difficulties Disorder of written expression
		315.5	Mixed development disorder
		315.8	Other specified delays in development
315.9	Learning Disorder NOS	315.9	Unspecified delay in development Learning disorder NOS
		313.83	Academic underachievement disorder
		309.23	Specific academic or work inhibition

Motor Skills Disorder

DSM-IV-TR		ICD-9-CM	
315.4	Developmental Coordination Disorder	315.4	Developmental coordination disorder

Communication Disorders

DSM-IV-TR		ICD-9-CM	
315.31	Expressive Language Disorder	315.31	Expressive language disorder Developmental aphasia Word deafness
315.31	Mixed Receptive–Expressive Language Disorder	315.32	Mixed receptive–expressive language disorder
315.39	Phonological Disorder	315.39	Other Phonological disorder
307.0	Stuttering	307.0	Stuttering
307.0	Communication Disorder NOS	307.9	Other and unspecified special symptoms or syndromes, not elsewhere classified

Pervasive Developmental Disorders

DSM-IV-TR		ICD-9-CM	
299.00	Autistic Disorder	299.00	Autistic disorder Infantile autism
299.80	Rett's Disorder	299.9	Unspecified pervasive developmental disorder Pervasive developmental disorder NOS
299.10	Childhood Disintegrative Disorder	299.1	Childhood disintegrative disorder
299.80	Asperger's Disorder	299.8	Asperger's disorder Other specified pervasive developmental disorders
299.80	Pervasive Developmental Disorder NOS	299	Pervasive developmental disorders (Enter the 5th digit as follows: 0, current or active state; 1, residual state)

Attention-Deficit and Disruptive Behavior Disorders

DSM-IV-TR		ICD-9-CM	
314.01	Attention-Deficit/Hyperactivity Disorder, Combined Type or Predominantly Hyperactive–Impulsive Type	314.01	Attention deficit disorder with hyperactivity
		314.1	Hyperkinesis with developmental delay
		314.2	Hyperkinetic conduct disorder
		314.8	Other specified manifestations of hyperkinetic syndrome
314.00	Attention-Deficit/Hyperactivity Disorder, Predominantly Inattentive Type	314.00	Attention deficit disorder without mention of hyperactivity
314.9	Attention-Deficit/Hyperactivity Disorder NOS	314.9	Unspecified hyperkinetic syndrome
312.81	Conduct Disorder, Childhood-Onset Type	312.81	Conduct disorder, childhood-onset type
312.82	Conduct Disorder, Adolescent-Onset Type	312.82	Conduct disorder, adolescent-onset type
312.89	Conduct Disorder, Unspecified Onset	312.89	Conduct disorder, unspecified onset
313.81	Oppositional Defiant Disorder	313.81	Oppositional defiant disorder
312.9	Disruptive Behavior Disorder NOS	312.9	Unspecified disturbance of conduct Juvenile delinquency Disruptive behavior disorder NOS
		312	Disturbance of conduct, not elsewhere classified (Options for the 5th digit of 312.0, 312.1, and 312.2: 0, unspecified; 1, mild; 2, moderate; 3 severe)

DSM-IV-TR	ICD-9-CM	
	312.0	Undersocialized conduct disorder, aggressive type
	312.1	Unsocialized conduct disorder, unaggressive type
	312.2	Socialized conduct disorder
	312.3	Disorders of impulse control, not elsewhere classified
	312.4	Mixed disturbance of conduct, not elsewhere classified
	312.8	Other specified disturbances of conduct, not elsewhere classified Conduct disorder of unspecified onset

Feeding and Eating Disorders of Infancy or Early Childhood

DSM-IV-TR		ICD-9-CM	
307.52	Pica	307.52	Pica
307.53	Rumination Disorder	307.53	Rumination disorder
		307.54	Psychogenic vomiting
307.59	Feeding Disorder of Infancy or Early Childhood	307.59	Other Feeding disorder of infancy or early childhood

Tic Disorders

DSM-IV-TR		ICD-9-CM	
307.23	Tourette's Disorder	307.23	Tourette's disorder
307.22	Chronic Motor or Vocal Tic Disorder	307.22	Chronic motor or vocal tic disorder
307.21	Transient Tic Disorder Specify if: Single Episode/ Recurrent	307.21	Transient tic disorder
307.20	Tic Disorder NOS	307.20	Tic disorder, unspecified Tic disorder NOS

Elimination Disorders

DSM-IV-TR		ICD-9-CM	
787.6	Encopresis With Constipation and Overflow Incontinence	307.7	Encopresis, continuous or discontinuous
307.7	Encopresis Without Constipation and Overflow Incontinence		
307.6	Enuresis (Not Due to a GMC) Specify type: Nocturnal Only/ Diurnal Only/Nocturnal and Diurnal	307.6	Enuresis, primary or secondary

Other Disorders of Infancy, Childhood, or Adolescence

DSM-IV-TR		ICD-9-CM	
309.21	Separation Anxiety Disorder Specify if: Early Onset	309.21	Separation anxiety disorder
		309.22	Emancipation disorder of adolescence and early adult life
313.23	Selective Mutism	313.23	Selective mutism
313.89	Reactive Attachment Disorder of Infancy or Early Childhood Specify type: Inhibited/Disinhibited Type	313.89	Other or mixed emotional disturbances of childhood or adolescence Reactive attachment disorder of infancy or early childhood
307.2	Stereotypic Movement Disorder Specify if: With Self-Injurious Behavior	307.3	Seterotypic movement disorder
313.9	Disorder of Infancy, Childhood, or Adolescence NOS	313.9	Unspecified emotional disturbance of childhood or adolescence Mental disorder of infancy, childhood, or adolescence NOS
		313.0	Overanxious disorder
		313.1	Misery and unhappiness disorder
		313.2	Sensitivity, shyness, and social withdrawal disorder
		313.22	Shyness disorder of childhood
		313.3	Relationship problems Sibling jealousy
		313.8	Other or mixed emotional disturbances of childhood or adolescence

29.5. Disorders Found in Children and Adolescents but Not Exclusive to Them

Adjustment Disorders

DSM-IV-TR		ICD-9-CM	
309.0	Adjustment Disorder With Depressed Mood	309.0	Adjustment disorder with depressed mood
		309.1	Prolonged depressive reaction
		309.2	Adjustment reaction with predominant disturbance of other emotions
		309.21	Separation anxiety disorder
		309.22	Emancipation disorder of adolescence and early adult life
309.24	Adjustment Disorder With Anxiety	309.24	Adjustment disorder with anxiety
309.28	Adjustment Disorder with Mixed Anxiety and Depressed Mood	309.28	Adjustment disorder with mixed anxiety and depressed mood
		309.29	Other Culture shock

DSM-IV-TR		ICD-9-CM	
309.3	Adjustment Disorder With Disturbance of Conduct	309.3	Adjustment disorder with disturbance of conduct
			Conduct disorder or destructiveness as adjustment disorder
309.4	Adjustment Disorder With Mixed Disturbance of Emotions and Conduct	309.4	Adjustment disorder with mixed disturbance of emotions and conduct
		309.8	Other specified adjustment reactions
309.9	Adjustment Disorder, Unspecified	309.9	Unspecified adjustment reaction

Anxiety Disorders

DSM-IV-TR		ICD-9-CM	
300.01	Panic Disorder Without Agoraphobia	300.01	Panic disorder without agoraphobia
300.21	Panic Disorder With Agoraphobia	300.21	Agoraphobia with panic disorder
			Panic disorder with agoraphobia
300.22	Agoraphobia Without History of Panic Disorder	300.22	Agoraphobia without mention of panic attacks
300.29	Specific Phobia	300.29	Other isolated or specific phobias
300.23	Social Phobia	300.23	Social phobia
300.3	Obsessive–Compulsive Disorder	300.3	Obsessive–compulsive disorders
309.81	Posttraumatic Stress Disorder	309.81	Posttraumatic stress disorder
			Posttraumatic stress disorder NOS
		309.82	Adjustment reaction with physical symptoms
		309.83	Adjustment reaction with withdrawal
		309.89	Other
308.3	Acute Stress Disorder	308	Acute reaction to stress
			Acute stress disorder
		308.0	Predominant disturbance of emotions
			Emotional crisis or panic state as acute reaction to exceptional (gross) stress
		308.1	Predominant disturbance of consciousness
		308.2	Predominant psychomotor disturbance
			Agitation or stupor
		308.3	Other acute reactions to stress
		308.9	Unspecified acute reaction to stress
300.02	Generalized Anxiety Disorder	300.02	Generalized anxiety disorder
		300.09	Other
		300.2	Phobic disorders
		300.20	Phobia, unspecified
293.89	Anxiety Disorder Due to . . . [Indicate the GMC]		
300.00	Anxiety Disorder NOS	300.00	Anxiety state, unspecified

Delirium, Dementia, and Amnestic and Other Cognitive Disorders

DSM-IV-TR		ICD-9-CM	
293.0	Delirium Due to . . . [Indicate the GMC]	293.0	Delirium due to conditions classified elsewhere
780.09	Delirium NOS		
294.1x	Dementia Due to Head Trauma		
294.1x	Dementia Due to . . . [Indicate other GMC]		
294.8	Dementia DOS	294.8	Dementia NOS
294.0	Amnestic Disorder Due to . . . [Indicate other GMC]	294.0	Amnestic syndrome
294.8	Amnestic Disorder NOS	294.8	Other persistent mental disorders due to condition classified elsewhere
			Amnestic disorder NOS
294.9	Cognitive Disorder NOS	294.9	Unspecified persistent mental disorders due to conditions classified elsewhere
			Cognitive disorder NOS
		310	Specific nonpsychotic mental disorders due to organic brain damage
		310.0	Frontal lobe syndrome

Dissociative Disorders

DSM-IV-TR		ICD-9-CM	
300.12	Dissociative Amnesia	300.12	Dissociative amnesia
300.13	Dissociative Fugue	300.13	Dissociative fugue
300.14	Dissociative Identity Disorder	300.14	Dissociative identity disorder
300.6	Depersonalization Disorder	300.6	Depersonalization disorder
			Derealization
300.15	Dissociative Disorder, NOS	300.15	Dissociative disorder or reaction, unspecified

Eating Disorders

DSM-IV-TR		ICD-9-CM	
307.1	Anorexia Nervosa Specify type: Restricting or Binge-Eating/Purging Type	307.1	Anorexia nervosa
		307.5	Other and unspecified disorders of eating
307.51	Bulimia Nervosa Specify type: Purging/Nonpurging Type	307.51	Bulimia nervosa
307.50	Eating Disorder NOS	307.50	Eating disorder, unspecified
			Eating disorder NOS

Factitious Disorders

DSM-IV-TR		ICD-9-CM	
		301.51	Chronic factitious illness with physical symptoms Munchausen syndrome
300.16	Factitious Disorder With Predominantly Psychological Signs and Symptoms	300.16	Factitious disorder with predominantly psychological signs and symptoms
300.19	Factitious Disorder With Predominantly Physical Signs and Symptoms	300.19	Other and unspecified factitious illness
300.19	Factitious Disorder With Combined Psychological and Physical Signs and Symptoms		Factitious disorder with combined psychological and physical signs and symptoms or with predominantly physical signs and symptoms
300.19	Factitious Disorder NOS		Factitious disorder NOS

Gender Identity Disorders

DSM-IV-TR		ICD-9-CM	
320.6	Gender Identity Disorder in Children	302.6	Gender identity disorder in children
	Gender Identity Disorder NOS		Gender identity disorder NOS
302.85	Gender Identity Disorder in Adolescents or Adults Specify if: Sexually Attracted to Males/Females/Both/Neither	302.85	Gender identity disorder in adolescents or adults

Impulse-Control Disorders Not Elsewhere Classified

DSM-IV-TR		ICD-9-CM	
312.34	Intermittent Explosive Disorder	312.34	Intermittent explosive disorder
		312.35	Isolated explosive disorder
312.32	Kleptomania	312.32	Kleptomania
312.33	Pyromania	312.33	Pyromania
312.31	Pathological Gambling	312.31	Pathological gambling
312.39	Trichotillomania	312.39	Disorders of impulse control, other Trichotillomania
312.30	Impulse-Control Disorder NOS	312.30	Impulse control disorder, unspecified
		312	Disturbance of conduct, not elsewhere classified

Mental Disorders Due to a GMC Not Elsewhere Classified

DSM-IV-TR		ICD-9-CM	
293.89	Catatonic Disorder Due to . . . [Indicate the GMC]	293.89	Other Catatonic disorder in conditions classified elsewhere
310.1	Personality Change Due to . . . [Indicate the GMC]	310.1	Personality change due to conditions classified elsewhere
		310.2	Postconcussion syndrome
		310.8	Other specified nonpsychotic mental disorders following organic brain damage
		310.9	Unspecified nonpsychotic mental disorder following organic brain damage
293.9	Mental Disorder NOS Due to . . . [Indicate the GMC]	293.9	Unspecified transient mental disorder in conditions classified elsewhere

Mood Disorders

DSM-IV-TR		ICD-9-CM	
300.4	Dysthymic Disorder Specify if: Early/Late Onset, With Atypical Features	300.4	Dysthymic disorder
		296	Episodic mood disorders (Use the following 5th digits for the 296 conditions: 0, unspecified; 1, mild; 2, moderate; 3, severe, without mention of psychotic behavior; 4, severe, specified as with psychotic behavior; 5, in partial or unspecified remission; 6, in full remission)
296.20	Major Depressive Disorder, Single Episode, Unspecified	296.2	Major depressive disorder, single episode
296.21	Major Depressive Disorder, Single Episode, Mild		Depressive psychosis
296.22	Major Depressive Disorder, Single Episode, Moderate		Endogenous depression
296.23	Major Depressive Disorder, Single Episode, Severe Without Psychotic Features		Involutional melancholia Manic–depressive psychosis or reaction, depressed type
296.24	Major Depressive Disorder, Single Episode, Severe With Psychotic Features		Monopolar depression
296.25	Major Depressive Disorder, Single Episode, In Partial Remission		Psychotic depression, all single episode or unspecified
296.26	Major Depressive Disorder, Single Episode, In Full Remission		

DSM-IV-TR		**ICD-9-CM**	
296.30	Major Depressive Disorder, Recurrent, Unspecified	296.3	Major depressive disorder recurrent episode (or any of those in 296.2, above)
296.31	Major Depressive Disorder, Recurrent, Mild		
296.32	Major Depressive Disorder, Recurrent, Moderate		
296.33	Major Depressive Disorder, Recurrent, Severe Without Psychotic Features		
296.34	Major Depressive Disorder, Recurrent, Severe With Psychotic Features		
296.35	Major Depressive Disorder, Recurrent, In Partial Remission		
296.36	Major Depressive Disorder, Recurrent, In Full Remission		
296.00	Bipolar I Disorder, Single Manic Episode, Unspecified	296.0	Bipolar I disorder, single manic episode
296.01	Bipolar I Disorder, Single Manic Episode, Mild		Hypomania (mild) NOS
296.02	Bipolar I Disorder, Single Manic Episode, Moderate		Mania (monopolar) NOS
296.03	Bipolar I Disorder, Single Manic Episode, Severe Without Psychotic Features		Manic–depressive psychosis or reaction, all single episode or unspecified
296.04	Bipolar I Disorder, Single Manic Episode, Severe With Psychotic Features		
296.05	Bipolar I Disorder, Single Manic Episode, In Partial Remission		
296.06	Bipolar I Disorder, Single Manic Episode, In Full Remission		
		296.1	Manic disorder (or any of those in 296.0, above) recurrent episode
296.40	Bipolar I Disorder, Most Recent Episode Manic, Unspecified	296.4	Bipolar I disorder, most recent episode (or current) manic
296.40	Bipolar I Disorder, Most Recent Episode Hypomanic		
296.41	Bipolar I Disorder, Most Recent Episode Manic, Mild		
296.42	Bipolar I Disorder, Most Recent Episode Manic, Moderate		
296.43	Bipolar I Disorder, Most Recent Episode Manic, Severe Without Psychotic Features		
296.44	Bipolar I Disorder, Most Recent Episode Manic, Severe With Psychotic Features		

DSM-IV-TR		**ICD-9-CM**	
296.45	Bipolar I Disorder, Most Recent Episode Manic, In Partial Remission		
296.46	Bipolar I Disorder, Most Recent Episode Manic, In Full Remission		
296.50	Bipolar I Disorder, Most Recent Episode Depressed, Unspecified	296.5	Bipolar I disorder, most recent episode (or current) depressed
296.51	Bipolar I Disorder, Most Recent Episode Depressed, Mild		
296.52	Bipolar I Disorder, Most Recent Episode Depressed, Moderate		
296.53	Bipolar I Disorder, Most Recent Episode Depressed, Severe Without Psychotic Features		
296.54	Bipolar I Disorder, Most Recent Episode Depressed, Severe With Psychotic Features		
296.55	Bipolar I Disorder, Most Recent Episode Depressed, In Partial Remission		
296.56	Bipolar I Disorder, Most Recent Episode Depressed, In Full Remission		
296.60	Bipolar I Disorder, Most Recent Episode Mixed, Unspecified	296.6	Bipolar I disorder, most recent episode (or current) mixed
296.61	Bipolar I Disorder, Most Recent Episode Mixed, Mild		
296.62	Bipolar I Disorder, Most Recent Episode Mixed, Moderate		
296.63	Bipolar I Disorder, Most Recent Episode Mixed, Severe Without Psychotic Features		
296.64	Bipolar I Disorder, Most Recent Episode Mixed, Severe With Psychotic Features		
296.65	Bipolar I Disorder, Most Recent Episode Mixed, In Partial Remission		
296.66	Bipolar I Disorder, Most Recent Episode Mixed, In Full Remission		
296.7	Bipolar I Disorder, Most Recent Episode Unspecified	296.7	Bipolar I disorder, most recent episode (or current) unspecified
296.80	Bipolar Disorder NOS	296.8	Bipolar disorder, unspecified Bipolar disorder NOS
		296.81	Atypical manic disorder
		296.82	Atypical depressive disorder

DSM-IV-TR		ICD-9-CM	
296.89	Bipolar II Disorder Specify (current or most recent episode): Hypomanic/Depressed	296.89	Other Bipolar II disorder Manic–depressive psychosis, mixed type
		296.9	Other and unspecified episodic mood disorder
296.90	Mood Disorder NOS	296.90	Unspecified episodic mood disorder Affective psychosis NOS Melancholia NOS
		296.99	Other specified episodic mood disorder Mood swings: brief, compensatory, rebound
301.13	Cyclothymic Disorder	301.13	Cyclothymic disorder Cyclothymic personality
293.83	Mood Disorder Due to ... [Indicate the GMC] Specify if: With Depressive Features/Major Depressive-Like Episode/Manic Features/Mixed Features		
311	Depressive Disorder NOS	311	Depressive disorder, not elsewhere classified Depression NOS

For children who have recently lost someone close to them, consider the DSM-IV-TR code V62.82, Bereavement.

Schizophrenia and Other Psychotic Disorders

DSM-IV-TR		ICD-9-CM	
		295	Schizophrenic disorder (Use the following 5th digits: 0, unspecified; 1, subchronic; 2, chronic; 3, subchronic with acute exacerbation; 4, chronic in acute exacerbation; 5, in remission)
		295.0	Simple type
295.30	Schizophrenia, Paranoid Type	295.3	Paranoid type
295.10	Schizophrenia, Disorganized Type	295.1	Disorganized type
295.20	Schizophrenia, Catatonic Type	295.2	Catatonic type
295.90	Schizophrenia, Undifferentiated Type	295.9	Unspecified schizophrenia Schizophrenia, undifferentiated type
		297	Delusional disorders Paranoid disorders
		297.0	Paranoid state, simple
295.60	Schizophrenia, Residual Type	295.6	Residual type Chronic undifferentiated schizophrenia

DSM-IV-TR		**ICD-9-CM**	
295.40	Schizophreniform Disorder Specify if: With/Without Good Prognostic Features	295.4	Schizophreniform disorder
295.70	Schizoaffective Disorder Specify type: Bipolar/Depressive Type	295.7	Schizoaffective disorder
		295.8	Other specified types of schizophrenia
297.1	Delusional Disorder Specify type: Erotomanic/ Grandiose/Jealous/Persecutory/ Somatic/Mixed/Unspecified Type	297.1	Delusional disorder Chronic paranoid psychosis
		297.2	Paraphrenia Involutional paranoid state
298.8	Brief Psychotic Disorder Specify if: With/Without Marked Stressors; With Postpartum Onset	298.8	Other and unspecified reactive psychosis Brief psychotic disorder
297.3	Shared Psychotic Disorder	297.3	Shared psychotic disorder Folie à deux
		297.8	Other specified paranoid states
		297.9	Unspecified paranoid state
		298.0	Depressive-type psychosis
		298.1	Excitative-type psychosis
		298.2	Reactive confusion
		298.3	Acute paranoid reaction
		298.4	Psychogenic paranoid psychosis
		298	Other nonorganic psychoses
293.81	Psychotic Disorder Due to . . . [Indicate the GMC], With Delusions		
293.82	Psychotic Disorder Due to . . . [Indicate the GMC], With Hallucinations		
298.9	Psychotic Disorder NOS	298.9	Unspecified psychosis Psychotic disorder NOS

Sleep Disorders

Dyssomnias

DSM-IV-TR		**ICD-9-CM**	
		307.40	Nonorganic sleep disorder, unspecified
		307.41	Transient disorder of initiating or maintaining sleep
307.42	Primary Insomnia Specify if: Recurrent	307.42	Persistent disorder of initiating or maintaining sleep

DSM-IV-TR		ICD-9-CM	
307.44	Primary Hypersomnia Specify if: Recurrent	307.44	Persistent disorder of initiating or maintaining wakefulness
347	Narcolepsy	347.0	Narcolepsy
780.59	Breathing-Related Sleep Disorder		
307.45	Circadian Rhythm Sleep Disorder Specify type: Delayed Sleep Phase/Jet Lag/Shift Work/ Unspecified Type	307.45	Circadian rhythm sleep disorder
307.47	Dyssomnia NOS	307.47	Other dysfunctions of sleep stages or arousal from sleep Dyssomnia NOS

Parasomnias

DSM-IV-TR		ICD-9-CM	
307.47	Nightmare Disorder	307.47	Nightmare disorder
307.46	Sleep Terror Disorder	307.46	Sleep arousal disorder
307.46	Sleepwalking Disorder		Night terror disorder Night terrors Sleep terror disorder Sleepwalking Somnambulism
307.47	Parasomnia NOS	307.47	Other dysfunctions of sleep stages or arousal from sleep Parasomnia NOS
		307.48	Other Subjective insomnia complaint

Sleep Disorders Related to Another Mental Disorder

DSM-IV-TR		ICD-9-CM
307.42	Insomnia Related to Disorder on Axis I or II	
307.44	Hypersomnia Related to Disorder on Axis I or II	

Other Sleep Disorders

DSM-IV-TR		ICD-9-CM
780.52	Sleep Disorder Due to . . . [Indicate the GMC], Insomnia Type	
780.54	Sleep Disorder Due to . . . [Indicate the GMC], Hypersomnia Type	

DSM-IV-TR		**ICD-9-CM**
780.59	Sleep Disorder Due to . . . [Indicate the GMC], Parasomnia Type	
780.59	Sleep Disorder Due to . . . [Indicate the GMC], Mixed Type	

Somatoform Disorders

DSM-IV-TR		**ICD-9-CM**	
300.81	Somatization Disorder	300.81	Somatization disorder
300.82	Undifferentiated Somatoform Disorder	300.82	Undifferentiated somatoform disorder
300.11	Conversion Disorder Specify type: With Motor Symptom or Deficit/With Seizures or Convulsions/With Sensory Symptom or Deficit/With Mixed Presentation	300.11	Conversion disorder
307.80	Pain Disorder Associated With Psychological Factors Specify if: Acute/Chronic	307.80	Psychogenic pain, site unspecified
307.89	Pain Disorder Associated With Both Psychological Factors and a GMC Specify if: Acute/Chronic	307.89	Other (Code first to site of pain)
300.7	Hypochondriasis Specify if: With Poor Insight	300.7	Hypochondriasis
300.7	Body Dysmorphic Disorder		
300.82	Somatoform Disorder NOS	307.89	Other somatoform disorders

Substance-Related Disorders

DSM-IV-TR		**ICD-9-CM**	
303.90	Alcohol Dependence	303.9	Other and unspecified alcohol dependence
305.00	Alcohol Abuse	305.0	Alcohol abuse
303.00	Alcohol Intoxication	303.0	Acute alcohol intoxication
291.81	Alcohol Withdrawal Specify if: With Perceptual Disturbances		
304.40	Amphetamine Dependence	304.40	Amphetamine and other psychostimulant dependence
305.70	Amphetamine Abuse	305.7	Amphetamine or related-acting sympathomimetic abuse
292.89	Amphetamine Intoxication		
292.0	Amphetamine Withdrawal		
305.90	Caffeine Intoxication	305.9	Caffeine intoxication
292.89	Caffeine-Induced Anxiety Disorder		

DSM-IV-TR		ICD-9-CM	
292.89	Caffeine-Induced Sleep Disorder		
304.30	Cannabis Dependence	304.3	Cannabis dependence
305.20	Cannabis Abuse	305.2	Cannabis abuse
292.89	Cannabis Intoxication Specify if: With Perceptual Disturbances		
304.20	Cocaine Dependence	304.2	Cocaine dependence
305.60	Cocaine Abuse	305.6	Cocaine abuse
292.89	Cocaine Intoxication		
292.0	Cocaine Withdrawal		
304.50	Hallucinogen Dependence	304.5	Hallucinogen dependence
305.30	Hallucinogen Abuse	305.3	Hallucinogen abuse
292.89	Hallucinogen Intoxication		
304.60	Inhalant Dependence	304.6	Other specified drug dependence Inhalant dependence Phencyclidine dependence Nonprescribed use of drugs or patent medicinals
305.90	Inhalant Abuse		
292.89	Inhalant Intoxication		
305.10	Nicotine Dependence	305.1	Tobacco use disorder
292.0	Nicotine Withdrawal		
304.00	Opioid Dependence	304.0	Opioid dependence
305.50	Opioid Abuse	305.5	Opioid abuse
292.89	Opioid Intoxication Specify if: With Perceptual Disturbances		
292.0	Opioid Withdrawal		

29.6. Other Conditions That May Be a Focus of Clinical Attention

Psychological Factors Affecting Medical Condition

DSM-IV-TR		ICD-9-CM	
316	... [Specified Psychological Factor] Affecting ... [Indicate the GMC] (Choose one of the following for [Specified Psychological Factor]: Mental Disorder, Psychological Symptoms, Personality Traits or Coping Style, Maladaptive Health Behaviors, Stress-Related Physiological Response, and Other or Unspecified Psychological Factors)	316	Psychic factors associated with diseases classified elsewhere Psychological factors in physical conditions classified elsewhere Use additional code to identify the associated physical condition

Relational Problems

	DSM-IV-TR		ICD-9-CM
V61.20	Parent–Child Relational Problem	V61.20	Parent–child relational problem
V61.8	Sibling Relational Problem	V61.8	Sibling relational problem
V62.81	Relational Problem NOS	V62.81	Relational problem NOS

Problems Related to Abuse or Neglect

	DSM-IV-TR	ICD-9-CM
V61.21	Physical Abuse of Child (Use 995.54 if focus of attention is on victim)	
V61.21	Sexual Abuse of Child (Use 995.53 if focus of attention is on victim)	
V61.21	Neglect of Child (Use 995.52 if focus of attention is on victim)	

Additional Conditions That May Be a Focus of Clinical Attention

	DSM-IV-TR		ICD-9-CM
V15.81	Noncompliance With Treatment	V15.81	Noncompliance with treatment
V71.02	Child or Adolescent Antisocial Behavior	V71.02	Child or adolescent antisocial behavior
V62.89	Borderline Intellectual Functioning (code on Axis II)		
V62.82	Bereavement	V62.82	Bereavement
V62.3	Academic Problem	V62.3	Academic problem
313.82	Identity Problem	313.82	Identity disorder Identity problems
V62.89	Religious or Spiritual Problem	V62.89	Religious or spiritual problem
V62.4	Acculturation problem	V62.4	Social maladjustment
V62.89	Phase of Life Problem	V62.89	Phase of life problem

Additional DSM-IV-TR Codes

300.9	Unspecified Mental Disorder (nonpsychotic)
V71.09	No Diagnosis or Condition on Axis I
799.9	Diagnosis or Condition Deferred on Axis I
V71.09	No Diagnosis on Axis II
799.9	Diagnosis Deferred on Axis II

29.7. Axis IV

Axis IV is a list of psychosocial or environmental problems a patient is currently experiencing that may affect the diagnosis, treatment, or course of a disorder. DSM-IV-TR groups these problems into the following categories (reprinted by permission of the American Psychiatric Association):

Problems with primary support group.
Problems related to the social environment.
Educational problems.
Occupational problems.
Housing problems.
Economic problems.
Problems with access to health care services.
Problems related to interaction with the legal system/crime.
Other psychosocial and environmental problems.

29.8. Axis V

Axis V is the Global Assessment of Functioning (GAF) Scale, a rating of a person's overall level of social, occupational, and psychological functioning. Ratings are made as follows, both for current functioning and for highest level of functioning during the last year. (The scale is reprinted by permission of the American Psychiatric Association.)

100–91   Superior functioning in a wide range of activities, life's problems never seem to get out of hand, is sought out by others because of his or her many positive qualities. No symptoms.

90–81   Absent or minimal symptoms (e.g., mild anxiety before an exam), good functioning in all areas, interested and involved in a wide range of activities, socially effective, generally satisfied with life, no more than everyday problems or concerns (e.g., an occasional argument with family members).

80–71   If symptoms are present, they are transient and expectable reactions to psychosocial stressors (e.g., difficulty concentrating after family argument); no more than slight impairment in social, occupational, or school functioning (e.g., temporarily falling behind in schoolwork).

70–61   Some mild symptoms (e.g., depressed mood and mild insomnia) OR some difficulty in social, occupational, or school functioning (e.g., occasional truancy, or theft within the household), but generally functioning pretty well, has some meaningful interpersonal relationships.

60–51   Moderate symptoms (e.g., flat affect and circumstantial speech, occasional panic attacks) OR moderate difficulty in social, occupational, or school functioning (e.g., few friends, conflicts with peers or co-workers).

50–41   Serious symptoms (e.g., suicidal ideation, severe obsessional rituals, frequent shoplifting) OR any serious impairment in social, occupational, or school functioning (e.g., no friends, unable to keep a job).

40–31   Some impairment in reality testing or communication (e.g., speech is at times illogical, obscure, or irrelevant) OR major impairment in several areas, such as work or school, family relations, judgment, thinking or mood (e.g., depressed man avoids friends, neglects family, and is unable to work; child frequently beats up younger children, is defiant at home, and is failing at school).

30–21   Behavior is considerably influenced by delusions or hallucinations OR serious impairment in communication or judgment (e.g., sometimes incoherent, acts grossly inappropriately, suicidal preoccupation) OR inability to function in almost all areas (e.g., stays in bed all day; no job, home, or friends).

20–11   Some danger of hurting self or others (e.g., suicide attempts without clear expectation of death, frequently violent, manic excitement) OR occasionally fails to maintain minimal personal hygiene (e.g., smears feces) OR gross impairment in communication (e.g., largely incoherent or mute).

10–1   Persistent danger of severely hurting self or others (e.g., recurrent violence) OR persistent inability to maintain minimal personal hygiene OR serious suicidal act with clear expectation of death.

0   Inadequate information.

30

Summary of Findings and Conclusions

30.1. General Information

The summary of findings and conclusions is the place to offer your integration of history, findings, or observations, as well as your understanding of the child's current and likely future functioning in the areas most relevant to the referrer's needs. If there is a referral question about assessment or diagnosis, it is likely to be answered here. However, for referral questions seeking a disposition, "Recommendations" (see Chapter 31) may be a more appropriate heading.

Summaries should be brief (ideally one to two paragraphs), although longer summaries are more common in lengthy neuropsychological evaluations. Summaries are almost always included in reports written for medical settings. Although the summary is otherwise considered optional, it is generally a good idea to include a review of the results, particularly if the report is lengthy. Because there will always be readers who need or want to read only a brief summary, be sure to include the information or conclusions with the most important implications for the client.

A summary should do the following:

- Restate the referral information and important identifying data (e.g., the child's name, age, and grade).
- Highlight the most pertinent findings.
- Be concise and easy to read.
- Not include any new information pertaining to the history.

Morrison and Anders (2001) provide the following outline for summarizing case formulation material:

- Briefly restate the material, such as identifying data, symptoms, course of illness, and mental status.
- List the differential diagnoses, with arguments for and against each diagnosis on the list.
- Indicate the best diagnosis.
- List the factors contributing to the patient's difficulties, such as family history and/or environment.
- Indicate any additional information that may be needed to confirm the diagnosis (records, consultation with other treating professionals, etc.).
- Provide an outline of the treatment plan.
- Indicate the prognosis, to the extent that this is possible.

A summary can also be structured by answering a series of questions such as these:

1. Why was the child seen in this clinic/office?
2. What does the cognitive/neuropsychological/academic testing reveal?
3. What strengths were noted in his/her cognitive/neuropsychological/academic profile?
4. What weaknesses were noted in her/his cognitive/neuropsychological/academic profile?
5. What do the personality and behavioral data reveal?
6. Is there evidence of a disability?
7. What can be done to help the child?

30.2. General Summary Paragraphs and Statements

Paragraphs Summarizing Findings and Diagnoses

The child is a ____-year old male/female with overall high/average/low intellectual functioning, who was referred for testing for _____ (state the referral reason). The child was/was not found to have a significant verbal–nonverbal discrepancy. His/her current performance and previous history indicate that he/she meets all of the primary criteria for _____ (state diagnosis), including _____ (list symptoms). The child also demonstrated associated impairment, such as _____ (list other symptoms).

The child is a(n) _____ (state positive adjective—e.g., enjoyable) ____-grade student. She/he was cooperative/uncooperative during the testing. The results are considered a valid measure of her/his functioning. Her/his strengths include _____ (list strengths). _____ (list weaknesses) are challenges for the child.

The child, age ____, was referred for _____ (state reason). He/she scored in the high-average/average/low-average/poor range in all/nearly all of the tests, with the exception of _____ (give names of tests and levels of performance). Strengths were exhibited in _____ (list strengths). According to the child's parent/teacher, testing results correlate with his/her performance in school. He/she is an excellent/quick/eager/motivated/thoughtful/interested/attentive/good/etc. learner who demonstrates difficulty with reading/attention/oppositional behaviors/hyperactivity/math/language processing/etc.).

The child is a ____-year-old female/male who is in the ____ grade at the _____ School in _____ (give city, state). She/he was referred for evaluation because of _____. Her/his overall intellectual abilities, as measured by the (give test name), are in the _____ range. There was/was not a significant difference between the child's scores on the _____ (specify two or more) scales/factors, indicating no evidence of a learning disability/evidence for dyslexia/a nonverbal learning disability/etc. Academic achievement skills were commensurate with/slightly/moderately/significantly discrepant from expectations. Tests of expressive vocabulary indicated _____, while tests of expressive vocabulary indicated _____. Auditory memory was found to be _____, and tests of attention were _____. Visual–spatial and visual–motor skills were _____. Behavior rating scales indicated _____. Results were consistent with a diagnosis of _____.

Treatment Summary Statements

Treatment was very successful/partially successful/minimally helpful.
The child has benefited considerably from therapeutic interventions.
The treatment has been successful in treating the following symptoms: _____.

The child did not benefit from treatment/had a negative treatment outcome.
The child's symptoms have worsened/stayed the same/shown no improvement/improved considerably.

The remainder of this chapter presents examples of summary paragraphs for some of the most commonly evaluated disorders seen in children. It is not meant to be an exhaustive or definitive guide, but rather to provide the reader with possible ways of structuring summaries for different diagnoses.

30.3. For ADHD

_____ is a ____-year-old female/male who is in the ____-grade. Her/his overall intellectual abilities, as measured by the _____ (give name of test), are in the average to high-average range. _____'s performance was stronger/weaker/about the same on tests requiring skills gained from the environment than/as on tests tapping visual–spatial and spatial reasoning skills. Academic achievement was commensurate with or exceeded expectations based on her/his cognitive ability. _____ was an area of considerable strength for her/him. Tests of visual–motor skills were within the average range. Results of this evaluation indicate that the child meets criteria for ADHD, Combined Type. This is not a specific learning disability, but a more pervasive disability that appears to affect her/his performance in a variety of settings. She/he demonstrates difficulties on tasks requiring sustained concentration and focus and presents with organizational difficulties and some impulsive responding. The child's performance on a number of tests of executive functions was below expectations based on his/her estimated ability.

The child is a ____-year-old boy/girl of overall average/low-average/etc. intelligence whose test protocol is indicative of strengths in _____, as well as relative weaknesses in _____. His/her background history, overall test protocol, behavioral observations, and parent teacher reports support a diagnosis of ADHD, which interferes with his/her ability to function in the classroom setting at a level commensurate with his/her abilities.

30.4. For Asperger's Disorder

The child is a ____-year-old male/female who is in the ____ grade and who was referred for evaluation due to problems with social awareness and poor social skills. His/her overall intellectual abilities as measured by the _____ (give name of test) are in the ____range. Factor scores indicated a strength in _____. Academic achievement in reading and spelling was _____, while performance on tests of math was _____. Tests of language were primarily within the _____ range. Tests of visual memory were _____, while tests of auditory memory were _____.
The child had difficulties on tasks that demanded spatial relationship ability/visual perception/visual–motor integration skills/organization/etc. Results from the testing, and previous history, also indicate that he/she meets criteria for an autism spectrum disorder such as Asperger's disorder. In review, the child's behavioral and social skills weaknesses, including problems with social awareness/poor social comprehension/poor emotional insight/inflexible adherence to routines/obsessional tendencies/stereotyped behaviors, etc. are all consistent with this diagnosis. In addition, his/her history of poor gross–motor coordination/sensory integration problems/dyscalculia/etc. is also frequently observed in people with Asperger's.

30.5. For Depression

The child is a ____-year-old girl/boy whose cognitive strengths fell in the _____ domain and whose cognitive weaknesses were within the _____ domain. Expressive language was _____, while attention and concentration were _____. Projective findings suggest that she/he is currently struggling with deep feelings of sadness and anxiety; has a tendency to be socially isolated and emotionally withdrawn; and is experiencing feelings of guilt and low self-worth. Results of projective and behavioral measures indicate that the child is suffering from major depression, a disorder that often manifests as increased sadness, irritability, and social difficulty in children.

30.6. For Disorder of Written Expression

The child is a ____-year-old right/left-handed boy/girl who was evaluated to address concerns regarding his/her current academic performance. His/her general intellectual abilities fell within the ____ range. Within the academic domain, a significant discrepancy was seen between _____'s general intellectual ability and his/her performance on academic measures of written language. His/her performance on these achievement measures was also ____ grade levels below his/her current academic placement. Thus this discrepancy meets the diagnostic criteria for a disorder of written expression. In contrast, the child's performance on tests of reading and math was consistent with his/her expected level of performance.

30.7. For Dyslexia/Reading Disorder

The child is a ____-year-old female/male who was found to have intellectual abilities in the average/below-average/above-average range. She/he appears to have a reading disability, in that her/his performance on a variety of reading measures was significantly discrepant from expectations based on IQ. The child's reading speed is slow when compared with individuals of his/her age; reading comprehension was significantly below expectations as well. In addition to these difficulties, she/he has marked difficulties reading nonsense words. The pattern of this child's scores and the types of errors she/he made are highly characteristic of individuals with dyslexia.

The child is a ____-year-old male/female of above-average/average/below-average intelligence who is in the ____ grade. Test results and history indicate that he/she has a reading disorder (dyslexia), as his/her achievement in reading and spelling is significantly below grade level and discrepant from what would be expected on the basis of his/her general intellectual ability. Timed reading tests and nonword reading were particularly difficult for him/her. It will be important for future instructors to be made aware of the nature of the child's learning disability, so that they can assist him/her in maximizing the development of strengths and not unduly penalize him/her for deficiencies.

30.8. For Mental Retardation

The child is a ____-year-old female/male who currently attends _____ school. She/he is currently functioning in the range of mild/moderate/severe/profound mental retardation, with widespread cognitive difficulties consistent with this picture. She/he shows executive/planning problems such as difficulty maintaining and switching cognitive set/

increased perseveration/a segmented approach to complexity/concreteness of thought/difficulty seeing the logical cause and effect between details/problems with planning ability/ etc.). Deficits were also seen in visual and auditory memory/expressive and receptive language/visual constructional ability/etc. On tests of achievement, the child's performance fell at the _____ level. Her/his social maturity as measured on the Vineland-II is equivalent to that of a ____-year-old.

30.9. For NLD

The child is a ____-year-old boy/girl of high/above-average/average/below-average/normal/limited intelligence who is in the ____ grade. Testing indicates that he/she meets all the primary criteria for a nonverbal learning disability (NLD), including a significantly lower nonverbal score than verbal IQ score; relative academic weaknesses in calculation and reading comprehension skills; relative difficulty in visual–motor tasks; a history of motor planning and graphomotor output difficulties; concreteness of thought; and problems in reading nonverbal/social cues that affect social reasoning. In addition, most children with NLD have associated executive function impairment, such as variable attention, impulsivity, perseverative tendencies, and organizational problems. This child shows evidence of sensory dysfunction as well, which is also often typical for children with NLD. Finally, like most individuals with NLD, he/she appears more adept at dealing with verbal information that is more rote in nature and experiences greater difficulty with organizing and conceptualizing verbal material.

31

Recommendations

The "Recommendations" section of a report is often the most important section, as the primary purpose of an evaluation is to determine how best to intervene in a particular case. This chapter provides lists of possible recommendations for common childhood psychological problems. They reflect the treatments that have been found effective for different disorders. Of course, each child is unique, and the recommendations chosen should reflect the child's particular pattern of strengths and weaknesses. Providing a comprehensive listing of treatment parameters is beyond the scope of this book; however, this chapter does include many of the most common strategies for particular disorders. These strategies are the ones that have been shown to be effective as treatment or compensatory measures and are often used in individualized education plans (IEPs). The reader is encouraged to consult the resources listed in Section 36.3 for comprehensive treatment information.

31.1. For ADHD

Classroom Strategies

- Assign preferential seating in the classroom (seating close to the teacher or work areas, and away from any visual or auditory distractions).
- Provide both written and oral directions for tests/projects.
- Give brief, concise directions.
- Break tasks into small components and provide clear, explicit step-by-step instructions, especially when new material is introduced.
- Use accompanying visual aids whenever possible in the classroom; use several sensory modalities of instruction to maintain attention and increase learning.
- Teach the child how to use an assignment book.
- Encourage the child to repeat, rephrase, and demonstrate instructions, to enhance comprehension and attention to tasks.
- Allow additional time if needed to complete assignments; provide homework modification in terms of the amount of work assigned and/or the amount of time an assignment should take.
- Reduce sources of distraction in the classroom.
- Have the child use attention-grabbing/self-monitoring devices, such as a highlighter.
- Provide consistency and structure through the use of daily schedules, standard seating arrangements, and clearly defined classroom expectations.
- Minimize unnecessary stressors; assign tasks that can be successfully completed.

- Remind the child at the beginning of the day to turn in homework or take homework out of his/her backpack/locker; remind the child at the end of the day about what he/she needs for school and home the next day.
- Offer one-to-one instruction time, especially before tests.
- Give a study sheet with key words/concepts prior to tests.
- Interact frequently with the child in the classroom to maintain her/his involvement; use voice, proximity, and touch.
- Frequently elicit questions and opinions from the child to maintain his/her involvement in an activity.
- Allow the child to tape-record lectures for later review.
- Schedule more frequent parent–teacher conferences to review progress.
- Tutor the child in specific course content when needed.

Homework Strategies

- Have the child check in once a day with a person who will supervise homework.
- Establish a system for monitoring the accomplishment of daily assignments through behavioral contracting.
- When assigning homework, be sure that the child can complete the amount of homework assigned.
- Schedule a "homework time" and help the child organize his/her free time to facilitate homework completion.
- Give the child an assignment sheet to complete each day, instead of having the child copy the entire assignment off the board; she/he circles or checks off each type of homework when it is finished. See the example below.

  Date: _4/10/06_

  1. Spelling: Write each spelling word in a sentence for Wednesday. ____
             Study spelling words for Friday test. ____

  2. Math: Do problems 7 through 15 on page 47 in math workbook. ____

  3. Geography: Read Chapter 6 and answer questions at end of chapter. ____

Other Strategies

- Refer the child to a physician for medication evaluation. Medications such as Ritalin and Metadate (methylphenidate); Adderall and Dexedrine (amphetamine compounds); and Strattera (atomoxetine) are frequently prescribed.
- Recommend behavior therapy and/or parent management training.

31.2. For Anxiety

- Recommend cognitive-behavioral therapy and instruction in self-regulation skills (e.g., coping skills to manage anxiety).
- Refer the child to a physician for medication evaluation.
- If the child has tendency to be withdrawn, pair her/him with a "study buddy" or encourage involvement in a small group.
- Provide the child with positive feedback and reassurance; offer constructive criticism in private.

- Reduce emphasis on competition and perfection.
- Provide structure, predictability, routines, and consistency.

31.3. For Asperger's Disorder

- Enroll the child in a class with a low student–teacher ratio, or provide a classroom aide when needed.
- Recommend therapies as appropriate; these may include occupational, sensory integration, speech and language, and/or physical therapies.
- Provide social skills training in a small-group setting, as well as social skills facilitation throughout the school day.
- Tutor the child in organizational and study skills.
- Provide special education or Section 504 support in areas of academic need (e.g., reading comprehension, math, written expression).
- Establish an organized environment that includes clear routines and schedules, with advance notice of changes.
- Recommend therapy to assist with social reasoning, anxiety reduction, and/or obsessive tendencies.

31.4. For Autism/Other Pervasive Developmental Disorders

- Recommend specialized therapies, such as speech and language, occupational, and/or physical therapies.
- Refer to a structured language-based program and/or specialized placement program specifically designed for children with autism or other pervasive developmental disorders.
- Provide behavior therapy to address concerns regarding self-stimulation, aggression, and/or disruptive behavior.
- Provide social skills training.
- Recommend parent support groups and other parent resources.
- Refer for medication evaluation.
- Recommend consultation with a pediatric neurologist, who may recommend follow-up tests such as genetic testing.

31.5. For Conduct Problems/ODD

- Provide a structured behavioral program both at home and at school.
- Recommend consistent, predictable behavior management (including a united parental front in regard to expectations and discipline).

31.6. For Depression (Unipolar and Bipolar)

- Recommend individual cognitive-behavioral therapy and/or family therapy.
- Structure the environment so that the child feels more competent, successful, and important; make the appropriate classroom/curricular adjustments to prevent unnecessary stress, frustration, or anger.
- Refer for medication evaluation.

31.7. For Disorder of Written Expression

- Provide tutoring that addresses prewriting components (e.g., brainstorming for ideas, verbal rehearsal, and outlining), writing clear sentences, developing a theme, proofreading, and revision of drafts.
- Provide the child with checklists for proofreading.
- Have the child use a computer as much as possible; teach typing skills necessary to become competent on the computer.
- Provide extra time on tests that involve writing.
- Reduce writing requirements; give the child the opportunity to express his/her creative ideas without the barrier of handwriting, such as permitting oral book reports.
- Have the child use AlphaSmart, or other hand-held spellers, or engage the help of a scribe.
- If the child is more successful using cursive writing than printing, encourage the use of cursive.
- Adjust expectations for fine motor activities to match the child's best efforts.
- Minimize copying activities by providing information or activities on worksheets or handouts rather than on the board.
- Assign follow-up activities that reduce a child's writing requirements (paired talking activities, cooperative small-group work, instructional games, short-answer/matching/multiple choice activity sheets, etc.).
- Access the support of an occupational therapist for specific treatment recommendations.
- Recommend direct instruction in a handwriting course, such as Handwriting without Tears.

31.8. For Dyslexia/Reading Disorder

Tutoring in a phonics-based, multisensory approach to reading (typically provided individually, multiple times per week) has been shown to be the most effective treatment for dyslexia. Approaches found to be effective in treating dyslexia include the Wilson (www.wilsonlanguage.com), Lindamood–Bell (www.lblp.com), and Orton–Gillingham (www.ortongillingham.com) programs.

Classroom Modifications

- Allow extra time on tests.
- Allow taking tests in an oral format when appropriate.
- Do not penalize the child for spelling errors.
- Assist with note taking and copying from the board, such as allowing the child to use teacher-made notes or to tape-record lectures for later review.
- Have the child use a word processor with spell-checking capabilities as much as possible, and/or a hand-held speller for in-class work.
- Allow exemption from a foreign language requirement, or, when this is not possible, encourage the child/adolescent to learn a foreign language that is phonetic (such as Spanish).

Strategies for a College-Age Student

- Encourage the student to take a reduced courseload.
- Allow extra time for taking tests and completing assignments.
- Have the student use Kurzweil Reader or other computerized reading assistance systems.
- Recommend books on tape.

Spelling Strategies

- Provide the child with consistent exposure to various word games or puzzles (e.g., crosswords, find-a-word games, Jumble, Scrabble).
- Provide the child with a spelling dictionary.
- Recommend commercially available spelling games to help practice encoding and rule use.
- Encourage the use of a word processor or a hand-held speller (see above).

Reading Comprehension Strategies

- Use scaffolded instruction, such as providing verbal prompts and visual examples/models.
- Prior to reading, provide focusing questions (e.g., "who," "what," "where," "when," "why," and "how") that direct the child's attention to salient formation and set a purpose for reading.
- Provide structural aids for reading assignments (e.g., comprehension questions prior to reading, a story map or web to be filled out while the child is reading, a skeletal outline of the reading).

31.9. For Eating Disorders

- Recommend individual and family therapy.
- Ensure medical stabilization.
- Recommend group therapy.

31.10. For Mathematics Disorder

- Provide direct special education services and/or tutoring support in mathematics.
- Provide compensatory strategies, such as written "recipes" for complex math problems, or the use of graph paper for the alignment of columns.
- Provide the student with a more concrete, hands-on approach to learning math concepts.
- Make math practically oriented, emphasizing real-life skills such as cooking and shopping.
- Provide child with instruction in evaluating which operations are required in calculations; in determining whether information given in a problem is pertinent or nonessential; and in estimating and checking answers against the estimates to evaluate their reasonableness.

31.11. For Memory Problems

- Create a system to help the child remember information, using things such as key words, mnemonic cues, or unique personal cues.
- Practice strategies of rehearsal and delayed control to gradually increase the amount of time the child must remember a command.
- Rehearse information frequently.

31.12. For Mental Retardation

- Recommend special education services, including educational services and vocational training.
- Provide direct instruction in safety, self-care, and social skills.

- Recommend math and other instruction that focuses on life skills training (e.g., use of money, time).
- Provide on-the-job training.
- Recommend occupational, speech, or physical therapy as needed.

31.13. For NLD

- Provide tutoring or resource room support in areas of weakness, such as math, reading comprehension, or written expression.
- Provide occupational therapy for problems with visual–spatial ability.
- Provide child with assistance in reading charts, graphs, and the like, if visual–spatial deficits are present.
- Recommend counseling or psychotherapy focusing on self-esteem and coping strategies.
- Provide group social skills training, as well as social skills facilitation throughout the school day.
- Provide child with opportunities to socialize with peers in appropriate ways (e.g., community recreational activities, sports, Scouts, etc.).
- Tailor course choices to accentuate strengths and avoid weaknesses.
- Use educational software to enhance skills in areas of weakness.
- Make classroom accommodations, such as those suggested for children with ADHD (*see Section 31.1*).
- Offer clear, concise information about tests and assignments.

31.14. For Obsessive–Compulsive Disorder

- Recommend cognitive-behavioral therapy.
- Refer for medication evaluation.

31.15. For Social Difficulties

- Provide group training in social skills group to learn skills for positive peer relationships.
- Encourage child to become involved in activities and school-related functions to promote positive relationships.

32

Closing Statements

32.1. Current Expectations

Prognostic statements are very rarely seen in child and adolescent reports. More typically seen are suggestions of what could be expected of the child in the near future in academic, social, and home settings. You should be extremely cautious about making long-range predictions, but when making such predictions you should do the following:

- Restate the child's level of functioning.
- Indicate, in light of the child's level of functioning, what he/she can be expected to accomplish with and without service interventions.
- Indicate the degree of confidence in your predictions.

The child's progress and prognosis are/may be limited by her/his diagnosis/condition/motivation/cognition/abilities/etc. However, positive prognostic indicators include motivation for treatment, cognitive/academic/etc. abilities, family/school/social support, history of progress, well-developed relationship with therapist, etc. I am quite confident that with the appropriate treatments (such as those mentioned in the recommendations) that he/she will continue to make excellent progress.

32.2. Value of the Information

I hope that this information is helpful to you.

I hope that this information proves useful to you as you support this child's education and development.

I hope this information will be useful to you as you consider this case's/child's/adolescent's needs and will aid you in your tasks/evaluation/treatment/decisions.

I hope that this information will be sufficient for you to judge this child's situation.

In the hope that these data will prove of assistance . . .

32.3. Thanking the Referrer

Thank you very much for the opportunity to see this very pleasant young man/young woman/ boy/girl. Please do not hesitate to call with any questions or concerns.

The consultant wishes to thank the staff at the _____ School for allowing this observation to take place.

Thank you for the opportunity to evaluate _____ (child's name).
Thank you for this interesting referral.
Thank you for the referral of this appealing young man/young woman/boy/girl.

32.4. Follow-Up Care

I would like to see him/her again in follow-up, in ____ months/years.
_____ should return in _____ for a follow-up evaluation. We will contact his/ her parents several months in advance, by mail, so they may call to schedule a follow-up appointment.
The child's family is asked to follow up with Dr. _____ in ____ days/weeks/months.
I have explained to the parents that I would be pleased to attend a team meeting at the child's school, if they would find that helpful.

32.5. Continued Availability

If I can be of any further assistance, please feel free to call me at _____ (give phone number).
If there are any questions regarding this evaluation or the content of this report, please feel free to contact the evaluator at the following number: _____.
I would be happy to assist this child and her/his family further in any way, but particularly in trying to secure the resources necessary to meet the above-mentioned recommendations.
I can be reached to answer any questions that this report may raise at the following number: _____.
Further discussions of these results are available upon request.
Please do not hesitate to contact me at _____ (insert contact information) if I can be of further assistance.
Please feel free to contact me if I can provide any further assistance, or can answer any questions you may have concerning this report.
I would be happy to answer any further questions you may have.
If there are questions about this report, please feel free to call me at _____ (insert phone number).
Given his/her parents' permission, I would be available to discuss the results of this evaluation.
Additional consultation and/or services are available upon request.
Please feel free to talk with me further about any questions or concerns, or if I can be of help in any way.
I would be pleased to discuss the results of this evaluation, given appropriate permission to do so.

32.6. Availability to Schools/Service Providers

I am happy to provide support to teachers or tutors as indicated.
This examiner would welcome any contact with _____'s school and/or service providers to help translate this evaluation into tangible terms.
I am available for discussion with _____'s parents or teacher(s) of specific findings from this examination.
I would be happy to share information from this evaluation with others working with this child, with appropriate consent, or to assist in monitoring the child's progress.

32.7. Concluding Statements

What follow are some positive statements that you can use to conclude the report. Of course, it is quite possible that the evaluation was not a pleasure for you. In that case, it is best either not to comment on this or to use a simple statement such as the following: **Thank you for the opportunity to evaluate _____.**

General Statements

It was a pleasure working with _____ and his/her family.
I have enjoyed working with this child and her/his parents/family over the course of this evaluation.
It was my pleasure to work with _____ and participate in his/her treatment.
In conclusion, it was a pleasure to meet and work with _____ and her/his parents.
It was a pleasure working with and getting to know _____.

Statements for Reevaluations

It was a pleasure to see _____ once again, and I hope that the information provided in this report is helpful in providing direction for his/her ongoing educational interventions and accommodations.
Once again, this child was a pleasure to evaluate.
It was a pleasure to work with _____ again and see the progress she/he has made.

32.8. Complimentary Closing and Signature

The signature is often preceded by one of the following types of statements:

Respectfully submitted,
Sincerely,
Yours truly,

The report should be signed by the person or persons who completed the evaluation. If the report was completed under the supervision of another professional, the supervisor should also sign the report. Underneath the signature(s) should be included the following:

- Typed name(s).
- Degree(s).
- Professional title(s) (e.g., Psychologist, School Psychologist, etc.).

Add any of these statements as appropriate:

I authorize that my name may be mechanically affixed to this report.
Dictated but not read, to facilitate mailing to you.
Typed and mailed in the doctor's absence.
If my initials do not follow this sentence, this printed report has not been reviewed/edited by me and may contain errors of typing or words that I would have changed.

Part III

Special Circumstances and Useful Resources

33

Writing for the Schools

This chapter addresses issues important to school evaluations. It includes information about the Individuals with Disabilities Education Act (IDEA) and individualized education plans (IEPs); it also includes information about observations of classroom behavior, as well as possible formats for reports of these observations. See Section 35.9 for a sample IEP, Section 35.10 for a sample classroom observation report, and Section 40.6 for a form for educational assessment of a student's current classroom functioning.

33.1. School versus Agency Referrals

The focus of school referrals generally differs from that of clinic referrals in a few important ways. The focus of a school evaluation is on determining how a child's psychological, learning, or developmental difficulties interfere with his/her ability to function and progress in school. The focus of a clinical evaluation is usually broader, in that the evaluator typically wants to diagnose and/or treat the child's difficulties in a variety of settings. For example, in a child exhibiting severe anxiety, a school psychologist will want to know why the child is anxious at school, whereas a clinical evaluator might want to determine the type of medication or psychotherapy that would be most beneficial. A multidisciplinary team (i.e., a team composed of professionals with diverse specialties, such as nurses, psychologists, special education teachers, general education teachers, the school principal, speech and language therapists, physical therapists, occupational therapists, etc.) is typically involved in school evaluations but is rarely involved in nonschool evaluations. Finally, triennial evaluations are required in the school setting to determine whether a child still qualifies for special education, whether the placement is appropriate, and what the child's current levels of functioning are.

33.2. Individuals with Disabilities Education Act (IDEA)

Under IDEA (1990, 1997, 2004) all children with disabilities are granted a free and appropriate education (FAPE). To qualify for special education and related services, IDEA specifies that a child must have a disability in one of the categories listed below. According to the law, a child is not eligible for special education services if her/his difficulties are due solely to a lack of instruction or to limited English proficiency.

Disability Categories

- Mental retardation.
- Hearing impairments (including deafness).
- Deafness/blindness.
- Multiple disabilities.
- Speech or language impairments.
- Visual impairments (including blindness).
- Emotional disturbance.
- Orthopedic impairments.
- Autism.
- Traumatic brain injury.
- Other health impairments.
- Specific learning disability.

Important Disability-Related Terms and Definitions

Americans with Disabilities Act (ADA): A law that makes it illegal to discriminate against anyone (a child or an adult) on the basis of a disability.

Behavioral intervention plan (BIP): An individualized plan created for students with behavior problems, which includes information about reinforcement schedules, behavioral interventions, strategies for managing behavior, classroom support, and other interventions as needed.

Early periodic screening, diagnosis, and treatment (EPSDT): Services that are provided to infants and children at risk.

Extended school year (ESY): Services provided outside the normal school year (e.g., during summer vacation) as needed for children with disabilities.

Free and appropriate public education (FAPE): As noted above, IDEA mandates an FAPE for every child.

Full inclusion: The education of children with disabilities in regular classrooms within their local schools.

Functional behavioral analysis (FBA): An assessment that provides information about how a child's situational, environmental, and behavioral factors may contribute to his/her problems.

Individualized education plan (IEP): The IDEA requires that every child with a disability have an IEP. (*See Section 33.3, below, for more information on the IEP.*)

Individualized education plan team (IEP team): The group of people who is responsible for developing, reviewing, and revising a child's IEP. It usually includes the child's parents and those responsible for implementing the IEP goals.

Individualized family service plan (IFSP): A plan for services for young children (under 3 years of age) and their families; it is similar to an IEP.

Individuals with Disabilities Education Act (IDEA): The current law requiring children with disabilities to be given an FAPE. This act replaced Public Law 94-142, the Education for All Handicapped Children Act of 1975 (*see below*). IDEA was originally enacted in 1990 and was amended in 1997 and 2004.

Least restrictive environment: According to Hallahan and Kauffman (1994), a legal term referring to the fact that exceptional children must be educated in as normal an environment as possible.

Office of Special Education and Rehabilitative Services (OSERS): The U.S. Department of Education agency that is responsible for enforcing IDEA in the public schools.

Public Law 94-142, the Education for All Handicapped Children Act: Superseded by IDEA (*see* *above*) in 1990, this law was passed in 1975 and mandated an FAPE for every child, regardless of ability or disability.

Regular education initiative (REI): The philosophy that regular education, as opposed to special education, should be the primary means of educating children with disabilities.

Section 504, Rehabilitation Act of 1973: Applies to students who have learning or performance weaknesses that could be deemed "disabilities," but who are not eligible for special education services.

Services plan: A plan developed for students in private school who are entitled to receive services.

33.3. Individualized Education Plan (IEP)

IDEA requires an IEP to be drawn up by an educational team for every child with a disability who meets the qualifying criteria. The IEP must include a statement of present educational performance, annual goals, special educational and related services to be provided, participation with nondisabled children, participation in statewide and districtwide tests, transition service needs, age of majority, and procedures for measuring progress (IDEA, 1997, 2004).

IEP Meeting

- The IEP meeting is conducted with the purpose of developing the child's IEP.
- The policy for providing an IEP (such as it relates to funding, administration, and implementation) is stated in IDEA, Part B.
- The meeting to develop a child's IEP must be held 50 calendar days after it has been determined that the child may need special services.
- Notice for the IEP meeting must include the purpose, time, place, and location of the meeting, as well as who will be in attendance. If the meeting will include transition services for the student, then the student must be invited to attend.
- The IEP team includes the child's parents; at least one of the child's teachers; at least one special education teacher; a representative who can provide or supervise special instructions; an individual who can interpret the educational implications of the results (this person may already be a member of the team); any other individuals who may have important information about the child or treatment services; and the child, when indicated.

Content of the IEP

The IEP includes the following components (IDEA, 1997, 2004):

1. A statement of the child's current level of performance, including information about how the child's disability may affect her/his ability to access the general curriculum.
2. Annual goals and short-term objectives that will address the child's educational needs.
3. The services, special education, and aids that will be provided to the child.
4. The extent (if any) to which the child cannot participate with nondisabled children.
5. Any modifications necessary for the child to participate in statewide or districtwide assessments. If it is indicated that the child will not participate in such assessments, then a statement is needed to describe why he/she will not participate.
6. The date services will begin, as well as the frequency, location, and duration of those services.
7. Beginning when the child is 14 years of age, and annually thereafter, a statement of transition needs that focus on the child's course of study. Beginning when the child is 16, a statement of transition services.

8. A statement of how the child's progress toward the goals will be measured.
9. A list of the members present.
10. Signatures of persons in attendance.

33.4. Observations of Classroom Behavior

Observations of children's behavior often constitute an important part of the diagnostic process. Furthermore, such observations are essential to FBA (*see Section 33.2*) and many types of behavioral treatment programs. In general, the following points are important to keep in mind when you are conducting a classroom observation:

- Do not interfere with normal events in the classroom.
- If the focus is on identifying a problem behavior, indicate when the problem behavior(s) occurs, what preceded the behavior, what happened immediately after the behavior occurred, and what affect (if any) it had on the environment.
- Conducting a thorough review of records and interviewing with classroom teacher(s) before the evaluation will help focus the observation.

According to Sattler (1992), the purpose of the school consultation should be to help teachers find solutions to students' problems. Sattler indicates that the consultations should help teachers do the following:

- Modify their behavior.
- Deal more effectively with children, parents, and other school personnel.
- Develop new teaching strategies or curriculum changes.
- Develop ways of documenting changes in behavior over time.

Formats for Classroom Observation Reports

Reason for referral.
Actions taken (e.g., classroom observation, review of records, teacher interview, etc.).
Classroom observation.
Conclusions.

Introduction.
Discussion with service providers.
Classroom observation 1.
    Impressions/analysis.
Classroom observation 2.
    Impressions/analysis.
Discussion with service providers of examiner's observations.
Overall analysis.

Reason for referral.
Evaluation methods.
Summary of record review.
Summary of observations.
Recommendations.

33.5. Behavior Management Plans

See Section 40.7 for a form that can be used in writing a behavior management plan.

Behavior management plans or behavior support plans are documents that define how a child's inappropriate behaviors will be remediated. O'Neill et al. (1997) indicate that a behavior support plan should include the following:

- Description of the problem behavior in operationalized terms.
- Summary statements from a functional assessment.
- Treatment strategies for extinguishing problem behaviors.
- Description of typical routines and difficult situations.
- Plan for monitoring and evaluation.

34

Treatment Planning

34.1. About Treatment Planning

Treatment plans identify a child's or adolescent's treatment needs, desired goals, and the strategies for achieving those goals. Such plans are typically written after a thorough assessment of needs has been completed. The assessment may include clinical interview(s), record review, testing, observation, and information from collateral sources.

The sequence of clinical practice suggests that a clinician goes from the initial assessment of the child or adolescent to selection of the interventions needed, and then to provision of those interventions, which should result in beneficial outcomes. Treatment planning, however, reflects the sequence for clinical thinking about a case. That sequence starts with assessment and diagnosis and then goes to desired goals; only then—looking at both starting points and desired ending points—does the clinician generate the interventions likely to achieve desired goals. The following discussion looks more closely at how a clinician thinks about treatment and treatment planning.

Assessment, Diagnosis, and Setting Priorities

Treatment planning begins with the assessment of the presenting problem or chief complaint, including the presenting symptoms, mental status, risks, background and history, testing results, and family expectations of treatment and outcome. This leads to diagnosis making. A single diagnosis, however, can encompass a number of different problems, symptoms, and deficits in functioning. The next step is therefore to set priorities (i.e., to rank the problems by importance) jointly with the parents or guardian, and also with an older child or adolescent if she/he is capable of participating in the planning process.

Goals and Objectives

Once there is agreement on the most important problems or symptoms to address, the planning process continues with a consideration of outcomes—goals, objectives, and desired benefits. Clinicians can ask themselves, "If we wish to achieve this goal by this date, what steps need to be taken before then?" Available resources, time, finances, and other considerations can impose limitations on what goals are realistic. Therefore, treatment goals and objectives often need to be selected and prioritized.

Among the criteria for "well-formed treatment goals" offered by Berg and Miller (1992) in regard to substance abuse treatment for adults, but readily adaptable to the present discussion, are the following:

- They must be important to the client (in the present context, the child or adolescent and his/her family).
- They should be small.
- They should be concrete, behavioral, and specific.
- They should focus on the presence rather than the absence of something (e.g., on desired behaviors rather than a lack of dysfunctional behaviors).
- They must focus on the first small steps—on what to do first, on a beginning rather than an end.
- They should be realistic and achievable within the context of the child's (and family's) life.

Once goals are selected, planning can proceed to the choice of interventions, efforts, methods, and means. Treatment planning should logically include the ending of treatment. Managed care (MCOs) organizations may ask what steps have been taken or will be taken to prepare the child and family for treatment termination. (*See Section 34.3, below, for a suggested treatment plan format for MCOs.*)

In writing a treatment plan, you may find yourself struggling between writing a plan that is too general and one that is too specific. A plan that is too general will be an empty exercise that offers no real guidance for treatment. An overly precise plan will require either following it rigidly or continually revising it in light of the realities of practice.

"Goals" are usually understood as long-term destinations, and "objectives" are the steps needed to reach those goals. But because there is no agreement in the field over the exact meaning of "objectives," you need not be precise in differentiating them from goals. Objectives are usually more behavioral and concrete than goals. Objectives are also shorter-term and more easily measurable. They are usually described in terms of the child's behavior or performance ("The child will be able to ... ").

Being able to assess change is absolutely crucial. Write desired outcomes in behavioral language. This means describing what a camera would see (actions and expressions), not invisible or intangible factors (e.g., emotions, cognitive processes, history, and intentions). Also avoid very broad or vague terms such as "increase," "communication skills," or "depression," because such terms do not make it clear what might count as change. Tie each objective and goal to the child's presenting limitations of functioning. Make these objectives observable or quantifiable. Frequency, duration, intensity, and latency are the classic dimensions for describing symptomatic behaviors. This objectification allows impartial evaluation.

Finally, avoid jargon, especially words understood only by professionals of a particular orientation. Either use common-language translations of theory, or (preferably) focus on specific symptoms and practical intervention strategies.

Interventions

You can specify interventions by asking yourself questions like these:

- What approaches have been shown to work for this problem?
- What are you trained to do with these kinds of problems? (If you lack the skill in these areas, do not try to fake it. Get the necessary training, or refer the child to a competent professional who has such training.)
- What techniques address the symptoms presented?
- How are these techniques implemented? (How often, for how long, with what tools?)
- What will you expect the child to do?

Offer specific descriptors of the mode of treatment (individual, group, family, school-based, etc.), the treatment orientation or modality (cognitive, interpersonal, psychodynamic, structural, etc.), particular techniques (social skills training, perspective training, systematic desensitization, etc.), and the clinical targets of treatment (problems in social relationships, fears/phobias, conduct problems, oppositional behaviors, etc.).

34.2. A Checklist of Strengths

Alternative terms for "strengths" include the following:

General:

> Assets, resources, capacities, talents, competencies, unrecognized resources, protective/generative factors.

Physical:

> Healthy, energetic, normal weight/size, eats/sleeps well, fit, in good physical shape, physical development is appropriate for age, active.

Cognitive:

> Can attend/concentrate/recall, has planning and organizational abilities, academic competence, strong intellectual skills, well-developed verbal/nonverbal/analytical skills, academic skills that are advanced for age, creative/imaginative/artistic/inventive/talented/adaptable/flexible/compliant/resourceful, common-sensical, accurately appraises demands.

Affective:

> Aware of feelings in self and others, comfortable with feelings, appropriately expressive, shows range of affects, tolerates emotional stress/distress, high frustration tolerance, can self-soothe.

Interpersonal:

> Socially skilled/competent, respectful/polite, tolerant of others, accepts/offers feedback, helpful/cooperative/accommodating, supportive/caring of others, popular/likeable/well-liked, admired by her/his peers, friendly, comfortable, outgoing/extroverted, sense of humor, shares, helpful, socially sensitive, aware of impact on others, good listener/empathic, shows concern for others, supports others.

34.3. A Treatment Plan Format for Managed Care Organizations (MCOs)

The following is adapted with permission from Zuckerman (2005, pp. 308–317).

    I. Identification of client(s) and providers.
       A. Purpose: Preauthorization for initial certification *or* concurrent review for reauthorization.
   II. Case formulation/overview.
       A. Presenting problem(s)/chief complaint/chief concern. *For questions to ask, see Chapters 1–4; for referral reasons, see Chapter 8.*
       B. Background of presenting problem(s) and current situation. *All elements needing clinical attention are conceived of as either stressors, diatheses, or abnormal behaviors. Behaviors may become new stressors. See Chapter 9 for current symptoms, Chapter 10 for medical and psychiatric background, Chapter 11 for developmental and family history, and Chapter 12 for academic and school history.*

C. Previous treatments. *Again, see Chapter 10 for medical and psychiatric background.*

D. Brief summary of mental status evaluation results.

E. Functional limitations and impairments.

F. Strengths.

G. Diagnoses. *See Chapter 29.*

H. Current assessment of knowable risks. *Suicide, homicide, and violence are risks of greatest concern to both clinicians and MCOs. Of only slightly less concern to MCOs are substance abuse and dependence.*

I. Recommended level of care. *See Chapter 31.*

III. Treatment concerns.

A. Progress in current treatment to date. *Use this section when seeking reauthorization for a continuation of your services. These concurrent reviews function like progress reports.*

B. Treatment plan.

1. Additional consultations or evaluations. *This section states what further information the treatment provider needs to know and how that information can be obtained. For example, additional testing or consultants may be necessary.*

2. Treatment objectives and goals. *For each problem or concern to be treated, specify:*

a. *The behaviors to be changed.*

b. *The planned interventions (who does what, how often, with what recourses; modality, frequency, duration).*

c. *Observable indicators of improvements (these are the behavioral goals; report expected number of session to achieve each indicator).*

d. *The level of problem behaviors expected at discharge.*

e. *Review date.*

3. Other current treatment providers. *(For each professional, list name, location, phone, and treatments being provided.)*

IV. Signature.

34.4. Tabular Treatment Plan Formats

Maxmen and Ward (1995) note that treatment plans should include the following:

1. Type of treatment (e.g., group, individual, family, etc.).
2. Frequency and amount of treatment (e.g., weekly/biweekly/etc.; number of weeks/months that therapy will continue).
3. Specific problems that will be the focus of the treatment.
4. Specific goals of treatment.
5. The timing of the treatments (e.g., focusing on acute problems before more chronic ones).

Each clinician, agency, funder, and monitor seems to have a different preferred format for treatment plans. Many of them use a tabular format—that is, a page turned sideways (if necessary) and divided into columns. For example, Wiger (1999) suggests a three-column format for the treatment plan:

(First column:) **Problems/Symptoms** (problems to be addressed in treatment)
(Second column:) **Goals/Objectives** (treatment outcomes in observable terms)
(Third column:) **Strategies** (treatment interventions to be used during therapy)

Below are other commonly used headings for such columns, plus a set of headings for a fourth column:

(First column:) **Behaviors to Be Changed, Diagnosis-Related Symptoms.**
(Second column:) **Outcome, Objective Sought/Desired/Expected, Output, Observable Indica-**

tors of Improvement, Symptom-Related Goals, Focus of Treatment, Short-Term Goal, Discharge Level of Problem Behavior, Performance.

(Third column:) Intervention, Resources to Be Employed, Methods, Treatments, Means, Tactics, Efforts, Inputs.

(Fourth column:) Time Frame, Date of Evaluation, Date of Initiation, Target Date, Completion Date, Expected Number of Sessions to Achieve Objective, Date of Review/Reevaluation/Progress Evaluation.

In the fourth (time frame) column, specify the target as a certain number of treatment sessions if you can, since clients may miss meetings during a specified time period. Similarly, it is preferable to offer a review date rather than an achievement or completion date.

Other columns may include the following:

Intensity, Frequency, Duration of Treatment.
Child's Strengths or Assets, Degree of Involvement.
Liabilities, Resistances/Barriers to Change (in the child or elsewhere).

Wilson's Social Work Model

Wilson's (1980) social work model can be applied to child psychotherapy. The model includes these elements:

The ideal means of meeting the needs of the child and family.
Realistic actions that can be taken to meet these needs.
The child's and/or the parent's willingness and ability to carry out these treatment plans.
Progress made or not made since the plan was written.
What you will now do differently.

The Analytical Thinking Model

This model (also described by Wilson, 1980) can be a useful way of thinking about and analyzing your work with a particular child or family.

1. Review in your mind everything you know about the case.
2. Make a list of the 10–15 key facts of the case.
3. Imagine what feelings the child or family might have about the situation, considering the perceptions of all involved parties:
   a. At whom or what might the feelings be directed?
   b. Why might each party feel that way?
   c. What would be the behavioral manifestations of those feelings?
4. Who are the child's/family's "significant others" (i.e., support network)?
5. Develop a treatment plan:
   a. List all the possible outcomes of treatment (whether realistic or not).
   b. Label each as realistic or not.
   c. For each realistic goal, list the subgoals or objectives to be achieved, and put them in any necessary sequence.
   d. State the exact treatment techniques that would accomplish the subgoals.
   e. Rank the goals in a time sequence, so that you know where to start.
   f. Estimate the time needed to achieve each goal.

Write a summary of the main thoughts of steps 2 through 4, and discard all the material except this and the lists developed in step 5.

34.5. A Children's Residential Agency Format

   I. Identifying information: Name, date of birth, date of admission, agency, primary worker.
  II. Data and needs.
     A. Education.
     B. Medical/physical status.
     C. Contacts (legal, family, etc.).
     D. Personal development (goals):
        1. Personal hygiene.
        2. Peer relationships.
        3. Adult relationships.
        4. Group relationships.
        5. Specialized treatments/therapies/support.
        6. Specific events.
 III. Treatment/program adjustments (to methods).
     A. Major incidents.
     B. Routine adjustments.
     C. Level changes (levels of programming).
     D. Attitude and motivation.
     E. Target summary (and changes in targets).
 IV. Family support and follow-up care.

35

Report Formats
and Sample Reports

This chapter provides formats for various types of reports, as well as some sample reports. For more information about school reports (as well as some school report formats) see Chapter 33, "Writing for the Schools." For more information on treatment plans (and some treatment plan formats), see Chapter 34, "Treatment Planning."

35.1. Standard Formats for Child Reports

A report should meet the needs of its readers, not the writer. The reader of child reports may include a varied population, such as the child's parents, school personnel, a pediatric neurologist, the child's tutor, and/or a pediatrician. Although it may be difficult to try to meet the needs of all the potential readers of a report, the evaluator can attempt to do this by providing (1) one or more concise referral questions; (2) describing the history in the client's (i.e., parent's and/or child's) language to the extent possible; (3) describing the results of the evaluation, using as little jargon as possible; and (4) providing recommendations that can be clearly understood by most persons who will read the report.

The sequential structure of Part II of this book can be used as a format for a child report. (*See also Table 1 in this book's Introduction.*) Use your agency's or your own letterhead with credentials of relevance. Give the title or type of report as the heading. Then provide the following:

> Name of child or adolescent; case/identification number; child's/adolescent's age, gender, and birth date.
> Date(s) of examination(s) and report.
> Evaluator's name (if not the same as the name on the letterhead), and supervisor's name if appropriate.
> Name of person or agency to whom the report is to be sent, if someone other than the parent or legal guardian.

Rivas-Vasquez, Blais, Rey, and Rivas-Vasquez (2001) recommend 12 content areas that should be covered in an initial evaluation. The 12 areas are listed below, with some additions and some comments on assessing them in children and adolescents.

> 1. Identifying information.
> 2. Chief complaint or concern.
>> In the client's language (usually the parent's language, but may also include the child's, depending on his/her age and cognitive ability).
>> Referral source and reason for referral.

3. History of present illness or problem.
   Symptoms, treatments, conflicts.
4. Medical history.
   Conditions, medications, treatments, treaters, nutrition.
5. Prior psychiatric history.
6. Substance abuse history.
   Typically only pertains to adolescent patients and is not usually commented on in children below the age of 13–14 years.
7. Family psychiatric and substance abuse histories.
8. Psychosocial history.
   Traumas, educational functioning, developmental history, legal issues.
9. Mental status examination.
   Appearance, behavioral observations.
   Mood and affect.
   Cognitive functions.
10. Psychometric database (when applicable).
    Summary of findings.
11. Diagnostic impression.
    Case formulation/summary.
    Reliability or cautions.
    Diagnoses.
12. Treatment plan or recommendations.
    Referrals.
    Resources.
    Motivation and barriers to treatment.

Rivas-Vasquez et al. (2001) state: "The outline presented above is intended to allow clinicians to structure the documentation of the initial diagnostic evaluation in order to produce a clinical and legal record that can attest to the work that was performed. It will also serve to outline the psychologist's diligence and thoroughness, serve as a communication between health care providers, and satisfy reimbursement requirements for third party payers" (p. 199).

Lewis (2002) points out that since the purposes of consultations differ, so should the content of reports, and that usually a limited number of the items listed above is more appropriate. He adds that the accepted practice in a given setting shapes the content.

Sattler (2001) indicates that a report should have nine sections, as listed below:

1. **Identifying information:** Include information such as child's name, date of birth, gender, age, grade in school, date(s) of assessment(s), and date of report.
2. **Assessment instruments:** List both formal and informal assessment measures.
3. **Reason for referral:** State the reason for the referral, as well as the referral source and relationship of referral source to the child.
4. **Background information:** Include pertinent information from the child's history that has been provided through interviews with the child, parents, teacher, and any others, as well as information provided from previous evaluations.
5. **Observations during the assessment:** Include your observations of the child during the assessment process.
6. **Assessment results and clinical impressions:** Provide a review of the assessment findings, including information about reliability and validity.
7. **Recommendations:** Provide recommendations based on your findings.
8. **Summary:** Give a short, integrated review of the findings of the evaluation.
9. **Signature:** Include your professional title and degree, along with your name and signature.

If you are completing this report under supervision, your supervisor's name, title, degree, and signature should also be included.

35.2. Child Assessment Format

Jenkins, Tinsley, and Van Loon (2001) offer this format for the psychiatric assessment interview of a child, which is adapted by permission. This format is also quite adaptable to report writing, and the same sequence can be used.

Beginning the Interview and Establishing Rapport

1. Meet the child and accompanying adult(s).
2. Find out why the child thinks she/he is being seen.
3. Discuss the nature and procedures of the interview.
4. Explain that information given is confidential, with the exception of protecting the child and others from imminent harm.

Developmental History

Note that the structure of the evaluation should include individual interviews with the parents.

Family

1. Child's attitude toward each parent.
2. Child's relationship with siblings.
3. Family psychiatric history.
4. History of each parent's childhood.
   a. Relationships with parents and siblings.
   b. Discipline methods used; evidence of abuse or dysfunction.
   c. Level of education and current occupation.
5. Circumstances of child's birth; if adopted, circumstances and motivation for adoption.

Developmental Milestones

1. Physical.
   a. Pregnancy, delivery, feeding, and weaning; neonatal illnesses.
   b. Early or significant medical illnesses or injuries.
   c. Neuromuscular development of speech and motor milestones (sitting, standing, walking, first words, play).
2. Behavioral.
   a. Toilet training and other training—response to discipline, methods used.
   b. Reactions to beginning day care and school.
   c. Sleep patterns, sleep disturbances.
   d. Phobias.
   e. Habit disorders (e.g., bedwetting and thumb sucking).

Significant Events

Ask about moves, parental illnesses/death/divorce, family violence, and so forth.

Current Level of Functioning

1. School performance.
2. Hobbies and extracurricular activities.

3. Peer relationships.
4. Relationships with adults other than parents.
5. Unusual habits and habit disorders.
6. Aims and ambitions.
7. Current health and medications.

Interview with the Child: Possible Topics of Discussion

Child's Ideas about the Problem

1. Expectations for outcome.
2. What the child would like to change in self or others.
3. "What problems have we not talked about yet?"

Symptom Review

1. Vegetative symptoms.
2. Anxiety symptoms.
3. Psychotic symptoms.
4. Suicidal ideation, other self-destructive acts.
5. Ruminations or acts of violence.
6. Substance abuse.
7. Victimization experiences.

Mental Status Exam

Drawings

1. House–Tree–Person.
2. Self-portrait.
3. Kinetic Family Drawing.
4. Person-in-the-Rain.

Other Information That May Be Sought

1. Psychological testing.
2. Medical consultations—pediatric, neurological.
3. School records, interview with teachers.
4. Interviews with other significant adults (noncustodial parents, grandparents, social worker).
5. Records of previous treatment or evaluations.

35.3. Psychiatric Evaluation Format

Psychiatric evaluations do not typically include formal test measures. Instead, there is an emphasis on mental status, psychiatric history, and diagnosis. The following is a possible format for a psychiatric evaluation:

Patient's name.
Date of birth.
Date(s) of evaluation(s).
Names of parents/guardians.
Telephone number of home where child resides.
Clinician(s): Name(s) and identifying information.

Sources of information.
History of present illness.
Previous medical history.
Previous psychiatric history.
Developmental history.
Social history.
Mental status exam.
   Appearance and behavior.
   Speech.
   Mood and affect.
   Thought processes.
   Thought content.
   Insight.
   Judgment.
Diagnostic formulation:
   Predisposing factors.
   Precipitating factors.
   Perpetuating factors.
   Protective factors.
DSM-IV-TR impressions.
   Axis I.
   Axis II.
   Axis III.
   Axis IV.
   Axis V.
Recommendations
Signature(s)/date(s).

35.4. Format for a Functional Behavioral Analysis (FBA) Report

An FBA is "an amalgamation of techniques that have the same purpose: identifying the variables that control a behavior and using that knowledge to design individualized interventions" (Watson & Steege, 2003, p. 5). Watson and Steege indicate that an FBA report should include the following (which is reprinted by permission):

Identifying information.
The reason for the referral.
The assessment procedures used.
The results of the assessment.
The identification of the interfering behaviors.
The description of the interfering behaviors.
The current level of occurrence of interfering behaviors.
Antecedent variables (e.g., "triggers").
Individual variables.
Consequence variables.
The hypothesized function(s) of the interfering behaviors.
Examples of how the variables influence the interfering behaviors.
Recommendations.

35.5. Neuropsychological Evaluation Formats and Sample Report

Report Format

Neuropsychological evaluation reports are typically lengthy documents that can vary considerably from clinician to clinician. A comprehensive report for a neuropsychological evaluation of a fictitious ten-year-old is given on pages 308–312. Immediately below is another possible format for a report of a comprehensive neuropsychological evaluation. Reports of briefer evaluations may only include only some of the following sections.

> Identifying information (e.g., child's name, date, etc.).
> Referral/background information.
> Current school program/status.
> Tests administered.
> Behavioral observations.
> Summary of neuropsychological findings.
>> Cognitive functioning.
>> Language skills.
>> Visual–spatial and visual–motor functioning.
>> Memory.
>> Attention/other executive functions.
> Summary of social and emotional functioning.
> Summary of educational findings.
>> Reading.
>> Written language.
>> Math.
> Summary and implications.
> Recommendations.

35.6. Progress Notes

Progress notes are typically completed at the end of each therapy session. Longer notes, sometimes titled "Progress Summary," are completed at various times during treatment (e.g., every 12 weeks), often at the request of an insurance company or agency policy. A sample progress summary for Jim Smith, a fictitious child, can be found on page 313. A sample format for progress notes follows. (*See also Section 40.8 for a reproducible blank progress note form.*)

Sample Format

1. Presenting problem or diagnosis (e.g., DSM-IV-TR diagnosis code).
2. Type of therapy (e.g., family, individual, group).
3. Description of client.
   a. Physical status.
   b. Psychological status.
4. General focus of interview.
   a. Topics discussed.
   b. Goals addressed.
   c. Behavior change in child or family, if any.
5. Plans for future sessions.
   a. Homework assigned, if any.
6. Plans for contacting other professionals, if relevant, and documentation of consent.

Mary Smith, PhD
Neuropsychologist
100 N. Main Street, Suite 301
Anytown, State 22222

Phone: (999) 555-5555
Fax: (999) 555-5556

State License #12345

Date of report: February 14, 2007

Neuropsychological Evaluation

Child's name: Larry Hall

Age: 10 years, 6 months

Date of birth: 11/25/96

Date(s) of evaluation: 2/11/07

Medical record #: 00111

PROCEDURES

Wechsler Intelligence Scale for Children—Fourth Edition (WISC-IV)
Wechsler Individual Achievement Test—Second Edition (WIAT-II)
Test of Written Language—Third Edition (TOWL-3)
Gray Oral Reading Tests, Fourth Edition (GORT-4)
Peabody Picture Vocabulary Test—Third Edition (PPVT-III)
Beery–Buktenica Developmental Test of Visual–Motor Integration, Fifth Edition (Beery VMI)
Rey–Osterrieth Complex Figure Test (ROCF)
Wide Range Assessment of Memory and Learning, Second Edition (WRAML2) subtests:
- Story Memory
- Sentence Memory
- Picture Memory
- Design Memory

Wisconsin Card Sorting Test (WCST)
Trail Making Test, Parts A and B
Stroop Color and Word Test
Behavior Assessment System for Children, Second Edition (BASC-2)
ADHD Rating Scale–IV
Clinical interview

IDENTIFYING INFORMATION

Larry Hall is a 10-year-old male who lives in Anytown, Anystate with his biological parents and a younger brother, age 6 years. He is in the fourth grade at the Foxboro School.

REASON FOR REFERRAL AND BACKGROUND INFORMATION

Larry was referred for psychological testing by his individual psychotherapist, Dr. Barbara Kelley, because of concerns regarding school performance and difficulties with attention and focusing. Particular difficulties have been noted in Larry's reading progress. Larry's medical care is handled by his pediatrician, Dr. Bill Webb.

(cont.)

Larry's parents, Albert and Deirdre Hall, describe him as having difficulty with transitions and with homework. They indicated that he needs to be asked many times to do what is requested of him. He does not appear to care about the quality of his work and would rather "get the task over quickly." His teacher reports that he has significant behavior problems at school, including difficulties sitting still, paying attention, following rules, and completing work. Larry also has a history of language and motor coordination delays; he currently receives speech and language therapy and occupational therapy at school and receives resource room support for his major academic subjects. He is otherwise placed in an integrated fourth-grade class in the public school system.

Larry has no history of head trauma or seizures. Developmental milestones were met within the appropriate time frames. Medical history is notable for chronic ear infections beginning at age 3. Larry is in good physical health and takes no medications. In his free time, he enjoys activities such as karate and soccer. He is reportedly a well-liked child who has no difficulty making friends.

BEHAVIORAL OBSERVATIONS

Larry presented as a friendly boy who cooperated well with the demands of the testing. He separated easily from his parents and conversed readily with the examiner without needing time to warm up. His eye contact was good, his affect was appropriate to the tasks, and he was animated in his interactions. No concerns were noted regarding prosody or pedantic speech. Larry was oriented to time, person, and place.

In this quiet setting, Larry remained appropriately focused, but he was impulsive at times in his response style. He frequently fidgeted in his chair and needed frequent breaks to maintain his attention. In spite of this, Larry put forth good effort on all the tests administered. Consequently, the results are felt to be valid.

TEST RESULTS

Cognitive Functioning

Larry achieved a WISC-IV Full Scale IQ of 95 (mean = 100, standard deviation = 15), which is in the average range of psychometric intelligence, and which falls at the 37th percentile. He achieved a Verbal Comprehension Index of 99 (47th percentile), a Perceptual Reasoning Index of 94 (34th percentile), a Working Memory Index of 84 (14th percentile), and a Processing Speed Index of 94 (34th percentile). Larry's subtest scores are as follows (mean = 10, standard deviation = 3):

Subtest	Scaled score	Percentile
Similarities	12	75th
Vocabulary	11	63rd
Comprehension	8	25th
Block Design	8	25th
Picture Concepts	9	37th
Matrix Reasoning	12	75th
Digit Span	6	9th
Letter–Number Sequencing	11	63rd
Coding	9	37th
Symbol Search	9	37th

A particular strength was noted on a test of nonverbal reasoning skills (Matrix Reasoning). Larry demonstrated the most difficulty on a task that relies heavily on sustained auditory attention (Digit Span).

Achievement Testing

Larry was administered subtests of the WIAT-II in order to assess his current academic abilities. He was also administered the GORT-4 to measure his ability to read both quickly and accurately and the TOWL-3 Sponta-

(cont.)

neous Formats subtests to examine his spontaneous writing ability. His achievement subtest scores are as follows:

WIAT-II subtests	Standard score	Grade equivalent	Percentile
Reading			
Word Reading	72	2.4	3rd
Reading Comprehension	68	1.6	2nd
Pseudoword Decoding	77	1.6	6th
Mathematics			
Numerical Operations	86	3.2	18th
Math Reasoning	95	4.2	37th
Written Language			
Spelling	76	2.1	5th

GORT-4 score	Standard score	Grade equivalent	Percentile
Rate	4	2.2	2nd
Accuracy	1	< 1.0	4th
Fluency	2	< 1.0	4th

TOWL-3 Spontaneous Format subtest	Scaled score	Percentile
Contextual Conventions	7	16th
Contextual Language	7	16th
Story Construction	7	16th

Based on these results, Larry was found to have a cluster of significant skills weaknesses in reading (familiar word decoding, novel word decoding, reading fluency, and reading comprehension). He was found to be 2–3 years delayed in these skills. In addition, his written expression skills were found to be in the low-average range and below grade level. His writing was significant for many dysphonetic spelling errors, poor sentence construction, and major organizational difficulties. These findings are consistent with a diagnosis of a reading disability, given the clustering of skills weaknesses in phonetic decoding, spelling, reading comprehension, and written expression.

Although Larry's conceptual math skills were found to be generally at grade level (WIAT-II Math Reasoning), he had difficulty with his calculation skills and math fact retrieval. He also made "careless" errors, such as adding when the sign indicated multiplication.

Language Skills

In general, Larry's language skills were found to be within the average range. On the WISC-IV Vocabulary subtest, Larry's performance fell at the 63rd percentile. The PPVT-III is a test in which the child is asked to decide which one of four pictures is the best depiction of a key word. The key word is usually an adjective or adverb and is not merely the name of an object. In this test, Larry achieved a standard score of 93 (mean = 100, standard deviation = 15), which carries a percentile rank of 32 and an age equivalent of 9 years, 4 months.

Visual–Motor/Spatial Skills

On the Beery VMI, a structured test of visual–motor integration, Larry obtained a standard score of 79 (8th percentile), which is in the borderline deficient range and has an age equivalent of 5 years, 10 months. On the

(cont.)

ROCF, a test of visual–motor integration, constructional skills, and organization, Larry obtained a copy score of 9 at the 1st percentile. Larry's reproduction was poorly organized and included errors of distortion, placement, perseveration, and orientation. Probably because of his difficulty in organizing the complex information, Larry's delayed-recall score after 30 minutes fell to 4, at the 1st percentile.

Executive Functioning

In regard to sustained auditory attention, Larry's skills were found to vary, as related test scores ranged from below average (WISC-IV Digit Span [see above]; WRAML2 Sentence Memory scaled score = 6, 9th percentile) to average (Story Memory scaled score = 12, 75th percentile). Visual memory and attention was also variable, in that Larry did much better on a test of Picture Memory (scaled score = 14, 92nd percentile), where he was asked to determine what changes were made to a picture, than on a test of Design Memory, where he was asked to reproduce designs (scaled score = 7, 16th percentile). Overall, tests of memory indicated difficulty with visual–spatial memory.

Though Larry was observed to be somewhat impulsive, he demonstrated adequate impulse control on the Stroop (Color–Word score = average range; Interference score = average range). On Trails A, a test of visual scanning, Larry scored in the average range (50th percentile) for his age. He had more difficulty on Trails B, which involves shifting set or cognitive flexibility, with a score at the 3rd percentile. Frustration probably contributed to Larry's poor performance on the WCST, a card-matching task that changes the rules during the course of the activity. After completing two matching categories, Larry had great difficulty figuring out a new matching principle; as a result, he scored below the 1st percentile for learning to learn from feedback ("right" or "wrong"). His overall performance on this test was in the deficient to low-average range and indicated general difficulty with complex problem solving and shifting set. Finally, organizational difficulties were noted in both the verbal (TOWL-3) and visual (ROCF) realms; concerns in this realm were also noted by Larry's parents and teachers.

Behavioral Functioning

Larry's parents and teacher completed the BASC-2 and the ADHD Rating Scale–IV, checklist in order to provide a quantification of his behavior. Results from the BASC-2 indicated that Larry is perceived as exhibiting significant symptoms of inattention and hyperactivity. Results from the ADHD Rating Scale–IV reflect that Larry meets DSM-IV-TR criteria for ADHD, Combined Type.

DIAGNOSTIC IMPRESSIONS

     315.00   Reading Disorder
     314.01   Attention-Deficit Hyperactivity Disorder, Combined Type

SUMMARY AND RECOMMENDATIONS

Larry Hall is a 10-year-old boy in the fourth grade who was found to have an estimated intelligence level in the average range. Achievement testing indicated that Larry is having significant difficulty in reading and language-based academic skills, including word decoding, spelling, reading comprehension, and written expression. The extent of his skills delays in these areas was found to be statistically significant with respect to his intelligence level; that is, Larry was found to have formal learning delays in these areas, which warrant the DSM-IV-TR diagnosis of Reading Disorder. Although Larry's understanding of math concepts was found to be on grade level, he demonstrated difficulty with math fact retrieval/retention and tended to make "careless" errors (e.g., misreading the operation sign).

Consistent with a DSM-IV-TR diagnosis of ADHD, Combined Type, Larry was found to be prone to variable attention, mild impulsivity, difficulty shifting set/gears, and organizational difficulties. Larry was also found to have a significant delay in visual–motor integration, which affects his handwriting and drawing abilities.

Based on the information acquired during this evaluation, the following recommendations are made:

(cont.)

1. Larry should receive intensive multisensory reading instruction in school, such as the Orton–Gillingham or Wilson approaches. Ideally, he should receive this service on a daily basis individually. He should also be provided with computer software (and time during the day to use it) that reinforces reading comprehension, spelling, and writing skills.
2. Larry should receive special education services to promote his math fact retention and retrieval skills. He should work with the learning specialist at least twice a week on this subject.
3. Larry should receive special education services for his written expression skills, though some of this will be covered through an appropriate reading program. An emphasis should be placed on sentence structure and organizational skills. General organizational skills tutoring should also be provided by the special education teacher at least twice a week.
4. Larry should receive extra time on tests and assignments as needed. Testing in an oral format, or oral defense of his written responses, is recommended when appropriate.
5. Larry will have difficulty with notetaking. Teachers can assist him by providing him with teacher-made notes.
6. Larry should receive an updated occupational therapy evaluation if one has not been completed within 2 years. These results support continued occupational therapy services.
7. Larry and his family should consult with his pediatrician as to whether medication is an appropriate treatment for his symptoms of ADHD.
8. To enhance Larry's attention and performance in school, the following accommodations are recommended:
   a. Provide preferential seating.
   b. Break tasks up into their smaller components.
   c. Provide both written and oral instructions for tests and assignments.
   d. Use multisensory teaching techniques.
   e. Allow for frequent motor breaks during the day.
   f. Reduce sources of distraction in the classroom.
   g. Maintain structure and routine.
   h. Help him maintain a homework notebook.
   i. Use visual checklists to help him with expected transitions.
   j. Give frequent 1:1 feedback and check-ins.
   k. Allow for extra time to complete work and proof it.
9. Larry should receive follow-up neuropsychological testing in 2 years to document his progress and amend his education plan as needed.

Mary Smith, PhD	*2/14/07*
Signature	Date

35.7. Treatment Summaries

A treatment summary reviews the client's current standing in treatment or summarizes a client's treatment at termination or upon her/his transfer to another clinician or program. A sample treatment summary for Cindy Pope, a fictitious adolescent, can be found on pages 314–315.

35.8. Formats for Discharge or Closing Summaries

Formats for Outpatient Treatment

Format 1

Child's name.
Date of summary.

Jane Brown, PhD
Psychologist
100 N. Main Street, Suite 301
Anytown, State 22222

Phone: (999) 555-5555
Fax: (999) 555-5556   State License #12345

Date of report: March 31, 2007

Progress Summary

Child's name: Jim Smith   **Date of birth:** 4/15/94

Parents: Bill and Linda Smith   **Date treatment initiated:** 11/5/06

Home address (mother):   **Date of summary:** 3/31/07

   5 Rintel Road
   Anytown, Anystate 12345

Home address (father):

   456 Elm Street
   Anytown, Anystate 12345

Jim Smith has been participating in individual 50-minute therapy sessions with his psychologist, Dr. Jane Brown (myself). These sessions are conducted at my office. Jim initially presented with symptoms of anxiety, panic attacks, and school refusal.

Jim's goals included (1) a significant decrease in his panic attacks and (2) better school attendance. In regard to the first goal, he has quickly acquired coping skills since his initial assessment in November; he can now control his panic attacks to the point where he is experiencing fewer than one a month. However, he continues to need cognitive-behavioral therapy to address his continued difficulties with consistent school attendance. One barrier to progress in these areas is a lack of consistent adherence to the treatment protocol by Jim's father. Jim's parents are divorced, and Jim stays with his father one week a month; although his mother has followed the suggestions by Jim's treatment team, his father does not consistently require Jim to go to school. In order for treatment to be successful, therapy will have to include a component that will assist Jim's father in acquiring the skills and knowledge he needs to help Jim successfully conquer his school refusal issues.

He demonstrates many excellent abilities, such as strong intellectual and cognitive skills and a desire to please. He is a true delight to work with and continues to make much improvement in the skills that are being addressed. It is recommended that Jim participate in 10–12 more therapy sessions targeting issues related to school refusal. It will probably be necessary to do an *in vivo* session or two in Jim's school on a day when he has spent the previous night at his father's house. An effort should be made to engage Jim's father in treatment; it would be extremely helpful if he could attend two sessions of therapy with Jim to help develop a plan that will address the school refusal on the weeks Jim lives with his dad.

_____   _____
         Jane Brown, PhD   *3/31/07*
           Signature   Date

Martin Dorn, PsyD
Psychologist
100 N. Main Street, Suite 301
Anytown, State 22222

Phone: (999) 555-5555
Fax: (999) 555-5556

State License #12345

Date of report: July 2, 2007

Treatment Summary

Name: Cindy Pope   **Date of birth:** 6/9/92   **Date of summary:** 7/2/07

IDENTIFYING INFORMATION

Cindy is a 15-year-old female who was referred to Dr. Martin Dorn (myself) for the treatment of depression.

BACKGROUND

Cindy's prenatal and birth histories were normal. She was born after a full-term pregnancy; her weight was 8 pounds, 4 ounces. Developmental milestones were within normal limits. Elementary and middle school histories indicated good academic achievement, and Cindy has never needed any special school accommodations.

Cindy's parents indicated that her symptoms began in eighth grade, subsequent to the parents' separation. Before then, according to her parents, she had been an "open-hearted, fun-loving girl who loved to be around people." About 3 months after her parents' separation, Cindy began spending large amounts of time by herself in her room. She lost interest in her friends and in gymnastics, a sport about which she was quite passionate. Her symptoms of sadness became worse once she began ninth grade, where she felt overwhelmed by the new academic demands and the "social scene" of high school.

ASSESSMENT

In an initial interview with Cindy, she reported a history of depressed mood, together with such symptoms as difficulty sleeping, decreased school performance, and a lack of energy. She felt that these symptoms had increased since she started high school and were impinging on daily functioning. Her primary concern was a lack of friends, while her parents' primary concern was her poor school performance. Her behavioral presentation in the initial interview was consistent with her report of depression, in that she was tearful and sad when discussing school and friendships. In addition to these symptoms, the patient endorsed a history of difficulties with concentration.

DIAGNOSIS

The results of the initial interview suggested that Cindy was suffering from major depression. She had few coping resources to deal with her negative emotions. Cognitive-behavioral therapy was recommended to address her symptoms. In terms of her strengths, Cindy presented with strong intellectual and vocabulary skills, a high motivation for treatment, the capacity for self-reflection, and a family who was obviously concerned about her.

    Axis I   296.21 (Major Depressive Disorder, Single Episode, Mild)
    Axis II   None
    Axis III   None
    Axis IV   Academic problems
    Axis V   GAF at intake, 58; GAF at discharge, 89

(cont.)

Treatment Summary
July 2, 2007
p. 2

TREATMENT

Cindy was treated over a 6-month period in 20 sessions of individual therapy and four family meetings. These sessions were primarily based on a cognitive-behavioral approach.

The purpose of the initial two sessions was to engage in discussions that would foster rapport. This included gathering information about Cindy's family history and emotional functioning. Cindy's response to these sessions indicated that she developed rapport quite easily and was very motivated to "get better."

The following two sessions focused on developing a set of treatment goals to address Cindy's depression. The goals included decreasing her feelings of sadness, as well as increasing her self-esteem, social relationships, school performance, and extracurricular activities. The patient was encouraged to collaborate in setting these goals—including helping to identify the specific behaviors that she wanted to change, such as "having more friends" and "doing better in algebra and biology."

The subsequent sessions were primarily devoted to teaching Cindy cognitive and behavioral strategies that would address her feelings of depression. In the final sessions before discharge, the focus was on reviewing what she had learned and how this had resulted in decreased symptoms of depression. We discussed the elements of her treatment that had enabled her to make these changes; Cindy indicated that cognitive restructuring was particularly helpful. Termination issues were explored in the last two sessions, and a plan was developed that Cindy could follow if she experienced any recurrence of depressive symptoms. The prognosis for Cindy is excellent.

Martin Dorn, PsyD	7/2/07
Name of Clinician	Date

Psychologist
License or Title

Date of birth.
Treatment dates.
Presenting problems.
Goals of therapy.
Achievement of goals.
Remaining problems.
Reason for termination.
Final diagnosis (Axis I–Axis V)
Disposition.
Signature and date.

Format 2

Child's name.
Date of birth.
Age.
Therapist's name.
Attending psychologist or psychiatrist (if any).
Medical record number.
Background information.
Treatment goals and mode of treatment.
Treatment attendance.

Course of therapy.
Family and environmental factors affecting treatment.
DSM-IV-TR diagnosis (Axis I–Axis V).
Impressions and recommendations.
Signature(s).

Format for Inpatient Treatment

Child's name.
Medical record number.
Date of birth.
Date of admission.
Date of discharge.
Treatment unit.
Treating physician.

History of present illness.
Mental status on admission.
Physical exam and laboratory data.
Consultations.
Hospital course.

Condition on discharge.
Aftercare plan.
Discharge medications.
Discharge diagnoses (Axis I–Axis V).
Signature.
Date.

35.9. Sample Individualized Education Plan (IEP)

Individualized Education Plan

IEP Dates: From _____ to _____

CHILD AND SCHOOL INFORMATION

Name: Bonnie O'Hara   **School ID #:** XX123

Date of birth: 03/07/1999   **School:** Grove Elementary

Grade: 1

Primary language: English   **Language of instruction:** English

PARENT/GUARDIAN INFORMATION

Name(s): John and Laura O'Hara   **Relationship to student:** Parents

Address: 16 Main Street

Home telephone: 400-222-2222

Primary language of parent(s): English

(cont.)

PARENT AND/OR STUDENT CONCERNS

It is often difficult for Bonnie to concentrate in the classroom. She has trouble attending during large-group activities. Transitions are difficult for her, and outbursts can occur when she is feeling frustrated. Her gross and fine motor skills are also quite weak.

STUDENT STRENGTHS

Bonnie is a caring and personable young child who is capable of thoughtfulness and compassion. She has become more serious about academics and works hard to complete her work. She is becoming more interested in fine and gross motor activities at home and at school. She has strengths in receptive and expressive vocabulary.

HOW DOES THE DISABILITY AFFECT PROGRESS?

Bonnie has difficulty being flexible in social and academic situations. She has a hard time stopping one activity to change to another. She often misses directions or instructions because she is distracted. Her impulsivity affects her interactions with others and her work in the classroom. Her poor motor skills are affecting her ability to learn writing skills.

CURRENT PERFORMANCE LEVELS/MEASURABLE ANNUAL GOALS

Goal 1

Current Performance Level

Bonnie is learning to write her name, but has trouble copying shapes, letters, and numbers.

Measurable Annual Goal

Bonnie will develop her small motor skills and visual–motor skills to a more age-appropriate level.

Objectives

- Bonnie will learn to write her name in appropriate upper- and lower-case letters.
- Bonnie will write the numbers 0–9 in correct formation.
- Bonnie will begin to write upper- and lower-case letters of the alphabet.

Goal 2

Current Performance Level

Bonnie is often distracted in large group teaching settings. She may miss directions or part of a lesson because she is not focused.

Measurable Annual Goal

Bonnie will pay attention in a large-group situation for an appropriate amount of time.

Objectives

- Bonnie will sit in a large group and actively participate for 10 minutes.
- Bonnie will raise her hand and answer questions appropriately in large-group settings.
- Bonnie will focus her attention on the teacher and other children speaking in a large-group setting.

SERVICE DELIVERY

Occupational therapy once a week for 30 minutes.

ASSESSMENT PARTICIPATION

No statewide or districtwide assessments are scheduled during this period.

35.10. Sample Classroom Observation Report

Mary G. Evaluator, PhD
School Psychologist
100 N. Main Street, Suite 301
Anytown, State 22222

Phone: (999) 555-5555
Fax: (999) 555-5556   State License #12345

Date of report: October 26, 2007

Classroom Observation Report

Name: Thomas Jones   **Date of birth:** 7/14/98

Parents: Mary/William Jones   **Age:** 9 years, 3 months

School: Valley Elementary   **Date of observation:** 10/26/07

Grade: 4th   **Evaluator:** Maria Ramirez

REASON FOR REFERRAL

To provide direct information about Thomas's adjustment and performance in his current grade setting.

BACKGROUND INFORMATION

A review of school records indicates that Thomas was found to be eligible for receipt of special education support services in first grade, as he presented with a reading disability. He was also diagnosed with ADHD by his doctor. On previous testing, Thomas scored within the average range on tests of intellectual ability, but weaknesses were seen on tests of word decoding, spelling, and attention/other executive functions. Thomas currently receives special reading assistance as well as classroom accommodations.

ACTION TAKEN

1. Reviewed school and medical records.
2. Consulted with classroom teacher.
3. Conducted classroom observation.

CONSULTATION WITH TEACHER

Discussion with Ms. Carley before the classroom observation indicates that Thomas is currently receiving four 45-minute individual reading tutoring sessions per week with the Wilson method. Ms. Carley indicated that she feels Thomas is making very good progress. Thomas also receives math support three times a week, as well as occupational therapy to help him with fine motor and writing skills.

CLASSROOM OBSERVATION

Fourth-grade classroom with Ms. Carley, 9:15 A.M.

(cont.)

Classroom Observation Report (cont.)

At the start of the observation, Thomas was seated at his desk, quietly reading a book as the students filed into the classroom. The classroom is set up in what appears to be a very comfortable arrangement. Couches and comfortable chairs surround the work area, which consists of desk clusters. Computer centers and blackboard centers are located around the room. When the teacher was ready to begin the day, she announced that all students should clear their desks and listen carefully to the schedule for the day. A discussion then transpired as to how the day would progress. The day would begin with activity centers where the children would rotate from one center to another, and the teacher asked the students to listen carefully to learn which activity center they would be working at.

Thomas complied with the instructions immediately. He waited patiently until he and four other children were directed to go to a table at the side of the room and work with the assistant teacher on a math activity. Each of the five students was given coins and asked to determine what kinds of coins would be needed to purchase various items that were placed on the table. Once the children found the correct answers they were asked to find other ways they could purchase the items, as well as how to purchase the items using the smallest number of coins. Thomas worked diligently and did an appropriate job of determining the correct answers. At one time, another group became quite loud, and Thomas became distracted; however, he came back to task with appropriate redirection from the teacher.

About 25 minutes into the center activities, it was time for Thomas to leave the classroom to go to the resource room for tutoring. He walked to the reading room, which is a short distance down the hallway. The work area consisted of a corner of a sunny room, which was set up in a typical Wilson fashion with a table, chairs, and cards. The teacher gave the observer a copy of her lesson for the day, which began with a review of the previous day's lesson. The reading tutor, Mrs. Ruppert, began with a traditional review of vowel sounds, and Thomas was asked to identify digraphs and blends from the felt board. He was then asked to read each base word, and then an analysis of the word itself was conducted. The tutoring continued according to Mrs. Ruppert's lesson plan. Thomas was very motivated and appeared quite pleased when he was recognized for a job well done. Thomas worked well with Mrs. Ruppert on a one-to-one basis.

CONCLUSIONS

1. Thomas followed all teacher directives as soon as they were given.
2. The Wilson implementation was of very high quality, and the combination of this approach and his specific reading teacher appear to be creating a very favorable reading experience for Thomas.
3. Thomas thrived when given positive reinforcement for the successes he received.
4. Thomas's classroom situation appears to be an ideal setting for him this year. The fact that the class does spend time in rotations seems quite favorable for Thomas, for several reasons. First of all, it allows him the opportunity to move around and not become overly stifled by sitting at his desk for the entire day. It also offers him a great opportunity to interact in both social and learning activities with his peers. He is exposed to consistent peer modeling, in conjunction with excellent teacher direction, and both factors are viewed as promoting his learning.
5. Thomas was easily distracted by the behaviors of his peers in the classroom, but was able to get back on task with a teacher directive.
6. Thomas did give the impression that he wanted very much to respond successfully to all requests that were given to him by his teachers, and he worked hard to achieve expected results on his assignments.

Overall, in the opinion of this observer/consultant, the current plan that is being implemented for Thomas does put him on a pathway that affords him the opportunity to begin compensating for his developmental dyslexia and simultaneously to remain abreast within a classroom situation that is both appropriate and stimulating to him.

Mary G. Evaluator, PhD	10/26/07
Signature	Date
School Psychologist	
Title	

36

Resources for Professionals

36.1. Professional Organizations

www.aacap.org

The website of the American Academy of Child and Adolescent Psychiatry provides information for the Academy's members, other professionals, and families about developmental, behavioral, and mental disorders in children. For professionals, the website provides information on current research, practice guidelines, managed care information, descriptions of awards and fellowships, and conference information. For parents, the website provides information on child and adolescent psychiatry, as well as fact sheets on various disorders.

www.aap.org

The website of the American Academy of Pediatrics provides information about issues relevant to the physical, mental, and social health of infants, children, and adolescents. It is useful for both parents and professionals who are interested in obtaining information about health and children.

www.academyofct.org

The official website of the Academy of Cognitive Therapy provides professionals with current information about cognitive therapy. It also provides assistance for consumers in finding a certified cognitive therapist.

www.nacbt.org

The official website of the National Association of Cognitive-Behavioral Therapists provides up-to-date information related to cognitive-behavioral therapy for professionals, as well as self-help cognitive-behavioral products and techniques for the general public.

www.psych.org

The website of the American Psychiatric Society provides information relevant to issues related to general psychiatric practice, including continuing educational opportunities, current research, and archival journal data.

www.apa.org

The official website of the American Psychological Association provides information for psychologists and other interested persons on current topics in psychology. The website provides information about conferences, continuing education, recent publications, and ethics.

www.psychologicalscience.org

The official website of the American Psychological Society provides information for professionals and students, including recent research and advocacy.

36.2. Test Publishers

American Guidance Service (now a division of Pearson Assessments)
4201 Woodland Road
Circle Pines, MN 55014-1796
http://ags.pearsonassessments.com

Consulting Psychologists Press
577 College
Palo Alto, CA 94306
www.cpp-db.com

DLM Teaching Resources
One DLM Park
Allen, TX 75002

Educational and Industrial Testing Service
P.O. Box 7234
San Diego, CA 92167
www.edits.net

Harcourt Assessment
19500 Bulverde Road
San Antonio, TX 78259
www.harcourtassessment.com

Harvard University Press
79 Gasden St.
Cambridge, MA 02138
www.hup.harvard.edu

Jastak Associates
(Products are now published by Psychological Assessment Resources, Inc.; see below)

Lafayette Instrument
P.O. Box 5729
Lafayette, IN 47903
www.lafayetteinstrument.com

Multi-Health Systems, Inc.
908 Niagara Falls Blvd.
North Tonawanda, NY 14120
www.mhs.com

National Rehabilitation Services
P.O. Box 1247
Gaylord, MI 49735

PRO-ED
8700 Shoal Creek Blvd.
Austin, TX 78757
www.proedinc.com

Psychological Assessment Resources, Inc.
16204 N. Florida Ave.
Lutz, FL 33549
www3.parinc.com

The Psychological Corporation
P.O. Box 839954
San Antonio, TX 78283-3954
www.harcourtassessment.com

Reitan Neuropsychology Laboratory
2920 South 4th Ave.
Tucson, AZ 85713
www.reitanlabs.com

Riverside Publishing
425 Spring Lake Dr.
Itasca, IL 60143-2079
www.riverpub.com

Western Psychological Services
12031 Wilshire Blvd.
Los Angeles, CA 90025
www.wpspublish.com

36.3. Treatment Resources

The resources listed in this section provide guidelines for treating particular populations or disorders.

Beidel, D. C., Turner, S. M., & Morris, T. L. (2000). Behavioral treatment of childhood social phobia. *Journal of Consulting and Clinical Psychology, 68,* 1072–1080.

Beidel, D. C., Turner, S. M., Young, B., & Paulson, A. (2005). Social effectiveness therapy for children: Three-year follow-up. *Journal of Consulting and Clinical Psychology, 73,* 721–725.

Bierman, K. L., Coie, J. D., Dodge, K. A., Greenberg, M. T., Lochman, J. E., McMahon, R. J., et al. (2002). Using the Fast Track randomized prevention trial to test the early-starter model of the development of serious conduct problems. *Developmental Psychopathology, 14,* 925–943.

Bos, C. S., & Vaughn, S. (2006). *Strategies for teaching students with learning and behavior problems* (6th ed.). Boston: Allyn & Bacon.

Crone, D. A., & Horner, R. H. (2003). *Building positive behavior support systems in schools.* New York: Guilford Press.

Curry, J. F., Wells, K. C., Lochman, J. E., Craighead, W. E., & Nagy, P. D. (2003). Cognitive-behavioral intervention for depressed, substance-abusing adolescents: Development and pilot testing. *Journal of the American Academy of Child and Adolescent Psychiatry, 42,* 656–665.

Dishion, T. J., & Kavanagh, K. (2003). *Intervening in adolescent problem behavior.* New York: Guilford Press.

Friedberg, R. D., & McClure, J. M. (2002). *Clinical practice of cognitive therapy with children and adolescents: The nuts and bolts.* New York: Guilford Press.

Kauffman, J. M., Mostert, M. P., Trent, S. C., & Hallahan, D. P. (2006). *Managing classroom behavior: A reflective case-based approach* (4th ed.). Boston: Allyn & Bacon.

Kazdin, A. E., & Weisz, J. R. (1998). Identifying and developing empirically supported child and adolescent treatments. *Journal of Consulting and Clinical Psychology, 66,* 19–36.

Kazdin, A. E., & Weisz, J. R. (Eds.). (2003). *Evidence-based psychotherapies for children and adolescents.* New York: Guilford Press.

Kearney, C. A. (2001). *School refusal behavior in youth: A functional approach to assessment and treatment.* Washington, DC: American Psychological Association.

Kearney, C. A. (2005). *Social anxiety and social phobia in youth: Characteristics, assessment and psychological treatment.* New York: Springer.

Kearney, C. A., & Albano, A. M. (2000). *When children refuse school: A cognitive behavioral therapy approach (Therapists' guide).* San Antonio, TX: Psychological Corporation.

Kendall, P. C. (Ed.). (2006). *Child and adolescent therapy: Cognitive-behavioral procedures* (3rd ed.). New York: Guilford Press.

Kendall, P. C., Safford, S., Flannery-Schroeder, E., & Webb, A. (2004). Child anxiety treatment: Outcomes in adolescence and impact on substance use and depression at 7.4 year follow-up. *Journal of Consulting and Clinical Psychology, 72,* 276–287.

Lochman, J. E., & Wells, K. C. (2004). The Coping Power Program for preadolescent aggressive boys and their parents: Outcome effects at the 1–year follow-up. *Journal of Consulting and Clinical Psychology, 72,* 571–578.

March, J. S., & Mulle, K. (1998). *OCD in children and adolescents: A cognitive-behavioral treatment manual.* New York: Guilford Press.

McMahon, R. J., & Forehand, R. L. (2003). *Helping the noncompliant child: Family-based treatment for oppositional behavior* (2nd ed.). New York: Guilford Press.

Orvaschel, H., Hersen, M., & Faust, J. (2001). *Handbook of conceptualization and treatment of childhood psychopathology.* Oxford: Elsevier Science.

Reinecke, M. A., Dattilio, F. M., & Freeman, A. (Eds.). (2003). *Cognitive therapy with children and adolescents* (2nd ed.). New York: Guilford Press.

Robin, A. L., & Foster, S. L. (1989). *Negotiating parent–adolescent conflict: A behavioral-family systems approach.* New York: Guilford Press.

Shaywitz, S. (2003). *Overcoming dyslexia: A new and complete science-based program for reading problems at any level.* New York: Knopf.

Spafford, C. S., & Grosser, G. S. (1995). *Dyslexia: Research and resource guide.* Boston: Allyn & Bacon.

Volkmar, F. R., Paul, R., Klin, A., & Cohen, D. J. (Eds.). (2005). *Handbook of autism and pervasive developmental disorders.* New York: Wiley.

36.4. Forensic Resources

Child Abuse

American Academy of Child and Adolescent Psychiatry. (1997). Practice parameters for the forensic evaluation of children and adolescents who may have been physically or sexually abused. *Journal of the American Academy of Child and Adolescent Psychiatry, 36,* 423–442.

Lubit, R., Hartwell, N., van Gorp, W. G., & Eth, S. (2002). Forensic evaluation of trauma syndromes in children. *Child and Adolescent Psychiatric Clinics of North America, 11,* 823–858.

Custody Evaluations

Ackerman, M. J. (2001). *Clinician's guide to child custody evaluations.* New York: Wiley.

Bernet, W. (2002). Child custody evaluations. *Child and Adolescent Psychiatric Clinics of North America, 11*(4), 781–804.

Brodzinsky, D. M. (1993). On the use and misuse of psychological testing in child custody evaluations. *Professional Psychology: Research and Practice, 24,* 213–219.

Galatzer-Levy, R. M., & Kraus, L. (Eds.). (1999). *The scientific basis of child custody decisions.* New York: Wiley.

Otto, R. K. (2000). The use of psychological testing in child custody evaluations. *Family and Conciliation Courts Review, 38,* 312–340.

Forensic Psychology (General)

Aldridge, M., & Wood, J. (1999). *Interviewing children: A guide for child care and forensic practitioners.* New York: Wiley.

Barsky, A. E., & Gould, J. W. (2002). *Clinicians in court: A guide to subpoenas, depositions, testifying, and everything else you need to know.* New York: Guilford Press.

Brodsky, S. L. (1991). *Testifying in court: Guidelines and maxims for the expert witness.* Washington, DC: American Psychological Associations.

Flynn, M. H. (1997). The good, the bad, and the useless: Writing reports that are helpful to the courts. *TCA Journal, 25,* 41–49.

Goldstein, A. M. (Ed.). (2003). *Handbook of psychology: Vol. 11. Forensic psychology* New York: Wiley.

Quinn, K. M. (1986). Competency to be a witness: A major child forensic issue. *Bulletin of the American Academy of Psychiatry and the Law, 14,* 311–321.

Ribner, N. G. (Ed.). (2002). *The California School of Professional Psychology handbook of juvenile forensic psychology.* San Francisco: Jossey-Bass.

Van Dorsten, B. (Ed.). *Forensic psychology: From classroom to courtroom.* New York: Kluwer Academic/Plenum.

36.5. Other Useful Websites

www.eric.ed.gov

The Education Resources Information Center (ERIC) is a national information system that is funded by the U.S. Department of Education. The organization provides a centralized bibliographic database of journal articles and other published and unpublished education materials. The website allows the reader to search the ERIC database.

www.nimh.nih.gov

The website of the National Institute of Mental Health provides information about clinical trials, funding opportunities, and recent research. It has information for the general public, for practitioners, and for researchers.

37

Resources for Parents

The number of websites and other useful resources for parents is quite large. This chapter is not meant to provide an exhaustive list.

37.1. General Resources

Braaten, E., & Felopulos, G. (2004). *Straight talk about psychological testing for kids.* New York: Guilford Press.

Faraone, S. V. (2003). *Straight talk about your child's mental health: What to do when something seems wrong.* New York: Guilford Press.

Wilens, T. E. (2001). *Straight talk about psychiatric medications for kids* (rev. ed.). New York: Guilford Press.

www.aboutourkids.org

A website of the New York University (NYU) Child Study Center, AboutOurKids provides information for parents and professionals, including articles about common mental health problems and parenting, current research news, and information regarding education for children with special needs.

www.ccbd.net

The Council for Children with Behavioral Disorders sponsors this website. The organization promotes educational services, provides professional support, encourages research, and disseminates current information about children with behavioral disorders.

www.cec.sped.org

The website of the Council for Exceptional Children is relevant not only for parents, but for teachers and other service professionals who are interested in issues regarding children with disabilities, exceptionality, or giftedness. The website provides information about public policy and advocacy, publications and products, and professional standards and accreditation.

www.cfw.tufts.edu

The Child & Family WebGuide site is operated by Tufts University and lists websites of interest to parents and professionals. All the sites on the WebGuide have been evaluated by graduate students or faculty members in child development. The WebGuide is organized by categories (family/parenting; education/learning; typical child development; health/mental health; resources/recreation) and by age.

www.childadvocate.net

The Child Advocate is a website that "serves the needs of children, families and professionals while addressing mental health, medical, educational, legal and legislative issues." It provides information on specific topics such as "ADHD and Brain Imaging," as well as a special link to disaster help for parents and children.

www.ffcmh.org

The website of the Federation of Families for Children's Mental Health provides information (including lists of publications, links to relevant websites, and a list of local chapters) about helping children with mental health difficulties.

www.nami.org

The Website of the National Alliance on Mental Illness provides general information about "severe" mental illnesses, such as schizophrenia and other psychotic disorders, bipolar disorders, anxiety disorders, pervasive developmental disorders, ADHD, and others. It also lists ways for people to become active in policies that affect persons with mental illness.

www.our-kids.org

The Our-Kids organization is a group of parents, caregivers, and others who are working with children with disabilities. Its website provides information about support lists, homemade equipment, recommended books, and other Internet resources for caregivers.

www.wpic.pitt.edu

The website of the Department of Psychiatry at the University of Pittsburgh School of Medicine includes information about clinical care, education, and research, as well as lectures and conferences that may be of interest to parents.

37.2. For ADHD

Barkley, R. (2000). *Taking charge of ADHD: The complete, authoritative guide for parents* (rev. ed.). New York: Guilford Press.

Hallowell, E., & Ratey, J. (1994). *Driven to distraction: Recognizing and coping with attention deficit disorder from childhood through adulthood.* New York: Pantheon Books.

Zeigler Dendy, C. A. (2006). *Teenagers with ADD and ADHD: A parents' guide* (2nd ed.)., Bethesda, MD: Woodbine House.

www.add.org

The website of the Attention Deficit Disorder Association provides information for individuals and families touched by ADHD, as well as the professionals who treat them. The website includes links to articles, lists of relevant conferences, and an ADDA Store.

www.chadd.org

The organization Children and Adults with Attention-Deficit/Hyperactivity Disorder (CHADD) operates this website, which is devoted to providing information about ADHD, including public policy, legal rights, answers to frequently asked questions, and current research.

37.3. For Anxiety Disorders

Chansky, T. E. (2000). *Freeing your child from obsessive–compulsive disorder: A powerful, practical program for parents of children and adolescents.* New York: Crown.

Dacey, J., & Fiore, L. (2000). *Your anxious child.* San Francisco: Jossey-Bass.

Last, C. G. (2006). *Help for worried kids: How your child can conquer anxiety and fear.* New York: Guilford Press.

Rapee, R., Spence, S., Cobham, V., & Wignall, A. (2000). *Helping your anxious child: A step by step guide for parents.* Oakland, CA: New Harbinger.

www.adaa.org
The website of the Anxiety Disorders Association of America includes members such as clinicians and researchers who treat and study anxiety disorders and individuals with anxiety disorders and their families. The website offers information about anxiety disorders, self-help tools, information about professional development and clinical trials, and information about support groups.

www.bu.edu/anxiety
The Center for Anxiety and Related Disorders at Boston University is one of the country's leading anxiety disorder research and treatment centers. Its website provides information about empirically validated treatment approaches.

www.ocfoundation.org
The website of the Obsessive Compulsive Foundation provides information about the organization and about obsessive–compulsive symptoms, medications, and treatment, as well as bimonthly newsletters with the very latest in information on research, resources, and recovery.

37.4. For Asperger's Disorder

Attwood, T. (1998). *Asperger's syndrome: A guide for parents and professionals.* London: Jessica Kingsley.

Bashe, P. R., & Kirby, B. L. (2005). *The OASIS guide to Asperger syndrome: Advice, support, insight, and inspiration* (rev. ed.). New York: Crown.

Ozonoff, S., Dawson, G., & McPartland, J. (2002). *A parent's guide to Asperger syndrome and high-functioning autism.* New York: Guilford Press.

www.asperger.org
This website provides information not only about Asperger's disorder, but about various related disorders (nonverbal learning disability, high-functioning autism, semantic–pragmatic disorder, and hyperlexia). The site provides numerous articles about these disorders and links to other relevant websites.

www.aspergersyndrome.org
The Online Asperger Syndrome Information and Support website provides a wealth of information, including papers and articles, diagnostic scales, message boards, schools and camps, adult issues, research projects, support groups, and lists of clinicians.

37.5. For Autism

Hart, C. (1993). *Parent's guide to autism.* New York: Pocket Books.

Seroussi, K. (2002). *Unraveling the mystery of autism and pervasive developmental disorders.* New York: Broadway Books.

Szatmari, P. (2004). *A mind apart: Understanding children with autism and Asperger syndrome.* New York: Guilford Press.

www.autism-society.org
The website of the Autism Society of America provides information about autism, autism resources, research, and local chapters. Information is also provided in Spanish.

www.feat.org

The Families for Early Autism Treatment (FEAT) website provides information for parents, as well as for educators and other professionals, about autism. Although this website is geared toward individuals in Northern California, it provides links to other FEAT websites in various areas of the United States.

www.info.med.yale.edu/chldstdy/autism

This website is operated by the Yale Child Study Center's Developmental Disabilities Clinic. Although the clinic serves children with a variety of developmental disabilities, the emphasis is on autism, Asperger's disorder, and other pervasive developmental disorders. The website is frequently updated and includes information about the clinic and the disorders it treats, research studies, resources, and publications.

37.6. For Bipolar Disorders

Demitri, F., Papolos, M., & Papolos, J. (2002). *The bipolar child: The definitive and reassuring guide to childhood's most misunderstood disorder* (rev. and expanded ed.). New York: Broadway Books.

Fristad, M. A., & Arnold, J. S. G. (2004). *Raising a moody child: How to cope with depression and bipolar disorder.* New York: Guilford Press.

www.cabf.org

This website is operated by the Child and Adolescent Bipolar Foundation, a parent-led web-based organization of families of children with bipolar disorders. The site provides information and resources for parents about bipolar disorders in children.

www.dbsalliance.org

This website is operated by the Depression and Bipolar Support Alliance; it provides information about mood disorders, as well as information about local support groups and chapters.

37.7. For Conduct Problems/ODD

Barkley, R. A., & Benton, C. M. (1998). *Your defiant child: Eight steps to better behavior.* New York: Guilford Press.

Greene, R. (2001). *The explosive child: A new approach for understanding and parenting easily frustrated, chronically inflexible children.* New York: HarperCollins.

Nichols, M. P. (2004). *Stop arguing with your kids: How to win the battle of wills by making your child feel heard.* New York: Guilford Press.

Riley, D. (2002). *The defiant child: A parent's guide to oppositional defiant disorder.* Cutten, CA: Taylor.

www.explosivekids.org

The Foundation for Children with Behavioral Challenges sponsors this website, which provides information about "explosive kids," support groups, resources for parents, and clinicians qualified to treat children with these types of difficulties.

37.8. For Depression

Koplewicz, H. (2002). *More than moody: Recognizing and treating adolescent depression.* New York: Putnam.

Mondimone, F. (2002). *Adolescent depression: A guide for parents.* Baltimore: Johns Hopkins University Press.

www.depression.org

This website is useful for those interested in getting more information about the symptoms of and treatment for depression.

37.9. For Drug Abuse

www.nida.nih.gov

This website is sponsored by the National Institute on Drug Abuse. It provides information for students and young adults, parents and teachers, and researchers and health professionals about how to prevent and treat addictions. It also provides information about publications and funding. The website is also available in Spanish.

37.10. For Dyslexia/Reading Disorder

Adelizzi, J. U., & Goss, D. B. (2001). *Parenting children with learning disabilities.* Westport, CT: Bergin & Garvey.

Clark, D. B., & Uhry, J. (1995). *Dyslexia: Theory and practice of remedial instruction.* Timonium, MD: York Press.

Shaywitz, S. (2003). *Overcoming dyslexia: A new and complete science-based program for reading problems at any level.* New York: Knopf.

www.interdys.org

The International Dyslexia Association operates this website, which provides a wealth of information on dyslexia for educators, parents, and individuals with dyslexia. One strength of the website is that it provides information for specific populations with dyslexia, such as college students, teens, children, and adults.

37.11. For Eating Disorders

Berg, F. M. (2001). *Children and teens afraid to eat: Helping youth in today's weight-obsessed world* (3rd ed.). Hettinger, ND: Healthy Weight Network.

Claude-Pierre, P. (1997). *The secret language of eating disorders.* New York: Vintage.

Lock, J., & le Grange, D. (2005). *Help your teenager beat an eating disorder.* New York: Guilford Press.

Neumark-Sztainer, D. (2005). *"I'm, like, so fat!": Helping your teen make healthy choices about eating and exercise in a weight-obsessed world.* New York: Guilford Press.

www.anred.com

Anorexia Nervosa and Related Eating Disorders, Inc., sponsors this website; it provides current information about anorexia nervosa, bulimia nervosa, and binge eating, including self-help tips and information about recovery and prevention.

37.12. For Giftedness

www.aagc.org

The website of the American Association for Gifted Children is devoted to understanding the needs and capabilities of these children. It provides news about current research in giftedness and resources for gifted children. The website is affiliated with Duke University.

37.13. For Learning Disabilities in General

Fisher, G., & Cummings, R. (1995). *When your child has LD (learning differences): A survival guide for parents.* Minneapolis, MN: Free Spirit.

www.advocacyinstitute.org

The Advocacy Institute describes itself as "dedicated to the development of products and services that work to improve the lives of people with disabilities, particularly learning disabilities." The website provides information about resources, services, and special subjects (e.g., choosing a college) for individuals with learning disabilities.

www.disabilityrights.org

This website is devoted to providing information about the rights of people with disabilities, including learning disabilities; it covers topics such as the Americans with Disabilities Act, "A Parent's Guide to Special Education," and taking action. The website is updated frequently and provides the reader with national news on topics relevant to those with disabilities.

www.ldanatl.org

This website is operated by the Learning Disabilities Association of America. It provides resources for parents and information about political and advocacy issues.

www.ldonline.org

This website calls itself "the world's leading website on learning disabilities and ADHD." It provides information about many types of learning disabilities, the latest research in the field, and issues related to parents and teachers.

www.ncld.org

This very comprehensive website provides information about many types of learning disabilities (including dyslexia, dyscalculia, dyspraxia, dysgraphia, and processing disorders), as well as ADHD. It also includes information about advocacy and research.

37.14. For Mental Retardation

Bogdan, R., & Taylor, S. (1994). *The social meaning of mental retardation: Two life stories* (Special Education No. 15). New York: Teachers College Press.
Cunningham, C. (1996). *Understanding Down syndrome: An introduction for parents.* Cambridge, MA: Brookline Books.

www.aamr.org

The American Association on Mental Retardation is an organization devoted to promoting research, policies, and practices for individuals with intellectual disabilities. Its website provides links to current policy research, news, and resources.

www.thearc.org

This website, operated by The Arc of the United States, is for people interested in developmental disabilities. It provides information about developmental disabilities, ways to get involved with the organization, and resources.

37.15. For NLD

Stewart, K. (2002). *Helping a child with nonverbal learning disorder or Asperger syndrome.* Oakland, CA: New Harbinger.

www.nlda.org
   This website is operated by the Nonverbal Learning Disorders Association and includes information about NLD, including diagnostic criteria and interventions.

37.16. For Written Expression Difficulties

Cicci, R. (1995). *What's wrong with me?: Learning disabilities at home and at school.* Toronto: York Press.
Richards, R. G. (1998). *Dysgraphia: The writing dilemma.* Riverside, CA: RET Center Press.

www.hwtears.com
   This is the website of Handwriting without Tears: A Complete Handwriting Curriculum for All Children. The website provides information about the curriculum and allows parents and clinicians to order the curriculum directly from the website.

38

Medications

38.1. Common Medications by Generic and Trade Names

This section lists some of the more common drugs used to treat psychiatric conditions in childhood and adolescence. It is not meant to be an exhaustive list. Also, do not assume that the uses listed are the only ones for these drugs.

Use this list to find both the generic and trade (or brand) names for a drug when you have only one name or the other, and to learn the drug's major uses. The first columns lists both generic and trade names in alphabetical order. The second column gives the trade name for each generic name, and the generic name for each trade name, listed in the first column. Uncapitalized words are generic names; capitalized words are trade or brand names. (For example, amitriptyline is the generic name for the trade name Elavil. It is used as an antidepressant and is one of the tricyclics.) The third column lists the drugs' major uses.

Medications by generic and trade names		Major uses
Adderall	amphetamine & dextroamphetamine	Stimulant
alprazolam	Xanax	Anxiolytic
Ambien	zolpidem	Miscellaneous hypnonanxiolytic
amitriptyline	Elavil	Tricyclic antidepressant
amphetamine & detroamphetamine	Adderall	Stimulant
Anafranil	clomipramine	Tricyclic antidepressant
Atarax	hydroxyzine	Antihistamine, anxiolytic
Ativan	lorazepam	Anxiolytic
atomoxetine	Strattera	Nonstimulant ADHD medication
Benadryl	diphenhydramine	Antihistamine, anxiolytic
bupropion	Wellbutrin	Atypical antidepressant
Buspar	buspirone	Hypnoanxiolytic
buspirone	Buspar	Hypnoanxiolytic
carbamazepine	Tegretol	Mood stabilizer
Catapes	clonidine	Antihypertensive anxiolytic
Celexa	citalopram	Selective serotonin reuptake inhibitor (SSRI) antidepressant
citalopram	Celexa	SSRI antidepressant
chlordiazepoxide	Librium	Anxiolytic
chlorpromazine	Thorazine	Antipsychotic
clomipramine	Anafranil	Tricyclic antidepressant

Medications by generic and trade names		*Major uses*
clonazepam	Klonopin	Hypnoanxiolytic
clonidine	Catapres	Antihypertensive, anxiolytic
clozapine	Clozaril	Antipsychotic
Clozaril	clozapine	Antipsychotic
Concerta	methylphenidate	Stimulant
Depakene	valproic acid	Mood stabilizer
Depakote	divalproex	Mood stablizer
desipramine	Norpramin	Tricyclic antidepressant
Desoxyn	methamphetamine	Stimulant
Desyrel	trazodone	Atypical antidepressant
Dexedrine	dextroamphetamine	Stimulant
dextroamphetamine	Dexedrine	Stimulant
diazepam	Valium	Hypnoanxiolytic
diphenhydramine	Benadryl	Antihistamine, anxiolytic
divalproex	Depakote	Mood stabilizer
Effexor	venlafaxine	Atypical antidepressant
Elavil	amitriptyline	Tricyclic antidepressant
Eskalith	lithium	Mood stabilizer
fluoxetine	Prozac	SSRI antidepressant
fluphenazine	Prolixin	Antipsychotic
fluvoxamine	Luvox	SSRI antidepressant
gabapentin	Neurontin	Mood stabilizer
Gabitril	tiagabine	Mood stabilizer
guanfacine	Tenex	Antihypertensive
Halcion	triazolam	Hypnoanxiolytic
Haldol	haloperidol	Antipsychotic
haloperidol	Haldol	Antipsychotic
hydroxyzine	Atarax	Anxiolytic
imipramine	Tofranil	Tricyclic antidepressant
Inderal	propranolol	Antihypertensive (used in treating ADHD and tics as well as sleep problems)
Klonopin	clonazepam	Hypnoanxiolytic
Librium	chlordiazepoxide	Anxiolytic
lithium	Eskalith, Lithonate	Mood stabilizer
Lithonate	lithium	Mood stabilizer
lorazepam	Ativan	Anxiolytic
Ludiomil	Maprotiline	Tricyclic antidepressant
Luvox	fluvoxamine	SSRI antidepressant
maprotiline	Ludiomil	Tricyclic antidepressant
Mellaril	thioridazine	Antipsychotic
Metadate	methylphenidate	Stimulant
methamphetamine	Desoxyn	Stimulant
methylphenidate	Metadate, Concerta, Ritalin	Stimulant
mirtazapine	Remeron	Atypical antidepressant
Moban	molidone	Antipsychotic
molidone	Moban	Antipsychotic
Navane	thiothixene	Antipsychotic
nefazodone	Serzone	Atypical antidepressant
Neurontin	gabapentin	Mood stabilizer
Norpramin	desipramine	Tricyclic antidepressant
nortriptyline	Pamelor	Tricyclic antidepressant
olanzapine	Zyprexa	Antipsychotic
Pamelor	nortriptyline	Tricyclic antidepressant
Parnate	tranylcypromine	Monoamine oxidase inhibitor antidepressant
paroxetine	Paxil	SSRI antidepressant

Medications by generic and trade names		*Major uses*
Paxil	paroxetine	SSRI antidepressant
perphenazine	Trilafon	Antipsychotic
Prolixin	fluphenazine	Antipsychotic
propranolol	Inderal	Antihypertensive
Prozac	fluoxetine	SSRI antidepressant
Remeron	mirtazapine	Atypical antidepressant
Risperdal	risperidone	Antipsychotic
risperidone	Risperdal	Antipsychotic
Ritalin	methylphenidate	Stimulant
Serzone	nefazodone	Atypical antidepressant
sertraline	Zoloft	SSRI antidepressant
Strattera	atomoxetine	Nonstimulant ADHD medication
Tegretol	carbamazepine	Mood stabilizer
Tenex	guanfacine	Antihypertensive
thioridazine	Mellaril	Antipsychotic
thiothixene	Navane	Antipsychotic
Thorazine	chlorpromazine	Antipsychotic
tiagabine	Gabitril	Mood stabilizer
Tofranil	imipramine	Tricyclic antidepressant
Topamax	topiramate	Mood stabilizer
topiramate	Topamax	Mood stabilizer
Tranylcypromine	parnate	Monoamine oxidase inhibitor antidepressant
triazolam	Halcion	Hypnoanxiolytic
Trilafon	perphenazine	Antipsychotic
trazodone	Desyrel	Atypical antidepressant
Valium	diazepam	Hypnoanxiolytic
valproic acid	Depakene	Mood stabilizer
venlafaxine	Effexor	Atypical antidepressant
Wellbutrin	bupropion	Atypical antidepressant
Xanax	alprazolam	Anxiolytic
Zoloft	sertraline	SSRI antidepressant
zolpidem	Ambien	Miscellaneous hypnonanxiolytic
Zyprexa	olanzapine	Antipsychotic

38.2. Finding Names of Street Drugs

The names of street drugs change frequently and are often local. A list is available online (http://en.wikipedia.org/wiki/List_of_street_names_of_drugs).

39

Abbreviations in Common Use

39.1. Assessments and Tests

ABAS	Adaptive Behavior Assessment System
ABS-RC:2	AAMR Adaptive Behavior Scales—Residential and Community: Second Edition
ABS-S:2	AAMR Adaptive Behavior Scales—School: Second Edition
ACTeRS	ADD-H Comprehensive Teacher Rating Scale
ASEBA	Achenbach System of Empirically Based Assessment (includes CBCL, TRF, YSR)
BASC-2	Behavior Assessment System for Children, Second Edition
BBCS-R	Bracken Basic Concept Scale—Revised
BDI-2	Battelle Developmental Inventory, Second Edition
BDI-II	Beck Depression Inventory–II
Beery VMI	Beery–Buktenica Developmental Test of Visual–Motor Integration, Fifth Edition
BNT	Boston Naming Test
BOT-2	Bruininks–Oseretsky Test of Motor Proficiency, Second Edition
BRIEF	Behavior Rating Inventory of Executive Functions
Bayley-III	Bayley Scales of Infant and Toddler Development, Third Edition
BVRT	Benton Visual Retention Test
CARS	Childhood Autism Rating Scale
CAT	Children's Apperception Test
CAVLT-2	Children's Auditory Verbal Learning Test–2
CBCL	Child Behavior Checklist (part of ASEBA)
CDI	Children's Depression Inventory
CELF-3	Clinical Evaluation of Language Fundamentals—Third Edition
CMS	Children's Memory Scale
COWAT	Controlled Oral Word Association Test
CPT II	Conners' Continuous Performance Test II
CRS-R	Conners' Rating Scales—Revised
CTONI	Comprehensive Test of Nonverbal Intelligence
CVLT-C	California Verbal Learning Test—Children's Version
CVLT-II	California Verbal Learning Test—Second Edition
DAS-II	Differential Ability Scales, Second Edition

DSMD	Devereux Scales of Mental Disorders
DTLA-4	Detroit Tests of Learning Aptitude—Fourth Edition
EOWPVT	Expressive One-Word Picture Vocabulary Test
EVT	Expressive Vocabulary Test
GADS	Gilliam Asperger's Disorder Scale
GORT-4	Gray Oral Reading Tests, Fourth Edition
ITPA-3	Illinois Test of Psycholinguistic Abilities—Third Edition
KABC-II	Kaufman Assessment Battery for Children, Second Edition
KAIT	Kaufman Adolescent and Adult Intelligence Test
LAC-3	Lindamood Auditory Conceptualization Test, Third Edition
LNNB-C	Luria–Nebraska Neuropsychological Battery—Children's Revision
LNNB-II	Luria–Nebraska Neuropsychological Battery—II
MAPI	Millon Adolescent Personality Inventory
MMPI-A	Minnesota Multiphasic Personality Inventory—Adolescent
MSE	Mental status exam
OWLS	Oral and Written Language Scales
PPVT-III	Peabody Picture Vocabulary Test—Third Edition
RAVLT	Rey Auditory Verbal Learning Test
RCMAS	Revised Children's Manifest Anxiety Scale
ROCF	Rey–Osterrieth Complex Figure Test
SB5	Stanford–Binet Intelligence Scales, Fifth Edition
SDMT	Symbol Digit Modalities Test
SIB-R	Scales of Independent Behavior—Revised
STAIC	State–Trait Anxiety Inventory for Children
TACL-3	Test for Auditory Comprehension of Language—Third Edition
TAT	Thematic Apperception Test
TED	Tasks of Emotional Development
TELD-3	Test of Early Language Development—Third Edition
TEMA-3	Test of Early Mathematics Ability—Third Edition
TOAL-3	Test of Adolescent and Adult Language—Third Edition
TOLD-I:3	Test of Language Development—Intermediate: Third Edition
TOLD-P:3	Test of Language Development—Primary: Third Edition
TONI-3	Test of Nonverbal Intelligence—Third Edition
TOVA	Test of Variables of Attention
TOWL-3	Test of Written Language—Third Edition
TPT	Tactual Performance Test
TRF	Teacher's Report Form (part of ASEBA)
TTFC	Token Test for Children
Vineland-II	Vineland Adaptive Behavior Scales, Second Edition
WAIS-III	Wechsler Adult Intelligence Scale—Third Edition
WASI	Wechsler Abbreviated Scale of Intelligence
WCST	Wisconsin Card Sorting Test
WIAT-II	Wechsler Individualized Achievement Test—Second Edition
WISC-IV	Wechsler Intelligence Scale for Children—Fourth Edition
WJ III	Woodcock–Johnson III
WMS-III	Wechsler Memory Scale—Third Edition
WPPSI-III	Wechsler Preschool and Primary Scale of Intelligence—Third Edition
WRAML2	Wide Range Assessment of Memory and Learning, Second Edition
WRAT-4	Wide Range Achievement Test, Fourth Edition
WRMT-R	Woodcock Reading Mastery Tests—Revised
YSR	Youth Self-Report (part of the ASEBA)

39.2. Associations

AACAP	American Academy of Child and Adolescent Psychiatry
AAMR	American Association on Mental Retardation
AAP	American Academy of Pediatrics
APA	American Psychological Association or American Psychiatric Association
APS	American Psychological Society
ASHA	American Speech–Language–Hearing Association
CHADD	Children and Adults with Attention-Deficit/Hyperactivity Disorder
NACBT	National Association of Cognitive-Behavioral Therapy

39.3. Academic Degrees

BSW	Bachelor of Social Work
CAGS	Certificate of Advanced Graduate Study
DO	Doctor of Osteopathy
EdD	Doctor of Education
MA	Master of Arts
MD	Doctor of Medicine
MS	Master of Science
MSW	Master of Social Work
PhD	Doctor of Philosophy
PsyD	Doctor of Psychology

39.4. Professional Titles, Certifications, and Licensures

Ψi	Psychiatrist
Ψo	Psychologist
ABMP	American Board of Medical Psychotherapists
ABPP	American Board of Professional Psychologists
LMFT	Licensed Marriage and Family Therapist
NCSP	Nationally Certified School Psychologist

Social Work

Titles may differ by state.

ACSW	Academy of Certified Social Workers
CSW	Clinical or Certified Social Worker
LCSW	Licensed Certified Social Worker
LGSW	Licensed Graduate Social Worker
LICSW	Licensed Independent Clinical Social Worker
LSW	Licensed Social Worker
LSWA	Licensed Social Work Associate

Counseling

Titles may differ by state.

CCC	Certified Communication Counselor
CCMHC	Certified Clinical Mental Health Counselor

CRC	Certified Rehabilitation Counselor
LPC	Licensed Professional Counselor
NBCC	National Board Certified Counselor
NCC	National Certified Counselor
NCCC	National Certified Career Counselor
NCSC	National Certified School Counselor

Chemical Dependency Work

Titles may differ by state.

CAC	Certified Alcoholism Counselor
CAS	Certified Addictions Specialist
CCDS	Certified Chemical Dependency Supervisor
CDA	Chemical Dependency Associate
CPS	Certified Prevention Specialist
LCDC	Licensed Chemical Dependency Counselor
MAC	Master Addictions Counselor

Nursing

APRN	Advanced Practice Registered Nurse
BSN	Bachelor of Science in Nursing
CRNP	Certified, Registered Nurse Practitioner
CS	Certified Specialist (in Psychiatric Nursing)
LPN	Licensed Practical Nurse
PHN	Public Health Nurse
RN	Registered Nurse

Allied Health Professions

LPE	Licensed Psychological Examiner
OT	Occupational Therapy/Therapist
OTR	Occupational Therapist, Registered or Licensed
PA	Physician's Assistant
PT	Physical Therapy/Therapist
SLP	Speech and Language Pathologist

39.5. Diagnoses and Conditions

Due to the multitude of abbreviations, only a small sample is included in this section.

A	Anxiety
ADHD	Attention-deficit hyperactivity disorder
AOD	Alcohol and other drugs
BD	Behavioral disorder
BD	Brain damage
BD, Bip	Bipolar disorder
CD	Conduct disorder
CHI	Closed head injury
CUS/CUSc	Chronic undifferentiated schizophrenia
CVA	Cerebral vascular accident
CD	Cerebral palsy
D	Depression

D + A	Drug and alcohol
D + H	Delusions and hallucinations
DM	Diabetes mellitus
EBD	Emotional or behavioral disorder
ED	Emotional disorder
EELD	Early expressive language delay
FAS	Fetal alcohol syndrome
GAD	Generalized anxiety disorder
GID	Gender identity disorder
h/a	Headache
HBP	Hypertension/high blood pressure
HI	Hearing impairment
HIV	Human immunodeficiency virus
LBP	Low back pain
LD	Learning disability
MDD	Major depressive disorder
MR	Mental retardation
MRELD	Mixed receptive–expressive language disorder
OCD	Obsessive–compulsive disorder
ODD	Oppositional defiant disorder
OSAS	Obstructive sleep apnea syndrome
$\underline{P}$	Panic
Pa	Paranoia
PD	Perceptual disturbance
PDD	Pervasive developmental disorder
PKU	Phenylketonuria
PTSD	Posttraumatic stress disorder
RAD	Reactive attachment disorder
SAD	Separation anxiety disorder
SLI	Speech and language impairment
sz	Seizures
TBI	Traumatic brain injury
tt	Temper tantrum
VI	Visual impairment

39.6 Educational Services and Educational Laws

AAC	Augmentative/alternative communication
CAI	Computer-assisted instruction
CRF	Community residential facility
EI	Early intervention
ES	Emotional support
ESL	English as a second language
FC	Facilitated communication
IAES	Interim alternative educational setting
IDEA	Individuals with Disabilities Education Act
IEP	Individualized education plan
IFSP	Individualized family service plan
LRE	Least restrictive environment
LS	Learning support
LSS	Life skills support

MDE	Multidisciplinary evaluation
MDT	Multidisciplinary team
NORA	Notice of recommended assignment
PS	Physical support
Section 504	Section 504 of the Rehabilitation Act of 1973
SIS	Sensory impairment support
SLS	Speech and language support
VI	Visually impaired

39.7. Legal Terms

CMM	Corrupting the morals of a minor
IA	Indecent assault
IDSI	Involuntary deviate sexual intercourse
IVDU	Intravenous drug use/user
UAD	Underage drinking/drinker

39.8. Medical Terms and Tests

CAT scan	Computerized axial tomography scan
CNS	Central nervous system
CT scan	Computerized tomography scan
EEG	Electroencephalogram
FMRI	Functional magnetic resonance imaging
MRI	Magnetic resonance imaging
PET scan	Positron emission tomography scan

39.9. Medication Regimens

b.i.d.	Twice a day	p.r.n.	Whenever needed
h.s.	At night/bedtime	q.d.	Every day
i.m.	Intramuscular	q.i.d.	Four times a day
i.v.	Intravenous	q.q.h.	Every 4 hours
o.m.	Every morning	q.s.	As much as required
p.c.	After meals	t.i.d.	Three times a day
p.o.	By mouth		

39.10. Family Relationships

B	Brother	H	Husband
bf	Boyfriend	HH	Household
bil	Brother-in-law	Mo	Mother
d	Daughter	S	Sister
Fa	Father	s	Son
gf	Girlfriend	Sil	Sister-in-law
GP[1]	Grandparent	W	Wife

[1]Grandparents may be further specified as follows: maternal grandmother/grandfather, MGM/MGF; paternal grandmother/grandfather, PGM/PGF.

39.11. Treatment-Related Terms

AMA	Against medical advice		P/A	Psychoanalysis
d/c	Discontinue/ed		P/T	Psychotherapy
d/ch	Discharge/ed		PTA	Prior to admission
Dx	Diagnosis		Px	Prognosis
h/o	History of		Rx	Treatment or prescription
HW	Homework		Σ	Summary
Hx	History		Sx	Symptom
I	Intelligence		Th	Therapist
IV	Interview		Tx	Treatment
NOS	Not otherwise specified		WNL	Within normal limits

39.12. General Aids to Recording

$\bar{a}$	Before (*ante*)		RTC	Return to clinic
@	At		RTS	Return to school
AO	Anyone		$\bar{s}$ or w/o	Without (*sine*)
c.	About (*circa*)		S+S	Signs and symptoms
$\bar{c}$	With (*cum*)		w/d	Withdrawal/withdrew
d or d/	Divorced		w/i or $\bar{c}$/in	Within
D	Died		1°	Primary
d/o	Disorder		2°	Secondary
DNKA	Did not keep appointment		× 3	Times 3
DNS	Did not show		~	Approximate
DOB	Date of birth		Δ	Change
DOD	Date of death		↓	Decreasing/-ed
EO	Everyone		↑	Increasing/-ed
f	Frequency		<	Less, lesser, smaller
FTKA	Failed to keep appointment		>	More, greater, larger
NO	No one		∅ or ⊖	Not present, absent
ntk	Intake		#	Number
$\bar{p}$ or s/p	After, by history (*post*)		⊕	Present, positive for
Q, ?	Question		∴	Therefore
R/O	Rule out			

40

Useful Forms

This chapter contains a number of blank forms that can be used for collecting or recording information. These forms may be reproduced on letterhead and used by clinicians in the course of their work with clients.

40.1. Release of Information Form

See Sections 1.1 and 1.4 for further information about use of this form. This form may be reproduced on your letterhead.

Release of Information

Child's/adolescent's name: _____ Date of birth: _____

When you complete and sign this form, it authorizes this clinic/therapist to release protected information from your and/ or your child's clinical records to the person or clinic named below, or to obtain information from this person or clinic. You have the right to revoke this authorization, in writing, at any time by sending notification of this revocation to my office address.

I, _____, give permission to my therapist, _____ (and/or his/her staff) to release/obtain the following information in regard to the above-named minor's psychological treatment and/or evaluation. The particular information to be disclosed/obtained is the following (please be specific):

_____

_____

_____

_____

The information should be disclosed to/obtained from the following (please provide full addresses and telephone numbers):

_____

_____

_____

_____

I understand the statements above, and I voluntarily consent to disclosing/obtaining this information to/from the person or agency named above. I release _____ from any liability that could arise from disclosing/obtaining this information, as long as she/he discloses/obtains the information in accordance with applicable laws.

This authorization shall remain in effect until _____.

Signature of parent or guardian: _____

Signature of child/adolescent (if appropriate): _____

Date: _____

40.2. Developmental History Form

See Chapters 1 and 2 for further information on interviewing parents or guardians. This form may be reproduced on your letterhead.

Developmental History Form

The purpose of this form is to obtain a detailed understanding of your child's growth and development. Please answer all of the questions below, to the best of your ability. If a question does not apply to your particular situation, leave it blank.

IDENTIFYING INFORMATION

Child's name: _____ Today's date: _____

Child's date of birth: _____ Child's age: _____ Sex: Male _____ Female _____

Home address: _____

_____

Home phone number: _____

PRESENTING PROBLEM

Why are you seeking this evaluation or treatment? _____

_____

When did these problems begin? _____

What are your goals for this evaluation or treatment? _____

_____

_____

PARENTS, SIBLINGS, AND OTHERS IN HOME

Mother's name: _____ Mother's age: _____

Address: _____

Home phone: _____ Work phone: _____

Occupation: _____ (Full-time/part time?)

Education/highest grade completed: _____

Father's name: _____ Father's age: _____

Address (if different from above): _____

Home phone: _____ Work phone: _____

Occupation: _____ (Full-time/part time?)

Education/highest grade completed: _____

(cont.)

Does your child have stepparents? No _____ Yes _____

If yes, please complete the following information:

Name(s): _____

Relationship(s) to child: _____

Address(es)/phone(s): _____

_____

Is the child adopted or being raised by persons other than his/her biological parents? No _____ Yes _____

If yes, explain: _____

Name of sibling	Age	Gender	Lives at home?	Nature of relationship with child?
1. _____	____	____	_____	_____
2. _____	____	____	_____	_____
3. _____	____	____	_____	_____

Please list any others living in the household:

Name: _____ Relationship to child: _____

Name: _____ Relationship to child: _____

FAMILY CIRCUMSTANCES

Who cares for the child when parents or caregivers are at work or gone? _____

With whom does the child currently live? _____

Are the parents divorced or separated?   No _____ Yes _____

If yes, who has custody? _____

How often does the noncustodial parent see the child? _____

Family's religious affiliation (optional): _____

How frequently does this child see her/his grandparents? _____

Has the family recently experienced any unusual or stressful events?   No _____ Yes _____

If yes, explain: _____

PREGNANCY

Did the mother receive prenatal medical care?   No _____ Yes _____

If yes, what kind? _____

Length of pregnancy: _____

Did the mother experience any emotional or medical difficulties during the pregnancy?   No _____ Yes _____

If yes, explain: _____

Length of labor: ____ hours Apgar scores: _____

Birth weight: ____ lbs. ____ oz. Length: ____ inches

(cont.)

DEVELOPMENT

Was this child breast-fed or bottle-fed? _____ Age weaned: _____

Did the child experience any of the following problems during infancy or toddlerhood? If yes, please explain.

Colic   No _____ Yes _____

Excessive crying   No _____ Yes _____

Delayed language development   No _____ Yes _____

Unclear speech   No _____ Yes _____

Eating problems   No _____ Yes _____

Delayed fine motor skills   No _____ Yes _____

Delayed gross motor skills   No _____ Yes _____

At what approximate age did your child begin exhibiting the following behaviors?

Crawled: _____ Sat alone: _____

Walked independently: _____ Spoke first words: _____

Spoke in sentences: _____ Was toilet trained: _____

For an adolescent, please indicate the following:

Age at onset of puberty: _____ Age at first menstruation (for a girl): _____

Which hand does your child use for writing? _____ Eating? _____

Throwing? _____ Other? _____

Has your child been the victim of abuse? No _____ Yes _____

If yes, please explain: _____

MEDICAL AND PSYCHIATRIC HISTORY

Name of child's primary care physician: _____

Address: _____

_____

Phone: _____

Date of most recent physical exam: _____ Results: _____

Date of most recent dental exam: _____ Results: _____

Date of most recent vision exam: _____ Results: _____

Date of most recent hearing exam: _____ Results: _____

Has the child experienced any of the following medical problems? If yes, please explain.

Frequent colds   No _____ Yes _____

Frequent ear infections   No _____ Yes _____

Asthma   No _____ Yes _____

Gastrointestinal problems   No _____ Yes _____

Muscle pain   No _____ Yes _____

Skin problems   No _____ Yes _____

Repetitive behaviors (head banging,   No _____ Yes _____
    rocking, etc.)

Allergies   No _____ Yes _____

(cont.)

Vision problems   No _____ Yes _____

Does your child wear glasses?   No _____ Yes _____

Hearing problems   No _____ Yes _____

Cerebral palsy   No _____ Yes _____

Lead poisoning   No _____ Yes _____

Seizures   No _____ Yes _____

Congenital problems   No _____ Yes _____

Please list any other health concerns: _____

Medication

Is your child currently taking any kind of medication?   No _____ Yes _____

If yes, indicate name, dose, and reason for medication: _____

Is your child experiencing any side effects from the medication(s)? _____

Alcohol or Drug Use

Does your child use alcohol or drugs?   No _____ Yes _____

If yes, explain: _____

Previous Evaluations

Has your child ever had any of the following evaluations? If yes, please indicate name of examiner, date of examination, and reason for exam.

Psychological or psychiatric evaluation: No _____ Yes _____

If yes, name of evaluator: _____ Date of valuation: _____

Reason for evaluation: _____

Neuropsychological evaluation: No _____ Yes _____

If yes, name of evaluator: _____ Date of valuation: _____

Reason for evaluation: _____

Neurological evaluation: No _____ Yes _____

If yes, name of evaluator: _____ Date of valuation: _____

Reason for evaluation: _____

Treatment History

Has your child ever received counseling or psychiatric treatment?   No _____ Yes _____

If yes, indicate dates, name of treating professional, reason for treatment, and effectiveness of treatment: _____

_____

_____

Family's Health

Mother's present health: _____

Father's present health: _____

Has anyone in your family experienced a mental, psychological, or academic problem, such as mental retardation, learning disabilities, schizophrenia, depression, epilepsy, or a bipolar disorder?   No _____ Yes _____

If yes, explain: _____

(cont.)

SOCIAL HISTORY

How does your child relate to other children? _____

Does your child prefer to play with younger or older children?   No ____   Yes ____

    If yes, indicate which (younger or older) and explain: _____

Does your child have a best friend?   No ____   Yes ____

How many friends does your child have? _____

RECREATIONAL INTERESTS

Does your child participate in sports or recreational activities outside of school?   No ____   Yes ____

    If yes, describe: _____

What does your child like to do in his/her free time? _____

_____

Have the child's interests in these activities changed recently?   No ____   Yes ____

    If yes, please explain: _____

What are your family's favorite activities? _____

BEHAVIORAL SYMPTOMS

Does your child have difficulty with any of the following problems? If yes, please explain.

Has trouble meeting new people; is shy or withdrawn	No ____ Yes ____
Is overly anxious	No ____ Yes ____
Seems sad or depressed	No ____ Yes ____
Has thought of suicide	No ____ Yes ____
Refuses to comply with adults' requests or violates parental rules	No ____ Yes ____
Has conduct problems	No ____ Yes ____
Is physically cruel to other people or animals	No ____ Yes ____
Is inattentive	No ____ Yes ____
Problems concentrating	No ____ Yes ____
Is restless	No ____ Yes ____
Makes careless mistakes	No ____ Yes ____
Has trouble playing quietly	No ____ Yes ____
Has frequent mood shifts	No ____ Yes ____
Frustrates easily	No ____ Yes ____
Has difficulty managing anger	No ____ Yes ____
Has eating problems	No ____ Yes ____
Has fears/phobias	No ____ Yes ____
Has hallucinations	No ____ Yes ____
Has experienced trauma	No ____ Yes ____

Has your child ever experienced difficulty with the law?   No ____   Yes ____

    If yes, explain: _____

(cont.)

EDUCATIONAL STATUS AND HISTORY

Current Status

Name of current school: _____ Grade: _____

Type of school: Private _____ Public _____ Home-schooled _____ Other _____

Teacher(s): _____

School address: _____

_____

School phone number: _____

Does your child currently receive any special education services? No _____ Yes _____

    If yes, please specify: _____

What grades does the child currently receive? _____

    Is this a change from previous years? No _____ Yes _____

    If yes, explain: _____

School History

Preschool: At what age? _____ For how many days/hours? _____

    Any problems? No _____ Yes _____ If yes, describe: _____

Did the child have difficulty or receive any special education services in any of the following grades? If so, please explain.

    Kindergarten   No _____ Yes _____

    Grades 1–3   No _____ Yes _____

    Grades 4–6   No _____ Yes _____

    Grades 7–8   No _____ Yes _____

    High school   No _____ Yes _____

Does your child dislike going to school? No _____ Yes _____

    If yes, why? _____

What are your child's favorite subjects? _____

What are your child's least favorite subjects? _____

What is your child's approach to her/his schoolwork (disorganized/organized, irresponsible/responsible, etc.)? _____

_____

WORK HISTORY

Does your child have a job, or is your child involved in a vocational program? No _____ Yes _____

If yes, who is the child's current employer? _____

Child's position: _____ Hours worked per week: _____

40.3. Teacher Questionnaire Form

See Chapter 4 for guidelines on interviewing teachers and obtaining information from them. This form may be reproduced on your letterhead.

Teacher Questionnaire

The purpose of this questionnaire it to obtain a more comprehensive understanding of the academic and social functioning of the child named below. Please answer these questions to the best of your ability. Please return this questionnaire, when completed, to _____.

Teacher's name: _____ Date: _____

Child's name: _____ Grade: _____

School: _____ School phone: _____

School address: _____

_____

What do you see as this child's major problem? _____

_____

_____

How long has this been a problem? _____

_____

_____

How serious do you perceive this child's problems to be? _____

What changes would you like to see happen as a result of this treatment/evaluation? _____

_____

_____

Does this child have any learning disabilities that you are aware of?   No ____   Yes ____

If yes, what are they? _____

(cont.)

Does this child receive special tutoring or support?   No _____ Yes _____

   If yes, please describe: _____

Is this child on a Section 504 plan or an IEP?   No _____ Yes _____

Has this child ever had special testing in school?   No _____ Yes _____

   If yes, please explain: _____

   _____

   _____

Does this child attend school regularly?   No _____ Yes _____

Does this child appear motivated for school? _____

Has this child ever had disciplinary action taken against him/her, such as being suspended or expelled?   No _____ Yes _____

   If yes, explain: _____

   _____

What was this child's highest grade on the last report card? _____

What was this child's lowest grade? _____

What do you see as this child's strongest and weakest areas of learning? _____

_____

_____

Does this child participate in extracurricular activities?   No _____ Yes _____

   If yes, describe: _____

   _____

In school, how many friends does this child have?   Many _____   A few _____   None _____

Do you have any concerns about this child's social relationships?   No _____ Yes _____

   If yes, describe: _____

   _____

Please list anything else about this child that would be helpful: _____

_____

40.4. Child Assessment Form for Professionals

Guidelines for obtaining information from other professionals can be found in Chapter 4. This form may be reproduced on your letterhead or in a letter format.

Child Assessment Form

Child's name: _____

Child's address: _____

_____

The above-named child has been referred to me for assessment/treatment (*indicate which*). Please fill out this form to the best of your knowledge and ability. If you would like to contact me for further information, my address and phone number are as follows:

My address: _____

_____

My phone: _____

In what capacity do you know this child? _____

For how long have you known this child? _____

Who initiated the referral for this child? _____

What are the referral questions? _____

_____

What do you see as the child's main difficulty? _____

_____

What type of evaluation/treatment do you think is necessary? _____

_____

Does this child carry any current or past DSM-IV-TR diagnoses?   No ____ Yes ____

    If yes, specify:

    Axis I: _____

    Axis II: _____

    Axis III: _____

    Axis IV: _____

    Axis V: _____

Are there any medical or neurological explanations for this child's current behaviors or symptoms? _____

Please list anything else about the child that would be helpful to know: _____

_____

Please describe any pertinent test results (e.g., psychiatric, psychological, medical, or neurological evaluations):

_____

_____

_____

40.5. Sentence Completion Test

See Section 27.8 for further information on sentence completion tests. This form may be reproduced on your letterhead.

Sentence Completion Test

1. When I see myself in the mirror, I _____.
2. When I'm by myself, _____.
3. The best things about boys is _____.
4. The best thing about me is _____.
5. When my schoolwork is poor, _____.
6. I can't _____.
7. The best thing about school _____.
8. My mother _____.
9. My friends think I _____
10. When I think about the future, _____.
11. The best thing about my body _____
12. Most dads _____.
13. No one knows _____.
14. The best thing about girls is _____.
15. The worst thing about school _____.
16. My life would be better if only _____.
17. My father _____.
18. The worst thing about my body _____.
19. Most moms _____.
20. I think most boys are _____.
21. I think most girls are _____.
22. If I had only one wish, _____.
23. When I'm with my family, _____.
24. If only my mom and dad would _____
25. When I see others do better than I'm doing, _____.
26. Someday I'd like to be _____.
27. I feel guilty when _____.
28. I wish I could forget about _____.
29. Other kids think I'm _____.
30. My family _____.
31. I learn best _____.
32. School is _____.
33. My teachers are _____.
34. My work has been _____.
35. It makes me sad when _____.
36. I am happiest when _____.
37. When I'm with other people, _____.
38. Adults are _____.
39. I feel nervous when _____.
40. I feel happy when _____.

40.6. Form for Educational Assessment of Student's Current Classroom Functioning

See Section 35.10 for an example of a completed classroom observation report. See also Chapter 33, "Writing for the Schools." This form may be reproduced on your letterhead.

Educational Assessment of Student's Current Classroom Functioning

Student's name: _____ Date of evaluation: _____

School: _____

Person completing form: _____

DESCRIPTION OF STUDENT'S CLASSROOM PERFORMANCE AND BEHAVIOR

1. Positive personal qualities:

   This student is capable of _____.

   She/he can demonstrate very good _____.

   He/she has shown him-/herself to be _____.

2. Student's self-confidence:

   This student's academic self-confidence is _____,

   which affects her/his ability to _____.

   Socially, he/she appears _____,

   while athletic confidence appears _____.

3. Class participation:

   This student makes his/her presence known in few/many/all activities.

   The nature of his/her participation is frequently _____.

4. Activity levels and patterns:

   This student has an extremely high/low activity level and is able/unable to sit and listen for extended periods of time.

   Verbal activity is _____.

   When seated at his/her desk, the student frequently _____.

   In less structured settings, her/his activity would be described as _____.

5. Attention to task:

   This student's ability to focus tends to be _____.

   His/her attention seems to be best in _____ circumstances.

   Problems with attention are often seen in _____.

6. Conditions under which performance improves:

   This student performs better at _____ times

   and in _____ settings.

   She/he shows her/his best performance in _____ subjects.

(cont.)

DESCRIPTION OF STUDENT'S BASIC SKILLS

1. Gross and fine motor coordination (body movements, balance, fine drawing, writing, etc.):

   This student has very coordinated/poorly coordinated gross motor skills.

   She/he is/is not a good athlete.

   His/her graphomotor output is _____.

   In the art center, she/he demonstrated the ability to _____.

   She/he is right/left handed and uses a _____ pencil grip.

2. Learning abilities observed:

   My observations would suggest that this student is most comfortable when material is presented verbally/visually didactically/through discussion/in small groups/multisensorially.

   When presented with material that has multiple steps, he/she loses focus/cannot process information/relates to the material in a disorganized fashion/is unable to handle _____.

   She/he appears to struggle most on _____ types of tasks.

3. Reading skills: Generally at/above/below grade level.

   a. Mechanics:

      This student is able/unable to decode, while fluency is _____.
      His/her reading is not/is somewhat/is quite effortful.

   b. Comprehension:

      In the context of a book discussion, this student shows _____
      ability to demonstrate understanding and appreciation of what she/he has read.

      When asked to write about what he/she has read, he/she demonstrates grade-appropriate/below-grade-level abilities.

   c. Conceptual skills:

      Although this student enjoys reading/being read to, she/he has/has not demonstrated an ability to deal with larger conceptual issues about what she/he has read/heard.

4. Language skills:

   a. Expressive language:

      Within the classroom, this student uses his/her verbal ability to _____.

      Her/his language skills are/are not at a level expected for a child her/his age, because _____.

   b. Written language skills:

      This student's writing tends to be _____.

      His/her sentence structure is _____,

      and his/her understanding of the writing process is _____.

      Writing is/is not a struggle for her/him because _____.

   c. Ability to follow simple and complex directions:

      Verbal directions do/do not present a problem for this student.

      When dealing with written directions, he/she typically reacts with _____.

(cont.)

5. Math skills:

   a. Computational skills:

   This student's skills in math computation could be described as _____.

   Basic facts (multiplication, addition, etc.) are automatic/not automatic.

   In multistep problems, she/he demonstrates _____.

   b. Problem-solving skills:

   This student's math problem-solving skills would be described as _____,

   because of _____.

6. Other academic areas (science, social studies, etc.): (*Describe.*) _____

   _____

   _____

   _____

   _____

7. Socialization skills:

   a. Group:

   In group situations, this student's typical behavior would be described as _____.

   b. Peers:

   This student has many/few/some friends.

   His/her play would be described as _____.

   c. Adults:

   With adults, the student has a tendency to _____.

   Her/his behavior with adults in 1:1 settings is typically _____.

   In the presence of peers, his/her behavior with adults is often _____.

SUMMARY OF CURRENT FUNCTIONING

In summary, this student's strengths are in the areas of _____

_____.

Her/his weaknesses appear to be _____

_____.

When both strengths and weaknesses are taken into account, his/her greatest needs in the classroom are _____

_____

_____.

40.7. Behavior Management Plan Form

See Section 33.5 for information about preparing behavior management plans. This form may be reproduced on your letterhead.

Behavior Management Plan

Behaviors of concern:

1. _____.
2. _____.
3. _____.
4. _____.
5. _____.

Baseline measurements:

1. _____.
2. _____.
3. _____.
4. _____.
5. _____.

Strengths, interests, and preferences:

1. _____.
2. _____.
3. _____.
4. _____.
5. _____.

Optimal environmental conditions:

1. _____.
2. _____.
3. _____.
4. _____.
5. _____.

(cont.)

Situations that cause unusual stress or that exacerbate negative behaviors:

1. _____.

2. _____.

3. _____.

4. _____.

5. _____.

Proactive teaching and environmental strategies likely to decrease inappropriate behaviors:

1. _____.

2. _____.

3. _____.

4. _____.

5. _____.

Responsive techniques likely to decrease inappropriate behaviors:

1. _____.

2. _____.

3. _____.

4. _____.

5. _____.

Measurements used to evaluate interventions:

1. _____.

2. _____.

3. _____.

4. _____.

5. _____.

40.8. Form for Psychotherapy Progress Notes

See Section 35.6 for information about progress notes and a sample progress summary. This form may be reproduced on your letterhead.

Psychotherapy Progress Notes

Client's name: _____ Date of birth: _____

Date of visit: _____ Type of visit: _____ Person present: _____

Content (list reviewed problems, symptom status, changes/interventions):

Mental status and risk factors:

Clinical impressions:

Diagnosis:

    Axis I:

    Axis II:

    Axis III:

    Axis IV:

    Axis V (GAF):

Treatment plan (list targeted problem/goal/intervention, homework assignment, date of next visit, collaboration, etc.):

_____ _____
      Therapist's signature   Date

References

Achenbach, T. M., & Rescorla, L. A. (2001). *Manual for ASEBA school-age forms and profiles.* Burlington: University of Vermont, Research Center for Children, Youth, and Families.

Adams, W., & Sheslow, D. (2003). *Wide Range Assessment of Memory and Learning.* San Antonio, TX: Psychology Corporation.

American Psychiatric Association. (2000). *Diagnostic and statistical manual of mental disorders* (4th ed., text rev.). Washington, DC: Author.

American Speech–Language–Hearing Association. (1982). Definitions: Communication disorders and variations. *Journal of Speech and Hearing Research, 24,* 949–950.

Anderson, R. N. (2002). Deaths: Leading causes for 2000. *National Vital Statistics Reports, 50*(16) [Electronic version]. Retrieved from www.cdc.gov/nchs/data/nvsr/nvsr50/nvsr50_16.pdf

Andrews, G., Craig, A., Feyer, A., Hoddinott, S., Howie, P., & Neilson, M. (1983). Stuttering: A review of research findings and theories circa 1982. *Journal of Speech and Hearing Disorders, 48,* 226–246.

Angold, A., Cox, A., Rutter, M., & Simonoff, E. (1996). *Child and Adolescent Psychiatric Assessment (CAPA): Version 4.2–Child Version.* Durham, NC: Duke Medical Center.

Apgar, V. (1953). A proposal for a new method of evaluation of the newborn infant. *Anesthesia and Analgesia: Current Researches, 32,* 26–267.

Baker, A. F. (1983). Psychological assessment of autistic children. *Clinical Psychology Review, 3,* 41–59.

Barker, P. (1990). *Clinical interviews with children and adolescents.* New York: Norton.

Barkley, R. A., & Murphy, K. R. (2006). *Attention-deficit hyperactivity disorder: A clinical workbook* (3rd ed.). New York: Guilford Press.

Bayley, N. (1969). *Bayley Scales of Infant Development.* New York: Psychological Corporation.

Bayley, N. (2005). *Bayley Scales of Infant and Toddler Development, Third Edition (Bayley-III).* San Antonio, TX: Psychological Corporation.

Bee, H. L. (1997). *The developing child* (8th ed.). New York: Longman.

Beery, K. E., Buktenica, N. A., & Beery, N. A. (2004). *Beery–Buktenica Developmental Test of Visual–Motor Integration–Fifth Edition.* Minneapolis, MN: NCS Pearson.

Bellak, L., & Bellak, S. S. (1949). *The Children's Apperception Test.* New York: C.P.S. Company.

Bender, L. (1938). *A visual motor gestalt test and its clinical use* (Research Monograph No. 3). New York: American Orthopsychiatric Association.

Benton, A. L. (1968). Differential behavioral effects in frontal lobe disease. *Neuropsychologia, 6,* 53–60.

Benton, A. L., Hannah, H. J., & Varney, N. R. (1975). Visual perception of line direction in patients with unilateral brain disease. *Neurology, 25,* 907–910.

Berg, I. K., & Miller, S. D. (1992). *Working with the problem drinker.* New York: Norton.

Berk, L. E. (1994). *Child development* (3rd ed.). Boston: Allyn & Bacon.

Boll, T. (1993). *Children's Category Test.* San Antonio, TX: Psychological Corporation.

Bowen, M. (1980). Key to the use of the genogram. In E. A. Carter & M. McGoldrick (Eds.), *The family life cycle: A framework for family therapy* (pp. 226–242). New York: Gardner.

Braaten, E. B., Biederman, J., DiMauro, A., Mick, E., Monuteaux, M. C., Muehl, K., et al. (2001) Methodological complexities in the diagnosis of major depression in youth: An analysis of mother and youth self-reports. *Journal of Pediatric Psychopharmacology, 11,* 395–408.

Braaten, E. B., & Handelsman, M. M. (1997). Client preferences for informed consent information. *Ethics and Behavior, 7,* 311–328.

Bracken, B. A. (1998). *Bracken Basic Concept Scale–Revised.* San Antonio, TX: Psychological Corporation.

Brown, J. I., Fishco, V. V., & Hanna, G. S. (1993). *Nelson–Denny Reading Test.* Chicago: Riverside.

Brown, L., Sherbenou, R. J., & Johnsen, S. K. (1997). *Test of Nonverbal Intelligence–Third Edition* (TONI-3). Austin, TX: PRO-ED.

Brown, T. E. (2001). *Brown Attention-Deficit Disorder Scales.* San Antonio, TX: Psychological Corporation.

Brownell, R. (2000a). *Expressive One-Word Picture Vocabulary Test–2000 Edition.* Novato, CA: Academic Therapy.

Brownell, R. (2000b). *Receptive One-Word Picture Vocabulary Test–2000 Edition.* Novato, CA: Academic Therapy.

Bruininks, R. H., & Bruininks, B. D. (2006). *Bruininks–Oseretsky Test of Motor Proficiency, Second Edition (BOT-2).* Circle Pines, MN: American Guidance Service.

Bruininks, R. H., Woodcock, R., Weatherman, R., & Hill, B. (1996). *Scales of Independent Behavior–Revised.* Chicago: Riverside.

Bukato, D., & Daehler, M. W. (1998). *Child development: A thematic approach.* Boston: Houghton Mifflin.

Butcher, J. N., Williams, C. L., Graham, J. R., Archer, R. P., Tellegen, A., Ben-Porath, Y. S., et al. (1992). *Minnesota Multiphasic Personality Inventory–Adolescent (MMPI-A): Manual for administration, scoring, and interpretation.* Minneapolis: University of Minnesota Press.

Campbell, R. J. (2003). *Campbell's psychiatric dictionary* (8th ed.). New York: Oxford University Press.

Carrow-Woolfolk, E. (1995). *Oral and Written Language Scales (OWLS).* Circle Pines, MN: American Guidance Service.

Carrow-Woolfolk, E. (1999). *Test for Auditory Comprehension of Language–Third Edition (TACL-3).* Austin, TX: PRO-ED.

Clark, L. A., Watson, D., & Reynolds, S. (1995). Diagnosis and classification of psychopathology: Challenges to the current system and future directions. *Annual Review of Psychology, 46,* 121–153.

Cohen, M. (1997). *Children's Memory Scale.* San Antonio, TX: Psychological Corporation.

Conners, C. K. (1997). *Conners' Rating Scales–Revised: Technical manual.* North Tonawanda, NY: Multi-Health Systems.

Delis, D. C., Kramer, J. H., Kaplan, E. F., & Ober, B. A. (1994). *California Verbal Learning Test–Children's Version (CVCL-T).* San Antonio, TX: Psychological Corporation.

Delis, D. C., Kramer, J. H., Kaplan, E., & Ober, B. A. (2000). *California Verbal Learning Test–Second Edition (CVLT-II).* San Antonio, TX: Psychological Corporation.

DiPerna, J. C., & Elliott, S. N. (2000). *Academic Competence Evaluation Scale.* San Antonio, TX: Psychological Corporation.

DiSimoni, F. (1978). *Token Test for Children.* Boston: Teaching Resources Corp.

Dunn, L. M., & Dunn, L. M. (1997). *Peabody Picture Vocabulary Test–Third Edition.* Circle Pines, MN: American Guidance Service.

DuPaul, G. J., Power, T. J., Anastopoulos, A. D., & Reid, R. (1998). *ADHD Rating Scale–IV: Checklists, norms and clinical interpretation.* New York: Guilford Press.

DuPaul, G. J., Rapport, M. D., & Periello, L. M. (1991). Teacher ratings of academic skills: The development of the Academic Performance Rating Scale. *School Psychology Review, 20,* 284–300.

Education for All Handicapped Children Act, Pub. L. No. 94-142, 20 U.S.C. 1400 et seq. (1975). [p. 622]

Elliott, C. D. (2006). *Differential Ability Scales, Second Edition (DAS-II): Administration and scoring manual.* San Antonio, TX: Psychological Corporation.

Exner, J. E. (2002). *A Rorschach workbook for the comprehensive system* (5th ed.). New York: Wiley.

Forrester, G., & Geffen, G. (1991). Performance measure to 15-year-old children on the Auditory Verbal Learning Test. *Clinical Neuropsychologist, 5,* 345–359.

Gilliam, J. E. (2001). *Gilliam Asperger's Disorder Scale.* Austin, TX: PRO-ED.

Ginsburg, H. P., & Baroody, A. J. (2003). *Test of Early Mathematics Ability (TEMA-3).* Austin, TX: PRO-ED.

Gioia, G. A., Espy, A., Isquith, P. K. (2003). *Behavior Rating Inventory of Executive Function–Preschool Version.* Lutz, FL: Psychological Assessment Resources.

Gioia, G. A., Isquith, P. K., Guy, S. C., Kenworthy, L. (2000). *Behavior Rating Inventory of Executive Function.* Lutz, FL: Psychological Assessment Resources.

Glutting, J. J., Adams, W., & Sheslow, D. (2000). *Wide Range Intelligence Test (WRIT).* Wilmington, DE: Wide Range.

Golden, C. J. (1978). *Stroop Color and Word Test.* Chicago: Stoelting.

Golden, C. J. (1987). Screening batteries for the adult and children's versions of the Luria–Nebraska Neuro-psychological Batteries. *Neuropsychology, 1,* 63–66.

Gordon, M. (1998). *The Gordon Diagnostic System.* DeWitt, NY: Gordon Systems.

Greenberg, L. M. (1990). *Test of Variables of Attention (TOVA).* Los Alamitos, CA: Universal Attention Disorders.

Gresham, F. M., & Elliott, S. N. (1990). *Social Skills Rating System (SSRS).* Circle Pines, MN: American Guidance Service.

Grunbaum, J. A., Kann, L., Kinchen, S. A., et al. (2002). Youth Risk Behavior Surveillance–United States, 2001. *Morbidity and Mortality Weekly Report, 51*(SS-4), 1–64.

Hallahan, D. P., & Kauffman, J. M. (1994). *Exceptional children: Introduction to special education.* Boston: Allyn & Bacon.

Hammill, D. D. (1998). *Detroit Tests of Learning Aptitude–Fourth Edition (DTLA-4).* Austin, TX: PRO-ED.

Hammill, D. D., Brown, V. L., Larsen, S. C., & Wiederholt, J. L. (1994). *Test of Adolescent and Adult Language–Third Edition (TOAL-3).* Austin, TX: PRO-ED.

Hammill, D. D., & Larsen, S. C. (1996). *Test of Written Language–Third Edition (TOWL-3).* Austin, TX: PRO-ED.

Hammill, D. D., Mather, N., & Roberts, R. (2001). *Illinois Test of Psycholinguistic Abilities–Third Edition (ITPA-3).* Austin, TX: PRO-ED.

Hammill, D. D., Pearson, N. A., & Wiederholt, J. L. (1997). *Comprehensive Test of Nonverbal Intelligence (CTONI).* Austin, TX: PRO-ED.

Handelsman, M. M. (2001). Accurate and effective informed consent. In E. R. Welfel & R. E. Ingersoll (Eds.), *The mental health desk reference* (pp. 453–458). New York: Wiley.

Harrison, P. L., & Oakland, T. (2000). *Adaptive Behavior Assessment System.* San Antonio, TX: Psychological Corporation.

Heaton, R. K. (1981). *Wisconsin Card Sorting Test manual.* Odessa, FL: Psychological Assessment Resources.

Hodges, K. (1993). *Child Assessment Schedule (CAS).* Ypsilanti, MI: Eastern Michigan University.

Hooper, H. E. (1983). *Hooper Visual Organization Test.* Los Angeles: Western Psychological Services.

House, A. E. (2002). *The first session with children and adolescents: Conducting a comprehensive mental health evaluation.* New York: Guilford Press.

Hresko, W. P., Reid, D. K., & Hammill, D. D. (1999). *Test of Early Language Development–Third Edition (TELD-3).* Austin, TX: PRO-ED.

Individuals with Disabilities Education Act (Pub. L. No. 101–476), 20 U.S.C. 1400 et seq.) (1990). (Regulations appear at 34 C.F.R. 300)

Individuals with Disabilities Education Act (IDEA) Amendments of 1997, Pub. L. No. 105-17, 20 U.S.C. 1400 et seq. (1997).

Individuals with Disabilities Education Improvement Act of 2004 (IDEA 2004), Pub. L. No. 108-446, 20 U.S.C. 1400 et seq. (2004). [p. 618]

Jarratt, C. J. (1994). *Helping children cope with separation and loss.* Boston: Harvard Common Press.

Jenkins, S. C., Tinsley, J. A., & Van Loon, V. A. (2001). *Pocket reference for psychiatrists* (3rd ed.). Washington, DC: American Psychiatric Press.

Kaplan, E. F., Goodglass, H., & Weintraub, S. (1983). *The Boston Naming Test* (2nd ed.). Philadelphia: Lea & Febiger.

Kaufman, A. S., & Kaufman, N. L. (1993). *Kaufman Adolescent and Adult Intelligence.* Circle Pines, MN: American Guidance Service.

Kaufman, A. S., & Kaufman, N. L. (2004). *Kaufman Assessment Battery for Children, Second Edition (KABC-II).* Circle Pines, MN: American Guidance Service.

Kaufman, J., Birmaher, B., Brent, D. A., Rao, U., & Ryan, N. (1996). *Schedule for Affective Disorders and Schizophrenia for School-Age Children–Present and Lifetime Version (K-SADS-PL).* Pittsburgh, PA: Western Psychiatric Institute and Clinic.

Knoff, H. M. (1986). The personality assessment report and the feedback and planning conference. In H. M. Knoff (Ed.), *The assessment of child and adolescent personality* (pp. 547–582). New York: Guilford Press.

Korkman, M., Kirk, U., & Kemp, S. (1998). *NEPSY: A developmental neuropsychological assessment.* San Antonio, TX: Psychological Corporation.

Kovacs, M. (1992). *Children's Depression Inventory (CDI).* North Tonawanda, NY: Multi-Health Systems.

Kramer, J. R. (1985). *Family interfaces: Transgeneration patterns.* New York: Brunner/Mazel.

Lachar, D., Wingenfeld, S.A., Kline, R. B., & Gruber, C. P. (2000). *Student Behavior Survey.* Los Angeles: Western Psychological Services.

Larry P. v. Riles, 343 F.Supp. 1306 (D.C. N.D. Cal., 1972), aff'd., 502 F.2d 963 (9th Cir. 1974), *further proceedings,* 495 F.Supp. 926 (D.C. N.D. Cal., 1979), aff'd., 502 F.2d 693 (9th Cir. 1984).

Lewis, B. L. (2002). Second thoughts about documenting the psychological consultation. *Professional Psychology: Research and Practice, 33*(2), 224–225.

Lezak, M. D. (1995). *Neuropsychological assessment* (3rd ed.). New York: Oxford University Press.

Lindamood, P. C., & Lindamood, P. (2004). *Lindamood Auditory Conceptualization Test, Third Edition (LAC-3).* Circle Pines, MN: American Guidance Service.

Maccoby, E. E., & Martin, J. A. (1983). Socialization in the context of the family: Parent–child interaction. In E. M. Hetherington (Ed.), *Handbook of child psychology* (4th ed.): *Vol. 4. Socialization, personality, and social development.* New York: Wiley.

MacGinitie, W. H., MacGinitie, R. R., Maria, K., & Dreyer, L. G. (2002). *Gates–MacGinitie Reading Tests, Fourth Edition (GMRT-4).* Itasca, IL: Riverside.

Matthews, C. G., & Kløve, H. (1964). *Instruction manual for the Adult Neuropsychology Test Battery.* Madison: University of Wisconsin Medical School.

Maxmen, J. S., & Ward, N. G. (1995). *Essential psychopathology and its treatment* (2nd ed.). New York: Norton.

McArthur, D. S., & Roberts, G. E. (1982). *Roberts Apperception Test for Children: Manual.* Los Angeles: Western Psychological Services.

McGoldrick, M., Gerson, R., & Shellenberger, S. (1999). *Genograms: Assessment and intervention* (2nd ed.). New York: Norton.

Merrell, K. W. (1999). *Behavioral, social and emotional assessment of children and adolescents.* Mahwah, NJ: Erlbaum.

Merrell, K. W. (2001). *Helping students overcome depression and anxiety: A practical guide.* New York: Guilford Press.

Millon, T., Green, C. J., & Meagher, R. B. (1982). *Millon Adolescent Personality Inventory.* Minneapolis, MN: National Computer Systems.

Morrison, J., & Anders, T. F. (2001). *Interviewing children and adolescents* (rev. ed.). New York: Guilford Press.

Murray, H. A. (1971). *Thematic Apperception Test: Manual.* Cambridge, MA: Harvard University Press.

Naglieri, J. A., LeBuffe, P. A., & Pfeiffer, S. I. (1994). *Devereux Scales of Mental Disorders.* San Antonio, TX: Psychological Corporation.

Newborg, J. (2004). *Battelle Developmental Inventory, Second Edition (BDI-2).* Itasca, IL: Riverside.

Newcomer, P. L., & Hammill, D. D. (1997a). *Test of Language Development–Intermediate: Third Edition (TOLD-I:3).* Austin, TX: PRO-ED.

Newcomer, P. L., & Hammill, D. D. (1997b). *Test of Language Development–Primary: Third Edition (TOLD-P:3).* Austin, TX: PRO-ED.

Nihira, K., Lel, H., & Lambert, N. (1993). *AAMR Adaptive Behavior Scales–Residential and Community: Second Edition (ABS-RC:2).* Austin, TX: PRO-ED.

Nuttall, E. V., & Ivey, A. E. (1986). The diagnostic interview process. In H. M. Knoff (Ed.), *The assessment of child and adolescent personality* (pp. 105–140). New York: Guilford Press.

O'Neill, R. E., Horner, R. H., Albin, R. W., Sprague, J. R., Storey, K., Newton, J. S. (1997). *Functional assessment and program development for problem behavior: A practical handbook.* Pacific Grove, CA: Brooks/Cole.

Orvaschel, H. (1995). *Schedule for Affective Disorders and Schizophrenia for School-Age Children–Epidemiological Version 5 (K-SADS-E5).* Fort Lauderdale, FL: Nova Southeastern University.

Parten, M. (1932). Social play among preschool children. *Journal of Abnormal and Social Psychology, 27,* 243–269.

Perry, L. A., & Vitali, G. J. (1991). Slosson Test of Reading Readiness. East Aurora, NY: Slosson Educational.

Powell, J., & Smith, C. A. (1997). *Developmental milestones: A guide for parents.* Manhattan, KS: Kansas State University Cooperative Extension Service. Retrieved from www.oznet.ksu.edu/library/famlf2/l834.pdf.

The Psychological Corporation. (1999). *Wechsler Abbreviated Scale of Intelligence (WASI).* San Antonio, TX: Author.

Quay, H. C., & Peterson, D. R. (1996). *Revised Behavior Problem Checklist, PAR Edition.* Odessa, FL: Psychological Assessment Resources.

Reitan, R. M., & Wolfson, D. (1985). *The Halstead–Reitan Neuropsychological Test Battery.* Tucson, AZ: Neuropsychology Press.

Reitan, R. M., & Wolfson, D. (1992). *Neuropsychological evaluation of young children.* Tucson, AZ: Neuropsychology Press.

Reitan, R. M., & Wolfson, D. (1993). *The Halstead–Reitan Neuropsychological Test Battery: Theory and clinical interpretation.* Tucson, AZ: Neuropsychology Press.

Reynolds, C. R., & Kamphaus, R. W. (2004). *Behavior Assessment System for Children, Second Edition (BASC-2).* Circle Pines, MN: American Guidance Service.

Reynolds, C. R., & Richmond, B. O. (1985). *Revised Children's Manifest Anxiety Scale (RCMAS).* Los Angeles: Western Psychological Services.

Rivas-Vasquez, R. A., Blais, M. A., Rey, G. J., & Rivas-Vasquez, A. A. (2001). A brief reminder about documenting the psychological consultation. *Professional Psychology: Research and Practice, 32*(2), 194–199.

Roid, G. (2003). *Stanford–Binet Intelligence Scales, Fifth Edition (SB5).* Itasca, IL: Riverside.

Root, R. W., II, & Resnick, R. J. (2003). An update on the diagnosis and treatment of attention deficit/hyperactivity disorder in children. *Professional Psychology: Research and Practice. 34*(1), 34–41.

Rorschach, H. (1942). *Psychodiagnostics* (5th ed.). Bern, Switzerland: Hans Huber. (Original work published 1921)

Rotter, J. B., & Rafferty, J. E. (1950). *Manual: The Rotter Incomplete Sentences Blank.* New York: Psychological Corporation.

Ryan, C. M., Hammond, K., & Beers, S. R. (1998). General assessment issues for a pediatric population. In P. J. Snyder & P. D. Nussbaum (Ed.), *Clinical neuropsychology* (pp. 105–123). Washington, DC: American Psychological Association.

Sacks, J. M., & Levy, S. (1950). The Sentence Completion Test. In L. E. Abt & L. Bellak (Eds.), *Projective psychology* (pp. 357–402). New York: Knopf.

Santrock, J. W. (1997). *Children* (5th ed.). Madison, WI: Brown & Benchmark.

Sattler, J. M. (1992). *Assessment of children* (3rd ed.). San Diego, CA: Author.

Sattler, J. M. (2001). *Assessment of children* (4th ed.): *Cognitive applications.* San Diego, CA: Author.

Sattler, J. M. (2002). *Assessment of children* (4th ed.): *Behavioral and clinical applications.* San Diego, CA: Author.

Satz, P., & Bullard-Bates, C. (1981). Acquired aphasia in children. In M. T. Sarno (Ed.), *Acquired aphasia* (pp. 399–426). New York: Academic Press.

Schaughnessy, M. F., & Nystul, M. S. (1985). Preventing the greatest loss—suicide. *Creative Child and Adult Quarterly, 10,* 164–169.

Schopler, E., Reichler, R. J., DeVellis, R. F., & Daly, K. (1980). Toward objective classification of childhood autism: Childhood Autism Rating Scale (CARS). *Journal of Autism and Developmental Disorders, 10,* 91–103.

Semel, E., Wiig, E. H., & Secord, W. A. (2003). *Clinical Evaluation of Language Fundamentals–Fourth Edition (CELF-4).* San Antonio, TX: Harcourt Assessment.

Shaffer, D. (1996). *Diagnostic Interview Schedule for Children, Version IV (DISC-IV).* New York: New York State Psychiatric Institute.

Shaffer, D., Garland, A., Gould, M., Fisher, P., & Trautman, P. (1988). Preventing teenage suicide: A critical review. *Journal of the American Academy of Child and Adolescent Psychiatry, 27,* 675–687.

Sivan, A. B. (1992). *Benton Visual Retention Test* (5th ed.). San Antontio, TX: Psychological Corporation.

Smith, A. (1982). *Symbol Digit Modalities Test (SDMT): Manual (rev. ed.).* Los Angeles: Western Psychological Services.

Snow, C. W. (1998). *Infant development* (2nd ed.). Upper Saddle River, NJ: Prentice Hall.

Sparrow, S. S., Cicchetti, D. V., & Balla, D. A. (2005). *Vineland Adaptive Behavior Scales, Second Edition (Vineland-II).* Circle Pines, MN: American Guidance Service.

Spreen, O., & Strauss, E. (1991). *A compendium of neuropsychological tests.* New York: Oxford University Press.

Stedman's medical dictionary (28th ed.). (2006). Baltimore: Lippincott Williams & Wilkins.

Stedman's psychiatry words (3rd ed.). (2002). Baltimore: Lippincott Williams & Wilkins.

Talley, J. L. (1993). *Children's Auditory Verbal Learning Test-2 (CAVLT-2).* Odessa, FL: Psychological Assessment Resources.

Tanner, J. M. (1978). *Fetus into man: Physical growth from conception to maturity.* Cambridge, MA: Harvard University Press.

Ullman, R. K., Sleator, E. K., & Sprague, R. L. (1991). *ACTeRS Teacher Form–Second Edition.* Champaign, IL: MetriTech.

U.S. Department of Health and Human Services. (1980). *International classification of diseases (9th rev.), clinical modification: Chapter 5. Mental and behavioral disorders* (DHHS Publication No. PHS 80-1260). Washington, DC: U.S. Government Printing Office.

Walker, H. M., & McConnell, S. R. (1988). *Walker–McConnell Scale of Social Competence and School Adjustment.* Austin, TX: PRO-ED.

Watson, T. S., & Steege, M. W. (2003). *Conducting school-based functional behavioral assessments.* New York: Guilford Press.

Wechsler, D. (1997a). *Wechsler Adult Intelligence Scale–Third Edition (WAIS-III).* San Antonio, TX: Psychological Corporation.

Wechsler, D. (1997b). *Wechsler Memory Scale–Third Edition (WMS-III).* San Antonio, TX: Psychological Corporation.

Wechsler, D. (2001). *Wechsler Individual Achievement Test–Second Edition (WIAT-II).* San Antonio, TX: Psychological Corporation.

Wechsler, D. (2002). *Wechsler Preschool and Primary Scale of Intelligence–Third Edition (WPPSI-III).* San Antonio, TX: Psychological Corporation.

Wechsler, D. (2003). *Wechsler Intelligence Scale for Children–Fourth Edition (WISC-IV).* San Antonio, TX: Psychological Corporation.

Wiederholt, J. L., & Bryant, B. R. (2001). *Gray Oral Reading Tests–Fourth Edition (GORT-4).* Circle Pines, MN: American Guidance Service.

Wiger, D. E. (1999). *The clinical document sourcebook.* New York: Wiley.

Wilkinson, G. S., Robertson, G. J. (2006). *Wide Range Achievement Test–Fourth Edition (WRAT4).* Lutz, FL: Psychological Assessment Resources.

Williams, K. T. (1997). *Expressive Vocabulary Test.* Circle Pines, MN: American Guidance Service.

Wilson, S. J. (1980). *Recording guidelines for social workers.* New York: Free Press.

Woodcock, R. W. (1998). *Woodcock Reading Mastery Tests–Revised (WRMT-R).* Circle Pines, MN: American Guidance Service.

Woodcock, R. W., McGrew, K. S., & Mather, N. (2001). *The Woodcock-Johnson III (WJ III).* Itasca, IL: Riverside.

World Health Organization. (1992). *International classification of diseases* (10th rev.): *Chapter V. Mental and behavioral disorders.* Geneva: Author.

Zuckerman, E. L. (2003). *The paper office* (3rd ed.). New York: Guilford Press.

Zuckerman, E. L. (2005). *Clinician's thesaurus* (6th ed.). New York: Guilford Press.

Index

Processing speed difficulties, as a referral reason, 70, 72
Procrastination, as a referral reason, 69, 72
Professional organizations
common abbreviations of, 337
resources for, 320–321
Professional titles, certifications, and licensures, common abbreviations of, 337–338
Professionals, consultations between, 6, 8
Professionals, questions for. *See* Questioning of teachers or other professionals
Prognostic statements, 286
Progress notes
form for, 359
overview, 307, 313
Projective assessments, questioning children and, 46
Proofreading reports, 10
Property destruction, conduct disorder and, 158
Proprioception
observations of for the report, 116
overview, 117
Psychiatric history
overview, 87
of parents, 95
Psychiatric symptoms, questioning children regarding, 43–46
Psychological factors, lists of DSM-IV-TR and ICD-9-CM codes for, 271
Psychosocial stressors, during pregnancy and birth, 82
Psychotic disorders
DSM-IV-TR and ICD-9-CM codes for, 175–176, 267–268
overview, 175–176
questions to elicit information regarding, 35–36
symptoms of, 176
Psychotic symptoms, as a referral reason, 71

Quality of affect, 133
Quality of moods, 134
Questioning of children
age of child and, 6
closing questions, 46
friends, 42
guidelines for, 37–38
home and family, 41
interests, 42
opening statements and questions, 39–40
preparing for an evaluation and, 6
projective assessments and, 46
psychiatric symptoms, 43–46
questions specific to adolescents, 43
responses to, 118–119
school-related questions, 40–41
Questioning of parents
anger and aggression, 29
anxiety, 29–30
bipolar disorders, 31
chief concern/problems from parents, 20–21

communication disorders, 31
depression, 31–32
developmental milestones or delays, 26
disruptive behavior disorders, 32
eating problems and disorders, 33
elimination problems, 33
history of patient, 20–27
interests and routines of child, 27–28
learning disabilities, 33–34
mental retardation, 34
movement and tic disorders, 35
obsessive–compulsive disorder, 35
obtaining identifying information during initial interview, 19–20
pervasive developmental disorders, 32
phobias, 35
schizophrenia and other psychotic disorders, 35–36
suicidality, 36
Questioning of teachers or other professionals, 47–50

Race, format of for report writing, 63
Range of affect, 133
Range of moods, 134
Range of motion, 117
Rapport
attitude toward testing and, 126–128
establishing during the interview, 17–18
initial contact and, 15
report writing and, 8
Reading difficulties, academic history and, 104
Reading disabilities. *See also* Learning disability
assessment instruments and, 165
DSM-IV-TR codes for, 165
overview, 165–167
questions to elicit information regarding, 34
recommendations section of a report and, 283–284
as a referral reason, 72
resources for parents regarding, 329
statements about, 165–167
summary of findings and conclusions and, 278
Reading skills
achievement measures, 211–218
descriptors of, 211
language functioning tests, 219–224
Receptive language difficulties, 156
Receptive One-Word Picture Vocabulary Test (ROWPVT), 2000 Edition, 222
Recommendations in reports, 9, 280–285
Recreational activities, 191–193
Referral reason, report writing and
behavioral and conduct concerns, 69–70
cognitive concerns, 70
emotional concerns, 70–71
family concerns, 71
learning and academic concerns and, 71–72

motor and physical concerns, 72
overview, 8, 67–73
social concerns, 72–73
speech and language concerns, 73
statement of referral reason, 67–68
summary of findings and conclusions and, 275
writing reports for the schools and, 291
Refusal of child to participate in testing, observations of for the report, 132
Regressive behaviors, as a referral reason, 69
Reitan–Indiana Neuropsychological Test Battery for Children, 234–235
Rejection, depression and, 144
Relapses, course of problems and, 78
Relational problems, lists of DSM-IV-TR and ICD-9-CM codes for, 272
Relationships
questions to elicit information regarding, 27
as a referral reason, 72–73
Release of information
form for, 343
informed consent and, 19
overview, 16
Reliability statements, including in report, 65–66
Remembering-in-play, questioning children and, 38
Remissions, course of problems and, 78
Remorse, lack of, as a referral reason, 71
Repetitive motor activities, as a referral reason, 72
Report writing
background information section, 77–78, 78–79
beginning the report, 61–66
common abbreviations to use in, 335–341
ending the report, 255–274, 275–279, 280–285, 286–288
formats of, 302–319
guidelines for, 10
referral reason, 67–73
for the schools, 291–295
suggested outline for, 8–9
Report writing, beginning
arrival for the evaluation, 64
consent and confidentiality statements and, 65
heading and dates for, 61
identifying information about client, 62–63
other sources of information for reports, 64
referral reason, 67–73
reliability statements and, 65–66
Report writing, ending
closing statements, 286–288
diagnoses and, 255
list of DSM-IV-TR and ICD-9-CM codes, 255–274
recommendations, 280–285
summary of findings and conclusions, 275–279